# Case Studies in Stroke

# Case Studies in Stroke

Editor: Morgan Campbell

AMERICAN
MEDICAL PUBLISHERS
www.americanmedicalpublishers.com

AMERICAN
MEDICAL PUBLISHERS
www.americanmedicalpublishers.com

**Cataloging-in-Publication Data**

Case studies in stroke / edited by Morgan Campbell.
p. cm.
Includes bibliographical references and index.
ISBN 979-8-88740-616-9
1. Cerebrovascular disease. 2. Cerebrovascular disease--Pathophysiology.
3. Cerebrovascular disease--Diagnosis. 4. Cerebrovascular disease--Treatment.
5. Brain--Diseases. 6. Neglect (Neurology). I. Campbell, Morgan.
RC388.5 .S873 2023
616.81--dc23



American Medical Publishers,
41 Flatbush Avenue,
1st Floor, New York,
NY 11217, USA

ISBN 979-8-88740-616-9 (Hardback)

# Contents

# Preface

A stroke is a medical condition that occurs when the blood supply to the brain is disrupted, leading to a lack of oxygen and nutrients. It can have severe consequences and is considered a medical emergency. It can cause sudden neurological deficits, such as paralysis, difficulty speaking, and loss of coordination. The most common cause of a stroke is a blockage or narrowing of blood vessels supplying the brain, known as ischemic stroke. Another type of stroke is hemorrhagic stroke, which occurs when a blood vessel in the brain ruptures, leading to bleeding. Various factors can increase the risk of stroke, including high blood pressure, smoking, diabetes, obesity, high cholesterol, atrial fibrillation, and a family history of strokes. This book contains some path-breaking studies on stroke. It will serve as a valuable source of reference for graduate and postgraduate students.

All of the data presented henceforth, was collaborated in the wake of recent advancements in the field. The aim of this book is to present the diversified developments from across the globe in a comprehensible manner. The opinions expressed in each chapter belong solely to the contributing authors. Their interpretations of the topics are the integral part of this book, which I have carefully compiled for a better understanding of the readers.

At the end, I would like to thank all those who dedicated their time and efforts for the successful completion of this book. I also wish to convey my gratitude towards my friends and family who supported me at every step.

**Editor**

# 1

# Noninvasive Ventilatory Correction as an Adjunct to an Experimental Systemic Reperfusion Therapy in Acute Ischemic Stroke

**Kristian Barlinn,[1,2] Clotilde Balucani,[1] Paola Palazzo,[1] Limin Zhao,[1] April Sisson,[1] and Andrei V. Alexandrov[1]**

[1] *Comprehensive Stroke Center, Department of Neurology, University of Alabama at Birmingham, RWUH M226, 619 19th Street South, Birmingham, AL 35249-3280, USA*
[2] *Dresden University Stroke Center, University of Technology Dresden, 01307 Dresden, Germany*

Correspondence should be addressed to Kristian Barlinn, kbarlinn@uab.edu

Academic Editor: Chelsea S. Kidwell

*Background.* Obstructive sleep apnea (OSA) is a common condition in patients with acute ischemic stroke and associated with early clinical deterioration and poor functional outcome. However, noninvasive ventilatory correction is hardly considered as a complementary treatment option during the treatment phase of acute ischemic stroke. *Summary of Case.* A 55-year-old woman with an acute middle cerebral artery (MCA) occlusion received intravenous tissue plasminogen activator (tPA) and enrolled into a thrombolytic research study. During tPA infusion, she became drowsy, developed apnea episodes, desaturated and neurologically deteriorated without recanalization, re-occlusion or intracerebral hemorrhage. Urgent noninvasive ventilatory correction with biphasic positive airway pressure (BiPAP) reversed neurological fluctuation. Her MCA completely recanalized 24 hours later. *Conclusions.* Noninvasive ventilatory correction should be considered more aggressively as a complementary treatment option in selected acute stroke patients. Early initiation of BiPAP can stabilize cerebral hemodynamics and may unmask the true potential of other therapies.

## 1. Introduction

Obstructive sleep apnea (OSA) is the most common form of sleep disordered breathing in patients with acute ischemic stroke and associated with early neurological deterioration, increased mortality rates, and poor functional outcomes [1, 2]. Given that the rate of neurological deterioration is the highest during the acute stroke setting [3, 4], urgent treatment with noninvasive ventilatory correction may provide a novel therapeutic target to improve outcomes [5].

## 2. Case Report

A 55-year-old female (weight 233 pounds, height 5 feet 7.75 inches, and body mass index 35.7) with a history of untreated OSA and arterial hypertension woke up with fluctuating right-hemispheric stroke symptoms. On admission, she had mild left-sided hemiparesis and facial palsy with dysarthria (National Institutes of Health Stroke Scale (NIHSS) Score 6). Cerebral computed tomography (CT) revealed early ischemic changes involving less than 1/3 of the right anterior middle cerebral artery (MCA) distribution and a hyperdense MCA sign (Figure 1). Transcranial Doppler (TCD) demonstrated a blunted flow of the right proximal/middle MCA (Thrombolysis in Brain Ischemia (TIBI) score 2, Figure 1) indicating an MCA occlusion. We initiated intravenous thrombolysis with tissue plasminogen activator (tPA) 200 minutes after symptom onset. After initiation of intravenous tPA infusion, the patient was enrolled in a thrombolytic research study (involving a direct thrombin inhibitor, permission of the sponsor was obtained to release this case report).

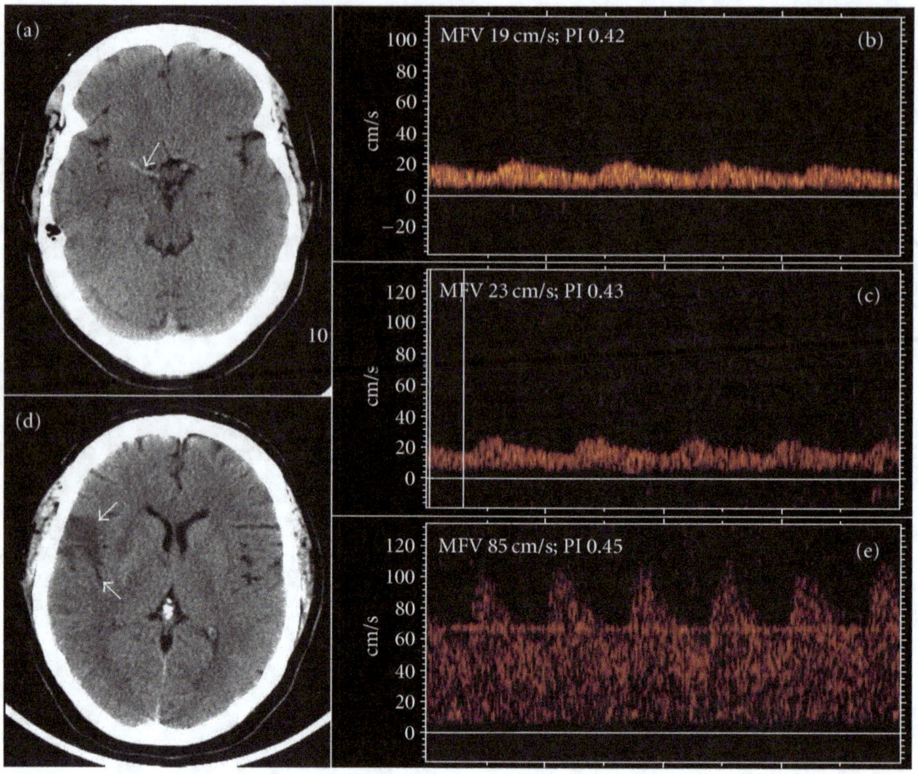


FIGURE 1: (a) Baseline noncontrast CT: a long thromboembolus within the right MCA trunk (arrow). (b) Baseline TCD: flattened systolic flow acceleration (TIBI 2) at a depth of 48 mm, indicating right proximal MCA occlusion. (c) One-hour TCD: improved flow velocities/waveforms (TIBI 2) at a depth of 58 mm suggestive of slow and partial recanalization. (d) Followup CT reveals a small cortical infarction (arrows). (e) 24-hour TCD: normal flow velocities and waveforms (TIBI 5) at a depth of 46 mm.

At the end of tPA infusion, the patient developed excessive sleepiness with repetitive episodes (each lasting approximately 30 seconds) of irregular breathing and desaturation (with oxygen saturation levels below 90% under 2 to 4 liters supplemental oxygen delivered by a nasal cannula), and her neurological symptoms worsened rapidly (in less than 1 minute) to complete left-sided hemiplegia (NIHSS score 24). Her blood pressure (BP) and heart rate ranged from 126/61 to 164/93 and 72 to 98 bpm, respectively, during the entire monitoring period, and did not drop significantly during the neurological worsening. There were no clinical signs or lab results suggestive of a systemic inflammatory response syndrome (e.g., elevated white blood cell count or CRP, abnormal body temperature). An urgent CT (within 15 minutes after neurological worsening) ruled out intracerebral hemorrhage and edema progression. TCD monitoring showed persisting right MCA occlusion (TIBI score 2) and paradoxical as well as transient velocity decreases (>10 cm/s) during hypoventilation episodes consistent with intracranial blood flow steal. Because of continuation of excessive sleepiness with apnea periods, the patient was placed on biphasic positive airway pressure (BiPAP). Within the next hour, the patient improved to an NIHSS score of 13, and TCD showed continuing improvement in flow velocities suggestive of slow and partial recanalization (Figure 1). Next day, CT demonstrated an infarction involving 1/3 of the MCA territory (Figure 1). On TCD, right MCA appeared completely recanalized (TIBI score 5, Figure 1). Further clinical workup revealed a moderate stenosis (50 to 69%) in the right internal carotid artery strongly suggesting large-artery thrombosis and artery-to-artery embolism as the likely mechanism of her stroke.

BiPAP was transitioned to night-time ventilation only, and her neurological status improved to an NIHSS of 6 at discharge. One month later, she had a residual minor left-sided hemiparesis and was functionally independent (NIHSS 3, modified Rankin Scale 1). An overnight sleep study in our sleep-wake disorder center four months later demonstrated a significant OSA (apnea-hypopnea index > 10/h), which improved on continuous positive airway pressure.

## 3. Discussion

In this paper, an early neurological deterioration was noticed that was not related to proximal vessel patency changes but coincidentally with the development of drowsiness and sleep apnea. Noninvasive ventilatory correction was applied in the hyperacute phase of ischemic stroke, and this could have improved cerebral hemodynamics distal to the occlusion. The latter is likely to have occurred as evident from her fast neurological improvement on BiPAP without complete vessel recanalization. Although tPA infusion was bridged with an experimental protocol that involves a direct thrombin inhibitor, the specific agent here was not at question. Our case highlights possible significance of ventilatory management in acute stroke, and the magnitude at which ventilatory compromise can affect both routine treatment and any hyperacute clinical trial.

OSA is frequently present in patients with acute ischemic stroke and associated with a higher likelihood of early clinical deterioration [1, 2]. However, the underlying pathophysiologic mechanism for irregular breathing and early neurological deterioration in acute ischemic stroke patients is poorly understood. Under ischemic conditions, cerebral vasomotor reserve may become exhausted with occurrence of an intracranial blood flow steal, and affected vessels are less responsive to vasodilator stimuli like carbon dioxide leading to an intracranial blood flow steal from the affected to the nonaffected side [6–8]. This intracranial hemodynamic steal phenomenon has been documented on continuous TCD monitoring in up to 14% of stroke patients, leading to clinical deterioration in 7% of cases (termed reversed Robin Hood syndrome) [7]. Moreover, patients with proximal arterial occlusion and excessive daytime sleepiness were more vulnerable to intracranial blood flow steal than patients without these conditions.

We cannot rule out that early neurological deterioration in our case simply reflected a natural course of proximal MCA occlusion and failure of collateral flow [9]. However, at the time of neurological worsening, our patient developed excessive sleepiness with recurrent and witnessed episodes of hypoventilation/apnea. Unfortunately, we did not measure arterial blood gases as arterial stick after intravenous tPA infusion was deemed risky. Nevertheless, early clinical recovery after application of BiPAP may represent a clinical surrogate of arterial carbon dioxide correction and increased blood flow in vessels supplying ischemic tissue. We considered that early clinical recovery might also have reflected a partial recanalization after intravenous thrombolysis. However, at the time of significant clinical improvement, MCA was still occluded.

In conclusion, noninvasive ventilatory correction should be considered more aggressively as a complementary treatment option in selected acute stroke patients. Further research is needed to determine whether early initiation of this treatment may improve functional outcomes and unmask the true potential of other therapies.

## Acknowledgment

Dr. A. V. Alexandrov and University of Alabama Hospital, Comprehensive Stroke Center are funded by the National Institute of Neurological Disorders and Stroke (NINDS) University of Texas-Houston Medical School to conduct studies on experimental combinatory therapies (SPOTRIAS Program). The other coauthors have no disclosures.

## References

[1] D. M. Hermann and C. L. Bassetti, "Sleep-related breathing and sleep-wake disturbances in ischemic stroke," *Neurology*, vol. 73, no. 16, pp. 1313–1322, 2009.

[2] A. Iranzo, J. Santamaría, J. Berenguer, M. Sánchez, and A. Chamorro, "Prevalence and clinical importance of sleep apnea in the first night after cerebral infarction," *Neurology*, vol. 58, no. 6, pp. 911–916, 2002.

[3] J. C. Grotta, K. M. A. Welch, S. C. Fagan et al., "Clinical deterioration following improvement in the NINDS rt-PA stroke trial," *Stroke*, vol. 32, no. 3, pp. 661–668, 2001.

[4] A. Dávalos, D. Toni, F. Iweins, E. Lesaffre, S. Bastianello, and J. Castillo, "Neurological deterioration in acute ischemic stroke: Potential predictors and associated factors in the European Cooperative Acute Stroke Study (ECASS) I," *Stroke*, vol. 30, no. 12, pp. 2631–2636, 1999.

[5] S. A. Broadley, L. Jørgensen, A. Cheek et al., "Early investigation and treatment of obstructive sleep apnoea after acute stroke," *Journal of Clinical Neuroscience*, vol. 14, no. 4, pp. 328–333, 2007.

[6] M. Silvestrini, F. Vernieri, P. Pasqualetti et al., "Impaired cerebral vasoreactivity and risk of stroke in patients with asymptomatic carotid artery stenosis," *Journal of the American Medical Association*, vol. 283, no. 16, pp. 2122–2127, 2000.

[7] A. V. Alexandrov, H. T. Nguyen, M. Rubiera et al., "Prevalence and risk factors associated with reversed robin hood syndrome in acute ischemic stroke," *Stroke*, vol. 40, no. 8, pp. 2738–2742, 2009.

[8] E. B. Ringelstein, C. Sievers, S. Ecker, P. A. Schneider, and S. M. Otis, "Noninvasive assessment of CO2-induced cerebral vasomotor response in normal individuals and patients with internal carotid artery occlusions," *Stroke*, vol. 19, no. 8, pp. 963–969, 1988.

[9] M. Saqqur, K. Uchino, A. M. Demchuk et al., "Site of arterial occlusion identified by transcranial Doppler (TCD) predicts the response to intravenous thrombolysis for stroke," *Stroke*, vol. 38, pp. 948–954, 2007.

2

# Playing Piano can Improve Upper Extremity Function after Stroke: Case Studies

**Myriam Villeneuve[1,2] and Anouk Lamontagne[1,2]**

[1] *School of Physical and Occupational Therapy, McGill University, Montreal, QC, Canada H3A OG4*
[2] *Feil and Oberfeld Research Centre, Jewish Rehabilitation Hospital, Research Site of the Montreal Center for Interdisciplinary Research in Rehabilitation (CRIR), 3205 Place Alton-Goldbloom, Laval, QC, Canada H7V 1R2*

Correspondence should be addressed to Anouk Lamontagne; anouk.lamontagne@mcgill.ca

Academic Editor: Majaz Moonis

Music-supported therapy (MST) is an innovative approach that was shown to improve manual dexterity in acute stroke survivors. The feasibility of such intervention in chronic stroke survivors and its longer-term benefits, however, remain unknown. The objective of this pilot study was to estimate the short- and long-term effects of a 3-week piano training program on upper extremity function in persons with chronic stroke. A multiple pre-post sequential design was used, with measurements taken at baseline ($week_0$, $week_3$), prior to ($week_6$) and after the intervention ($week_9$), and at 3-week follow-up ($week_{12}$). Three persons with stroke participated in the 3-week piano training program that combined structured piano lessons to home practice program. The songs, played on an electronic keyboard, involved all 5 digits of the affected hand and were displayed using a user-friendly MIDI program. After intervention, all the three participants showed improvements in their fine (nine hole peg test) and gross (box and block test) manual dexterity, as well as in the functional use of the upper extremity (Jebsen hand function test). Improvements were maintained at follow-up. These preliminary results support the feasibility of using an MST approach that combines structured lessons to home practice to improve upper extremity function in chronic stroke.

## 1. Introduction

Persistent contralateral motor impairments are common following a stroke. It is estimated that 80% to 95% of patients experience sensorimotor upper extremity impairments as well as activity and participation limitations, which persist beyond 6 months after stroke onset [1]. This is a major concern as in order to manage daily activities, chronic stroke survivors often use nonoptimal compensation strategies that can lead to a pattern of learned disuse of the paretic arm and further exacerbate the level of disability. Existing therapies that aim at improving upper extremity function show modest to moderate improvements [2], possibly due to insufficient training intensity [3] and lack of adherence. It was also shown that well beyond the optimal recovery window that occurs within the first 6 months after a stroke, rehabilitation still has the potential to induce neurological and functional changes [4, 5]. There is a need to develop and implement interventions that will meet the patient's interests to actively engage them during and beyond the supervised rehabilitation period so that long-term improvements in upper extremity function can be achieved.

Music-supported therapy (MST) is an innovative approach that has been shown to yield larger improvements in fine and gross motor dexterity compared to conventional rehabilitation and constraint-induced movement therapy in acute stroke survivors [6]. MST was also shown to yield enhanced motor skills and neuroplastic changes of auditory-motor network in chronic stroke participants [7]. In addition to integrating key principles of motor learning and providing instantaneous auditory feedback on performance, the rapid establishment of auditory-motor coupling during music playing would underlie the efficacy of MST [7, 8]. Such coupling can be observed within 20 minutes of musical training and is largely enhanced after 5 weeks of training in nonmusicians [9]. Existing MST

TABLE 1: Initial participant characteristics.

| | Participant 1 | Participant 2 | Participant 3 |
|---|---|---|---|
| Age (years) | 60 | 67 | 58 |
| Gender (male/female) | Male | Male | Male |
| Time since stroke (months) | 9 | 10 | 16 |
| Side of stroke (left/right) | Right | Left | Right |
| Type of stroke (ischemic/hemorrhage) | Ischemic | Ischemic | Hemorrhage |
| CMSA arm/hand score (max = 7) | 3/3 | 3/3 | 4/5 |
| Piano experience (years) | 0 | 0 | 0 |
| Handedness | Right | Right* | Left* |

*Affected hand is the dominant hand; CMSA: Chedoke-McMaster Stroke Assessment.

programs, however, involve 5 days/week of training and may be difficult to implement in an outpatient and community rehabilitation settings. Furthermore, no previous MST program has focused on finger movement accuracy, timing, and speed, which are important determinants of finger coordination. We have developed, using a user-friendly computerized piano program, a piano training paradigm that provides feedback on note accuracy, timing and speed while allowing participants to progress through finger sequences of increasing complexity. The purpose of this study was to investigate the feasibility of an individually tailored piano training intervention that targeted finger movement coordination and combined structured piano lessons to home practice. The specific objective was to estimate the short-term and retention effects of a 3-week piano training program on manual dexterity, finger movement coordination, and functional use of upper extremity in persons with chronic stroke.

## 2. Methods

Three male participants with a mild to moderate deficits of upper extremity motor function due to a first supratentorial chronic stroke (6 to 24 months duration) in the middle cerebral artery territory were recruited after being discharged from rehabilitation (Table 1). Participants had (1) some capacity of dissociation of upper extremity movements as reflected by scores of 3 to 6 on the arm and hand components of the Chedoke-McMaster Stroke Assessment and (2) the ability to follow simple instructions. They had corrected to normal vision and were free of visual field defects (Goldman perimetry), hemineglect (<6 omissions, Bell's test), and cognitive deficits (scores > 23, Montreal Cognitive Assessment). None had musical experience. The study was approved by the Ethics Committee of the Centre for Interdisciplinary Research in Rehabilitation (CRIR), and informed consent was obtained from each participant.

Subjects participated in a step-by-step musical training consisting of three individual 1-hour sessions per week for 3 consecutive weeks, for a total of 9 sessions. The individual sessions were complemented with a home program consisting of biweekly piano exercises of 30 min duration. Synthesia, an MIDI piano program, was used to program and display the musical pieces played by the participants on the electronic piano keyboard (Yamaha P155) during the training sessions. The musical pieces involved all 5 fingers of the paretic hand, and participants were cued to press the piano key(s) indicated by the visual stimuli (illuminated, blue dot) presented on the computer screen. Nine musical pieces were created and were introduced to the participants in an increasing order of difficulty: (1) *simple*, or "following notes" involving movements of consecutive fingers; (2) *intermediate*, or third, fourth, and fifth intervals involving movements of nonconsecutive fingers; and (3) *complex*, which involves chords, that is 2 fingers played at the same time. Within each musical piece, the participants started at a tempo of 30 bpm. When reaching a note accuracy and timing score of 80%, as measured in Synthesia, the tempo increased by steps of 10% until reaching a tempo of 60 bpm. Home piano exercises were executed on a roll up flexible piano (Hand Roll Piano 61 K).

Changes in fine motor (nine hole peg test (NHPT)) and gross motor dexterity (box and block test (BBT)) were measured at multiple baseline time points ($week_0$, $week_3$), immediately prior to ($week_6$) and after the intervention ($week_9$), and at a 3-week follow-up ($week_{12}$). The Jebsen hand function Test (JHFT), which reflects the functional use of the hand, is time-consuming and was administered only at pre- and post-intervention, as well as follow-up. Piano performance measures, including timing and note accuracy, were collected with Synthesia throughout the training sessions. Participants recorded their home practice duration and frequency in a logbook.

## 3. Results

All participants showed improvements in note accuracy and timing accuracy within and across the training sessions. Participant 3 completed 3 musical pieces and the two others completed 5 pieces during the 3-week intervention. They progressed through finger sequences of increasing complexity, involving movements of consecutive fingers followed by movements of nonconsecutive fingers (intervals). Each musical piece started at 30 bpm and were practiced on an average of 25 times over 2 to 3 training sessions before reaching a note accuracy > 80% at 60 bpm. When considering a tempo of 60 bpm, the duration of musical pieces also increased from 17 s to 48 s (participants no. 1 and no. 2) and from 17 s to 32.5 s (participant no. 3) between the first and last training session.

A mean increase of 6 blocks (range: 4–10 blocks) and a mean reduction of 24.8 s (16–31 s) were observed on the BBT and NHPT, respectively, between pre- and post-intervention (Figure 1). At variance, little variations were observed between baseline measurements at week$_0$ (BBT = 23.3; NHPT = 139.2 s) and week$_3$ (BBT = 24.7; NHPT = 134.8 s) and pre-intervention (BBT = 23.7; NHPT = 138.1 s). None of the participants were able to complete the writing subtest of the JHFT. The 3 participants, however, showed larger scores on all other subtests of the JHFT at post-intervention compared to pre-intervention, with mean increments ranging from 36.2% to 44.2% (Figure 1). Post-intervention scores for the BBT, NHPT, and JHFT were maintained at the 3-week follow-up. Average home practice duration was 50 minutes per session, which exceeded the 30 minutes practice time required. All participants reported enjoying the piano training program, and they all expressed the desire to continue piano lessons after their participation in the study. No adverse reactions to the intervention were reported, with the exception of one participant (no. 2) displaying occasional "hand stiffness" typical of spasticity during the intervention, as well as a fatigue described as a "general fatigue" after the training sessions. The stiffness was going away with frequent breaks, and the fatigue resolved within a few hours after the sessions.

## 4. Discussion

This case study is, to our knowledge, the first to report the immediate and retention effects of a structured piano training program combined to home practice in chronic stroke survivors. Improvements in fine and gross manual dexterity, as well as in the functional use of the hand, were observed in all three participants immediately after, but also at the 3-week follow-up. These changes were accompanied by improvements in the speed of execution, as well as in the timing accuracy and note accuracy for each musical piece. Such positive training effects are especially remarkable, considering that participants involved in this study were suffering from a chronic stroke and were exposed to an intervention of short duration. Similar improvements in manual dexterity were observed in a 3-week MST program involving piano and drum pad playing in acute stroke survivors [6], although changes in fine dexterity in the present study (NHPT: +24.8 s) do appear to exceed those reported in the combined drum-piano MST paradigm (NHPT: +13 s). Present results contrast, however, with findings from a case report involving the combined drum pad and piano playing intervention in chronic stroke survivors, where no changes on the NHPT and BBT were observed following the intervention [10]. We hypothesize that the impact on manual dexterity observed in the present study is attributed to the intensity and specificity of the piano exercises that were specifically designed to target dissociated and coordinated finger movements, with an emphasis on note and timing accuracy, as well as speed of execution. Rich feedback was provided to the participants throughout the supervised training session using a computerized program that provided knowledge of performance (note accuracy and timing) and knowledge of result (final speed and error score).

Comparison of present training effects with other existing upper extremity interventions in chronic stroke such as constraint-induced movement therapy is difficult, due to the use of different outcome measures and inclusion of participants with different characteristics. Present findings, however, can be interpreted in the light of the smallest real differences, or true changes, for the BBT (6 blocks) and the NHPT (32.8 s) [11]. Despite of their chronic stage, our participants either approached (nos. 1 and 3) or exceeded (no. 2) the smallest real difference on the BBT. Similarly, one participant (no. 1) almost reached the smallest real difference for the NHPT while the two others made more modest gains. These observations suggest that MST has the potential to yield real improvements in upper extremity function in chronic stroke participants with different levels of hand and arm motor recovery. The presence of an enhanced functional use of the upper extremity post-intervention also suggests that a better coordination of finger movements can impact on the upper extremity as a whole, and may be a prime target for rehabilitation. Finally, the persistence of positive effects at follow-up further indicates that improvements can be maintained even after the cessation of the training. Compared to other therapies such as constraint-induced movement therapy MST may be less time consuming and labor intensive. It has the potential to be safely self-managed and pursued well beyond the rehabilitation period, such that gains can be maintained or further enhanced.

MST relies on key principles of motor learning, including repeated and task-specific practice as well as the involvement of multisensory feedback, which gives instantaneous knowledge of result and performance. It would further take advantage of a rapid establishment of auditorimotor coactivation induced by the musical training [8], while engaging the participants in an individually tailored and rewarding program. Participant's remarkable adherence to the home practice sessions, which led to practice times beyond expectations, indicates high levels of motivation. This motivation, as well as a perception of being engaged in an enjoyable, socially valued leisure activity, are factors that may help patients pursuing musical lessons beyond the usual rehabilitation time frame.

The small sample size in this pilot study limits the generalization of results. Present results, however, support the feasibility of MST in chronic stroke and provide useful information that can be used to generate further hypotheses and design larger intervention studies. Longer-term benefits of the training on upper extremity function and quality of life should also be investigated.

## 5. Conclusion

This study provides preliminary evidence indicating that a piano training program combined to home practice is feasible and can lead to meaningful improvements in manual

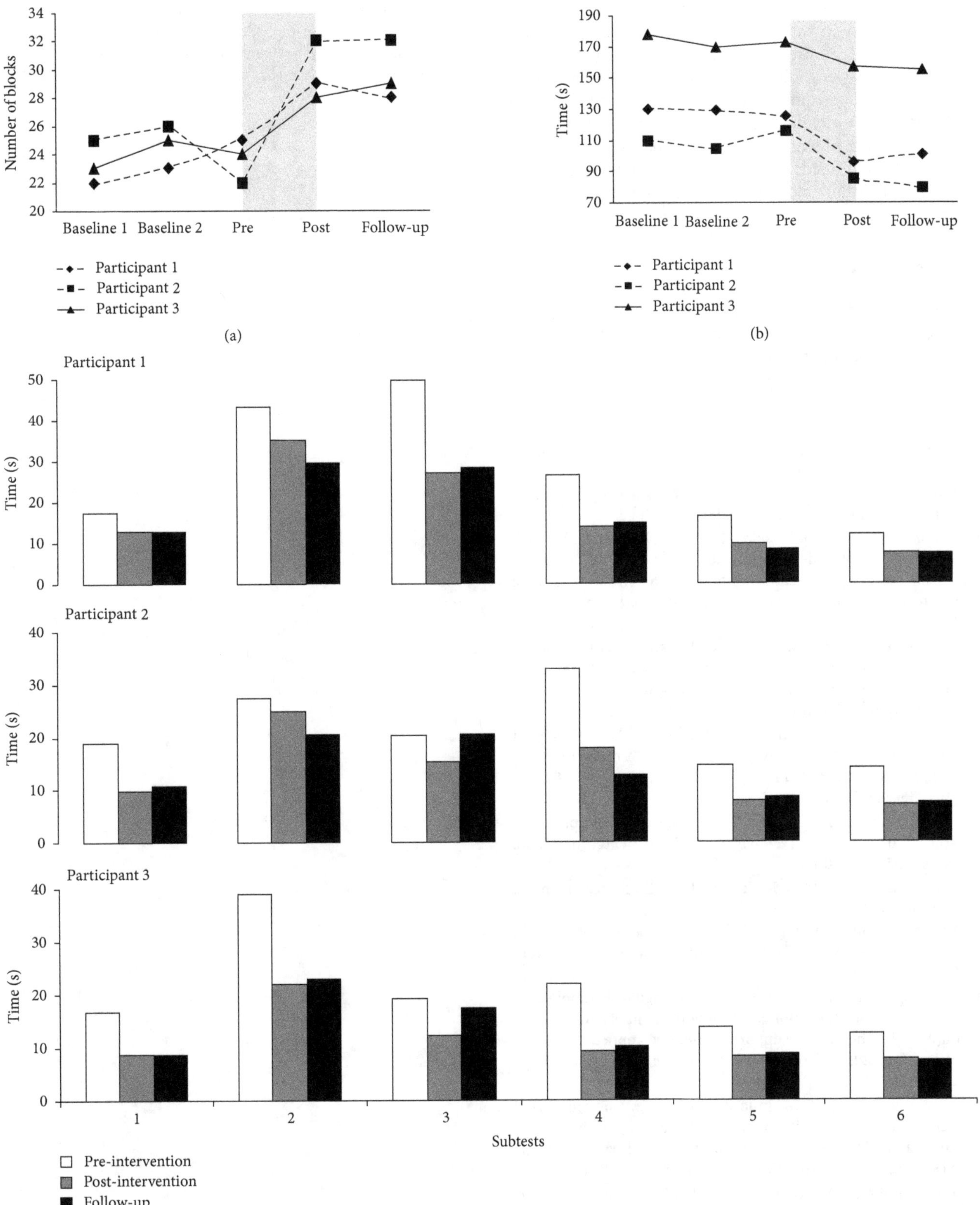


FIGURE 1: Scores of the three participants at different time points on the box and block test (a), nine hole peg test (b), and the Jebsen hand function test (c). For the box and block test, the scores represent the maximum number of blocks transported from one box to the other in 60 seconds. For the nine hole peg test, the time required to place and remove nine dowels into a nine holes is represented. For the Jebsen hand function test, the time required to complete the following subtests is shown: (1) simulating page turning; (2) lifting small common objects; (3) simulated feeding; (4) stacking checkers; (5) lifting large, light objects; (6) lifting large, heavy objects.

dexterity, finger movement coordination, and functional use of upper extremity in chronic stroke survivors. For the first time, it was also demonstrated that MST training effects are maintained at a 3-week follow-up. This unique intervention, which targeted finger movement coordination, engaged the participants in an individually tailored and highly motivating program. It has the potential to be self-managed and pursued on the long term, outside the rehabilitation setting, and lead to further and sustainable improvements in upper extremity function.

## Acknowledgments

The authors want to thank all the participants who took part in this study. This project was supported by the Foundation of the Jewish Rehabilitation Hospital.

## References

[1] G. Kwakkel, B. J. Kollen, J. V. Van der Grond, and A. J. H. Prevo, "Probability of regaining dexterity in the flaccid upper limb: impact of severity of paresis and time since onset in acute stroke," *Stroke*, vol. 34, no. 9, pp. 2181–2186, 2003.

[2] R. P. S. Van Peppen, G. Kwakkel, S. Wood-Dauphinee, H. J. M. Hendriks, P. J. Van der Wees, and J. Dekker, "The impact of physical therapy on functional outcomes after stroke: what's the evidence?" *Clinical Rehabilitation*, vol. 18, no. 8, pp. 833–862, 2004.

[3] E. V. Cooke, K. Mares, A. Clark, R. C. Tallis, and V. M. Pomeroy, "The effects of increased dose of exercise-based therapies to enhance motor recovery after stroke: a systematic review and meta-analysis," *BMC Medicine*, vol. 8, article 60, 2010.

[4] F. Ferrarello, M. Baccini, L. A. Rinaldi et al., "Efficacy of physiotherapy interventions late after stroke: a meta-analysis," *Journal of Neurology, Neurosurgery and Psychiatry*, vol. 82, no. 2, pp. 136–143, 2011.

[5] P. M. Rossini and G. Dal Forno, "Neuronal post-stroke plasticity in the adult," *Restorative Neurology and Neuroscience*, vol. 22, no. 3-4, pp. 193–206, 2004.

[6] S. Schneider, T. Münte, A. Rodriguez-Fornells, M. Sailer, and E. Altenmüller, "Music-supported training is more efficient than functional motor training for recovery of fine motor skills in stroke patients," *Music Perception*, vol. 27, no. 4, pp. 271–280, 2010.

[7] A. Rodriguez-Fornells, N. Rojo, J. L. Amengual, P. Ripollés, E. Altenmüller, and T. F. Münte, "The involvement of audio-motor coupling in the music-supported therapy applied to stroke patients," *Annals of the New York Academy of Sciences*, vol. 1252, pp. 282–293, 2012.

[8] N. Rojo, J. Amengual, M. Juncadella et al., "Music-Supported Therapy induces plasticity in the sensorimotor cortex in chronic stroke: a single-case study using multimodal imaging (fMRI-TMS)," *Brain Injury*, vol. 25, no. 7-8, pp. 787–793, 2011.

[9] E. Altenmüller, J. Marco-Pallares, T. F. Münte, and S. Schneider, "Neural reorganization underlies improvement in stroke-induced motor dysfunction by music-supported therapy," *Annals of the New York Academy of Sciences*, vol. 1169, pp. 395–405, 2009.

[10] M. Bangert and E. O. Altenmüller, "Mapping perception to action in piano practice: a longitudinal DC-EEG study," *BMC Neuroscience*, vol. 4, article 26, 2003.

[11] H. M. Chen, C. C. Chen, I. P. Hsueh, S. L. Huang, and C. L. Hsieh, "Test-retest reproducibility and smallest real difference of 5 hand function tests in patients with stroke," *Neurorehabilitation and Neural Repair*, vol. 23, no. 5, pp. 435–440, 2009.

3

# Cardiac Fibroelastoma: A Rare Cause of Stroke in Young Adults

**Ahmad Mirdamadi,[1] Mohsen MirmohammadSadeghi,[2] Mahfar Arasteh,[3] and Mojgan Gharipour[4]**

[1] *Medical School, Islamic Azad University, Najafabad Branch, Isfahan, Iran*
[2] *Hypertension Research Center, Isfahan Cardiovascular Research Institute, Isfahan University of Medical Sciences, Isfahan, Iran*
[3] *Isfahan University of Medical Sciences, Isfahan, Iran*
[4] *Isfahan Cardiovascular Research Center, Isfahan Cardiovascular Research Institute (WHO Collaborating Center), Isfahan University of Medical Sciences, Isfahan, Iran*

Correspondence should be addressed to Mojgan Gharipour; gharipour@crc.mui.ac.ir

Academic Editors: R. Bornemeier, M.-R. Chen, A. J. Mansur, and C. S. Snyder

A 26-year-old man presenting with a transient episode of dysarthria and dizziness, 3 weeks prior to admission, was referred to our center to be evaluated for transient ischemic attack (TIA). The patient had been previously admitted to a different hospital and echocardiography was reported normal at that center, but upon presenting to our institution strand-like masses in the left ventricle (LV) were detected. Transesophageal echocardiography (TEE) revealed two distinct mobile LV masses suggesting a diagnosis of papillary fibroelastoma. CT angiography and histopathological studies confirmed this diagnosis.

## 1. Case Report

A 26-year-old man presenting with an episode of dysarthria and dizziness 3 weeks prior to admission was referred to our center to be evaluated for transient ischemic attack (TIA). His past medical history showed no evidence of previous illness. On admission, physical examination showed that he was in sinus rhythm, had a pulse rate of 75 bpm, and a blood pressure of 100/60 mm Hg. On auscultation, he had no murmur or carotid bruit. Laboratory tests were normal. He had a normal electrocardiogram and chest X-ray. Initial cardiac evaluation was also normal. The patient had been previously admitted to a different hospital which had performed transthoracic echocardiogram and reported it as normal. The patient was referred for transesophageal echocardiography (TEE) to rule out of patent foramen ovale (PFO). We performed another transthoracic echocardiogram (TTE), but mobile strand-like masses in left ventricular (LV) were detected (Figure 1). TEE also revealed two distinct highly mobile filamentous LV masses, suggesting papillary fibroelastoma (Figures 2(a) and 2(b)). One mass measuring $5 \times 0.6$ cm originated from the posterior wall, near the apex, and another mass measuring $3 \times 0.6$ cm originated from the mitral valve (MV) annulus just beside the posterior MV leaflet. Both of the masses extended toward LV outflow tract. Both aortic and mitral valve were spare, but chordae tendina was suspected to be involved. CT angiography confirmed the diagnosis. The patient was given anticoagulant therapy and referred for surgery. At operation, two large beading tumors were found in the LV (Figure 3). One of the tumors was attached to posterior leaflet of the MV and the other one was attached to the posterior papillary muscle adjacent to the chordae tendina. The tumors were successfully excised via mitral valve approach. Chordae reconstruction and MV annuloplasty were performed for the patient. The postoperative recovery was uneventful. Follow-up TEE revealed no residual tumor.

## 2. Discussion

Fibroelastomas are small, avascular, and usually solitude lesions (in 91% of cases) [1]. This tumor is a very rare tumor with an incidence of 0.001–0.3% at autopsy [2, 3], and most fibroelastomas are often diagnosed incidentally [4–7]. In

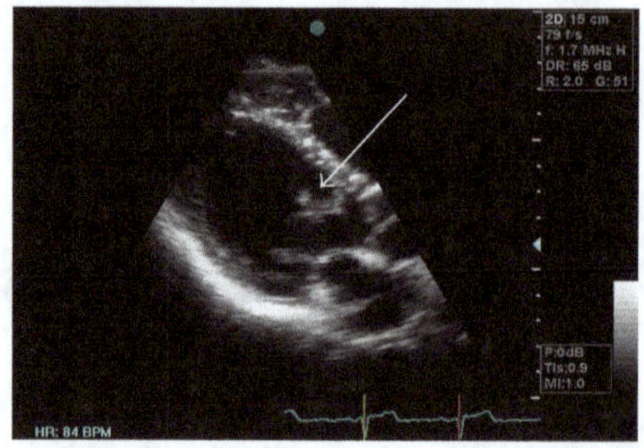

FIGURE 1: Evidence of strand-like LV masses, as shown by TTE.

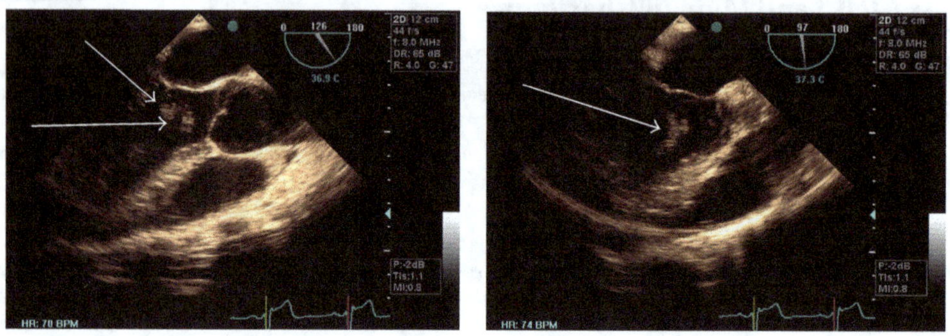

(a) (b)

FIGURE 2: Transesophageal echocardiographic image showing mobile LV masses attached to the mitral valve and the posterior wall extending to LV outflow tract.

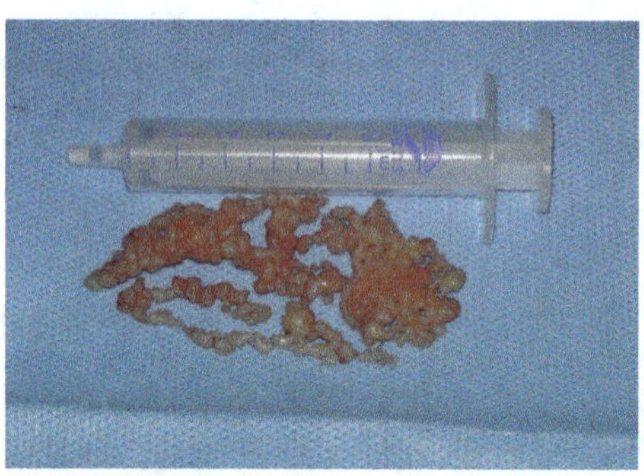

FIGURE 3: Gross specimen of papillary fibroelastoma demonstrating two large beading tumors.

symptomatic patients, the clinical presentation depends on the location of tumor [8]. The most common clinical presentation is stroke or transient ischemic attack (TIA) caused by cerebral emboli, originating from a thrombus on the tumor, or by a piece of the tumor itself. Unfortunately, the cerebral ischemia could also result in completed strokes [8]. They have multiple papillary fronds resembling sea anemones. Since the symptoms may mimic other conditions and the fibroelastoma has a similar echocardiographic appearance to thrombus and other various types of cardiac mass, the tumor may be not considered as a diagnosis or it may erroneously be regarded as a thrombus, vegetation, or degenerative valve tissue [9, 10].

In our case, the first transthoracic echocardiogram was not able to correctly diagnose the fibroelastoma and only after meticulous image acquisition, in a second echocardiogram, a correct diagnosis was made. The diagnosis of the fibroelastoma was confirmed by CT angiography and histology after surgery. In cases of cardiac tumor, TEE has an important role in making the diagnosis [11, 12]. Echocardiographic diagnosis can be very difficult, particularly when there is no definitive characteristic to distinguish fibroelastomas from other masses or when the acoustic window is not adequate. When the tumor is larger than 0.2 cm, the sensitivity and specificity of TTE are 88.9% and 87.8%, respectively [10]. Additionally, multiple fibroelastomas are only detected in 8.6% of cases by TEE [10]. Therefore, there should be high clinical suspicion to consider the possibility of a cardiac tumor and careful attention should be paid in order to find these masses in echocardiography. TEE should be performed to make the appropriate diagnosis.

## References

[1] R. S. Saad, C. O. Galvis, W. Bshara, J. Liddicoat, and D. J. Dabbs, "Pulmonary valve papillary fibroelastoma: a case report and review of the literature," *Archives of Pathology and Laboratory Medicine*, vol. 125, no. 7, pp. 933–934, 2001.

[2] J. Walkes, M. Ci, W. Smythe, and M. Reardon, "Cardiac neoplasms," in *Cardiac Surgery in the Adult*, L. Cohn, Ed., pp. 1479–1510, McGraw-Hill, New York, NY, USA, 2008.

[3] D. M. Sahian, S. B. Labib, and G. Chang, "Cardiac papillaryfibroelastoma," *The Annals of Thoracic Surgery*, vol. 59, pp. 538–541, 1995.

[4] E. Czekajska-Chehab, A. Tomaszewski, M. Wójcik, and A. Drop, "Papillary fibroelastoma as an accidental findding in multislice computed tomography scan of coronary arteries," *Canadian Journal of Cardiology*, vol. 22, no. 13, pp. 1155–1157, 2006.

[5] S. Uchida, N. Obayashi, H. Yamanari, K. Matsubara, D. Saito, and S. Haraoka, "Papillary fibroelastoma in the left ventricular outflow tract," *Heart and Vessels*, vol. 7, no. 3, pp. 164–167, 1992.

[6] G. LiMandri, S. Homma, M. R. Di Tullio et al., "Detection of multiple papillary fibroelastomas of the tricuspid valve by transesophageal echocardiography," *Journal of the American Society of Echocardiography*, vol. 7, pp. 315–317, 1994.

[7] L. Cohn, *Cardiac Surgery in the Adult*, McGraw-Hill Medical, New York, NY, USA, 2008.

[8] R. M. Gowda, I. A. Khan, C. K. Nair, N. J. Mehta, B. C. Vasavada, and T. J. Sacchi, "Cardiac papillary fibroelastoma: a comprehensive analysis of 725 cases," *American Heart Journal*, vol. 146, no. 3, pp. 404–410, 2003.

[9] E. Vizzardi, P. Faggiano, E. Antonioli et al., "Thrombus or tumor? A case of fibroelastoma as indicated during the submission process," *Cases Journal*, vol. 2, no. 1, article 31, 2009.

[10] J. P. Sun, C. R. Asher, X. S. Yang et al., "Clinical and echocardiographic characteristics of papillary fibroelastomas: a retrospective and prospective study in 162 patients," *Circulation*, vol. 103, no. 22, pp. 2687–2693, 2001.

[11] J. Butany, V. Nair, M. S. Ahluwalia, D. El Demellwy, S. Siu, and C. Fiendel, "Papillary fibroelastoma of the interatrial septum: a case report," *Journal of Cardiac Surgery*, vol. 19, no. 4, pp. 349–353, 2004.

[12] S. Mohammadi, A. Martineau, P. Voisine, and F. Dagenais, "Left atrial papillary fibroelastoma: a rare cause of multiple cerebral emboli," *Annals of Thoracic Surgery*, vol. 84, no. 4, pp. 1396–1397, 2007.

4

# Clinicoradiological Correlation of Macropsia due to Acute Stroke: A Case Report and Review of the Literature

**Mayra Johana Montalvo[1] and Muhib Alam Khan[2]**

[1]*Neuromodulation Center, Spaulding Rehabilitation Hospital, Harvard Medical School, 96/79 13th Street, Boston, MA 02129, USA*
[2]*Department of Neurology, Warren Alpert Medical School at Brown University, 110 Lockwood Street, Suite 324, Providence, RI 02903, USA*

Correspondence should be addressed to Mayra Johana Montalvo; jmonta2@gmail.com

Academic Editor: José Luis González-Gutiérrez

Dysmetropsia (macropsia, micropsia, teleopsia, or pelopsia) most commonly results from retinal pathologies, epileptic seizure, neoplastic lesions, viral infection, or psychoactive drugs. Vascular lesions are an uncommon cause of dysmetropsia. Vascular hemimicropsia, although rare, has been more frequently described in the literature, whereas hemimacropsia from acute ischemic injury is exceedingly rare. We describe a patient presenting in the emergency room (ER) with visual perception disturbances characterized by a distorted perception of the size of objects, compatible with left hemimacropsia. Magnetic resonance imaging (MRI) of the brain showed an acute occipitotemporal ischemic injury corresponding to the posterior cerebral artery (PCA) territory. The location of the lesion is consistent with previous case reports that suggest that hemimacropsia is associated with the occipitotemporal projection, which plays a decisive role in the visual identification of objects by interconnecting the striate, prestriate, and inferior temporal areas. The difference of our case as compared to previous case reports is that the lesion in our patient spared Brodmann area 17 (calcarine cortex) and therefore did not present symptoms of quadrantanopsia. Instead, the patient presented isolated hemimacropsia, therefore suggesting that the anatomical lesion causing hemimacropsia is located in the ventral portion of the occipitotemporal projection, more specifically Brodmann areas 18 (parastriate) and 19 (peristriate).

## 1. Introduction

Dysmetropsia refers to the collective group of perceptual alterations including macropsia, micropsia, teleopsia, and pelopsia [1, 2]. These alterations result in objects being perceived as too large, too small, too far away, and too close, respectively. Comprehensively, these visual distortions can be symptomatic of the so-called Alice in Wonderland or Todd Syndrome [2–4]. Dysmetropsia primarily results from retinal pathologies but may also be a manifestation of migraine, epileptic seizure, or neoplastic lesions, which usually involve the occipital lobe or associated cortices, such as parietal-occipital or temporal-occipital regions. Dysmetropsia is also attributed to Epstein-Barr and influenza infection, use of psychoactive drugs such as mescaline [1, 2, 5–8], toxic and metabolic disorders, and psychiatric illnesses. Less commonly, lesions of the brainstem may be associated with these phenomena [3, 9]. Reports of these symptoms have also been made in otherwise healthy children and adolescents [2, 4]. Vascular lesions associated with dysmetropsia are exceedingly rare; in a recent retrospective clinical study regarding the clinical features of 232 patients with posterior circulation infarctions, the most common symptoms were sensory deficits and hemianopia, 51.3% and 41.4%, respectively, and none of the patients presented with dysmetropsia [10].

## 2. Case Presentation

A 58-year-old male patient with history of hypertension and diabetes mellitus presented to the ER with 2 days history of visual perception disturbances characterized by distortion of the size and shape of objects, which he described as perceiving

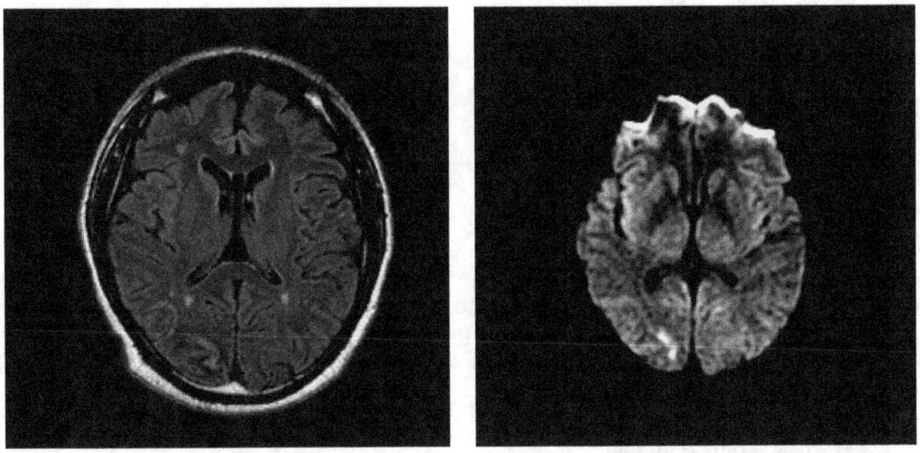

FIGURE 1: MRI 2 days after onset of symptoms, presenting acute occipitotemporal ischemic injury, corresponding to PCA territory sparing Brodmann area 17, and involving ventral portion of occipitotemporal projection; Brodmann areas 18 (parastriate) and 19 (peristriate).

a basketball player's hand as larger than normal when visualized in the left visual field. The altered visual perception lasted 2 days. He also complained of bifrontal headache and transient horizontal diplopia, which had subsequently resolved. In the ER the patient did not present with headache, scintillating scotomas, vision loss, nausea, or vomiting. He did not refer to twitching of face or extremities and had no loss of consciousness.

Neurological examination revealed full visual fields. Visual acuity was 20/20 in both eyes. Pupils are equal, round, and reactive to light and accommodation, and extra ocular movements are intact. There was no hemianopia or diplopia. EEG showed slowing to 6 Hz in the right occipital region but no spike wave discharges suggesting an interictal epileptic focus.

Magnetic resonance imaging of the brain showed an acute occipitotemporal ischemic injury corresponding to the PCA territory, affecting Brodmann areas 18 and 19 involving the cuneus (Figure 1). An angiomagnetic resonance revealed approximately 50% luminal stenosis involving the proximal right internal carotid artery. Surface echocardiogram was normal. Transesophageal echocardiogram was unremarkable except for a 2 mm × 6.8 mm layered immobile plaque involving the aortic arch without thrombus. The etiology of the stroke was thought to be cryptogenic at that point. Patient received 325 mg of ASA (aspirin) for 2 days while he was in the hospital and was then discharged on 81 mg of ASA (aspirin) and a simvastatin 20 mg daily. Six months later he had an acute infarct in the right parietal lobe.

## 3. Discussion

Micropsia is more frequently reported than macropsia, but both are rather infrequent phenomena, even more so if occurring as isolated symptoms [8]. It has been shown that cortical irritation or temporo-occipito-parietal epilepsy can be a transient cause of bilateral dysmetropsia [6]. Nevertheless, the anatomical location causing isolated hemidysmetropsia is not very well understood. Case reports describe that hemimicropsia can result from damage from a lesion affecting the lower part of Brodmann areas 18 and 19. Lesions causing left hemimicropsia involve the inferior portion of the right parastriate area but spare both the calcarine region and the geniculostriate projections [5]. Isolated hemimacropsia is extremely uncommon. To our knowledge, there has only been one case report of an ischemic lesion causing hemimacropsia due to a lesion in the ventral portion of the occipitotemporal projection, including the lingual and fusiform gyri that corresponded to the medial aspect of Brodmann areas 17, 18, and 19 [11]. Due to the anatomic location in Brodmann area 17, the patient also presented left homonymous upper quadrantanopsia. After one month, the macropsia resolved completely. In our case report the patient did not present any other visual field deficits besides left hemimacropsia. The location of the lesion is consistent with previous case reports that suggest that hemimicropsia is associated with the lateral aspect of the occipitotemporal projection, whereas hemimacropsia is associated with the ventral portion of the occipitotemporal projection, which plays a decisive role in the visual identification of objects by interconnecting the striate, prestriate, and inferior temporal areas [5, 11, 12].

The difference between our case and previous case reports presenting hemimacropsia is that the lesion in our patient spared Brodmann area 17 (calcarine cortex), which was consistent with symptoms because the patient did not present quadrantanopsia (would be expected with a lesion in this location). Instead, the patient presented isolated hemimacropsia, therefore suggesting that the anatomical lesion causing hemimacropsia is located in the ventral portion of the occipitotemporal projection, more specifically Brodmann areas 18 (parastriate) and 19 (peristriate).

## Conflict of Interests

The authors declare that there is no conflict of interests regarding the publication of this paper.

## References


[1] M. Ganssauge, E. Papageorgiou, and U. Schiefer, "Facial dysmorphopsia: a notable variant of the "thin man" phenomenon?" *Graefe's Archive for Clinical and Experimental Ophthalmology*, vol. 250, no. 10, pp. 1491–1497, 2012.

[2] N. S. Thaler, D. N. Allen, and J. G. Scott, "Neuropsychological assessment of Asian-American children and adolescents," in *Guide to Psychological Assessment with Asians*, pp. 407–425, Springer, 2014.

[3] T. M. Laudate and A. P. Nelson, "Macropsia," in *Encyclopedia of Clinical Neuropsychology*, pp. 1506–1506, Springer, New York, NY, USA, 2011.

[4] A. M. Liu, J. G. Liu, G. W. Liu, and G. T. Liu, ""Alice in wonderland" syndrome: presenting and follow-up characteristics," *Pediatric Neurology*, vol. 51, no. 3, pp. 317–320, 2014.

[5] F. Frassinetti, P. Nichelli, and G. Di Pellegrino, "Selective horizontal dysmetropsia following prestriate lesion," *Brain*, vol. 122, no. 2, pp. 339–350, 1999.

[6] D. Gersztenkorn and A. G. Lee, "Palinopsia revamped: a systematic review of the literature," *Survey of Ophthalmology*, 2014.

[7] Y. H. Hong, T. S. Lim, S. W. Yong, and S. Y. Moon, "Ipsilateral visual illusion after unilateral posterior cerebral artery infarction: a report of two cases," *Journal of the Neurological Sciences*, vol. 295, no. 1-2, pp. 114–116, 2010.

[8] J. Kassubek, M. Otte, T. Wolter, M. W. Greenlee, T. Mergner, and C. H. Lücking, "Brain imaging in a patient with hemimicropsia," *Neuropsychologia*, vol. 37, no. 12, pp. 1327–1334, 1999.

[9] K. Donnelly, "Metamorphopsia," in *Encyclopedia of Clinical Neuropsychology*, pp. 1585–1586, Springer, New York, NY, USA, 2011.

[10] A. Arboix, G. Arbe, L. García-Eroles, M. Oliveres, O. Parra, and J. Massons, "Infarctions in the vascular territory of the posterior cerebral artery: clinical features in 232 patients," *BMC Research Notes*, vol. 4, article 329, 2011.

[11] M.-G. Park, K.-D. Choi, S. K. Ji et al., "Hemimacropsia after medial temporo-occipital infarction," *Journal of Neurology, Neurosurgery and Psychiatry*, vol. 78, no. 5, pp. 546–548, 2007.

[12] N. E. Parks, H. B. Rigby, G. J. Gubitz, J. J. Shankar, and R. A. Purdy, "Dysmetropsia and cotard's syndrome due to migrainous infarction—or not?" *Cephalalgia*, vol. 34, pp. 717–720, 2014.

5

# Acute Ischemic Stroke Secondary to Iron Deficiency Anemia: A Case Report

**Preema J. Mehta,[1,2] Sherita Chapman,[1] Annapurni Jayam-Trouth,[1] and Mohankumar Kurukumbi[1]**

[1] *Department of Neurology, Howard University Hospital, 2041 Georgia Ave., Washington, DC 20060, USA*
[2] *Department of Neurology, Howard University College of Medicine, Washington, DC 20059, USA*

Correspondence should be addressed to Mohankumar Kurukumbi, mohan311@gmail.com

Academic Editors: J. E. Cohen, J. L. González-Gutiérrez, Y. Iwasaki, and H. Kocaeli

A rare case of acute ischemic stroke in a young patient with iron deficiency anemia (IDA) is reported. IDA has been suggested to have an association with stroke, but few cases have proven it thus far. Three physiological mechanisms explaining IDA to ischemic stroke include a hypercoagulable state secondary to IDA, thrombocytosis secondary to IDA, and anemic hypoxia induced by IDA. Our paper shows an example of a hypoxia-induced stroke secondary to IDA in a young woman with menorrhagia. Thrombus formation was ruled out as the Magnetic Resonance Angiogram (MRA) showed no evidence. As all other known causes for stroke were ruled out, the patient's IDA is a reasonable cause for her stroke. Iron deficiency decreases the amount of hemoglobin, which consequently decreases the amount of oxygen in the blood resulting in low-oxygen delivery to the brain. This causes hypoxic conditions in the brain, leading to death of brain tissue. Thus, we suggest a possible relationship between IDA and ischemic stroke in young adults. Considering IDA as one of the risk factors for ischemic stroke and treating with timely transfusions would be an important step one can take to prevent stroke.

## 1. Introduction

Strokes are often considered a consequence of hypertension and atherosclerosis. Some rare causes of stroke also include systemic hypoperfusion, sickle cell anemia, cerebral venous sinus thrombosis, arterial fibrillation, and cocaine abuse. Iron deficiency anemia as a risk factor for acute ischemic stroke has been reported in only a few case reports [1]. The majority of these few cases show thrombosis secondary to IDA causing ischemic stroke [1], but in our case it was hypoxia-induced stroke secondary to IDA.

## 2. Case Presentation

A forty-seven-year-old female presented to the emergency department with complaints of weakness and numbness of two-hour duration in the left upper extremity as well as slurred speech. Her past medical history was remarkable for iron deficiency anemia and menorrhagia due to a uterine fibroid. She also had a history of chronic pulmonary heart disease and asthma. She denied taking any medications for these conditions and was also not taking any oral contraceptives. Her family history was negative for any neurological or hematological conditions.

The clinical examination in the emergency room included mild dysarthria and decreased repetitive finger movements in her left upper extremity. The rest of the detailed neurological examination was normal. The patient was initiated with stroke protocol and CT of the head was done, which revealed an old bifrontal encephalomalacia with left greater than right, possibly secondary to previous trauma (Figure 1). MRI of the brain showed acute infarction in right middle cerebral artery (MCA) distribution (Figures 2(a) and 2(b)). MRA revealed no evidence of thrombus formation or carotid dissection (Figures 2(c) and 2(d)).

Laboratory analysis showed the patient's hemoglobin 7.6 g/dL, hematocrit 23%, ferritin 4.6 ng/mL, RBCs3.16 $\times 10^6$/uL, MCV 72.8 fL, and MCH 24.1 pg/cell, which were all below normal limits, and along with the peripheral blood smear, displayed microcytic hypochromic anemia. The

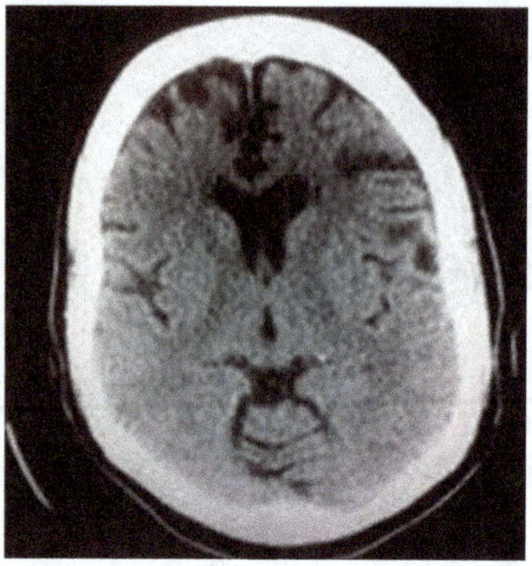

FIGURE 1: CT scan of the head without contrast showing old bifrontal encephalomalacia (left greater than right).

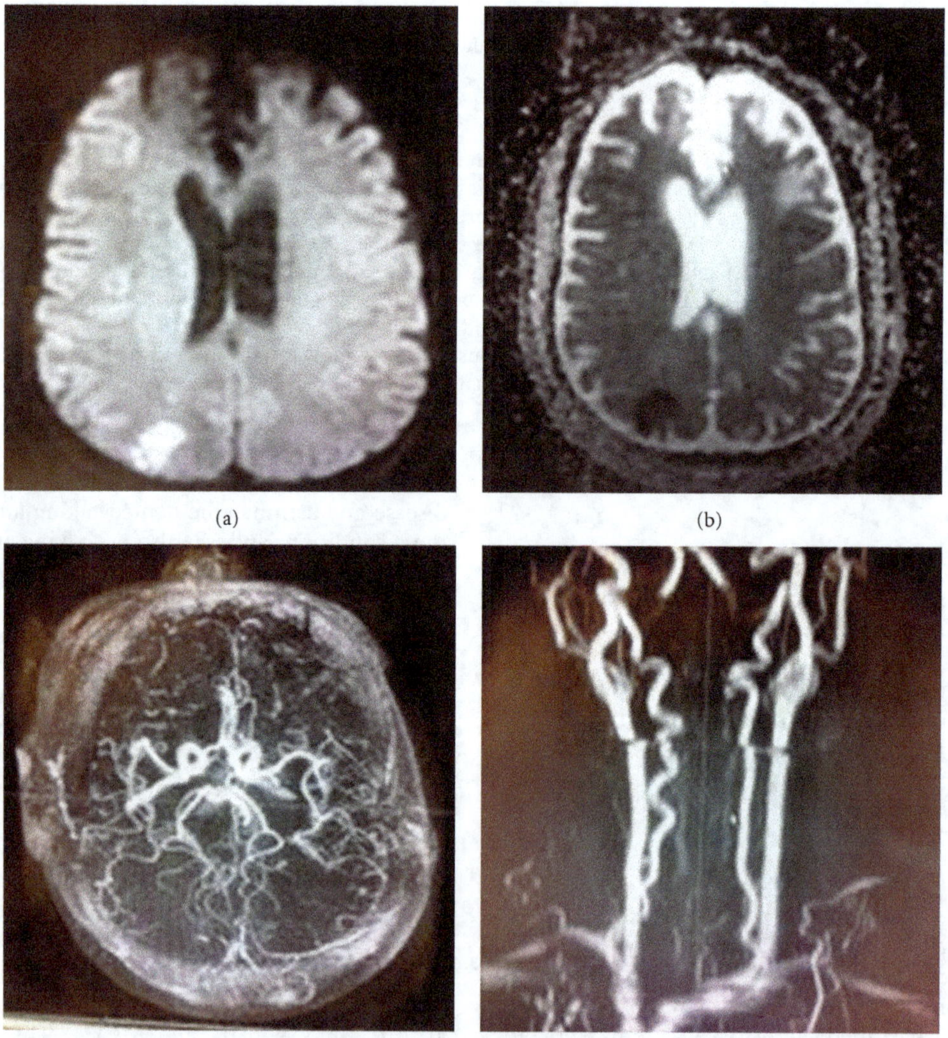

(a) (b) (c) (d)

FIGURE 2: MRI Brain (a) DWI showing hyperintense lesion in the right MCA territory. (b) ADC showing mismatch in the same region confirming acute infarction. (c) and (d) MRA showing no evidence of thrombus formation or carotid dissection.

patient also had thrombocytosis with a platelet count of 512,000. The patient's lipid panel was normal, consisting of LDL 67 mg/dL and HDL 42 mg/dL. The other laboratory parameters including white blood count, chemistry panel, urea, creatinine, and anion gap were also within normal limits.

During the hospital stay, the patient was found lying on the floor unresponsive, with bowel incontinence. The patient's eyes deviated to the right side, left face weakness, and left upper extremity with 0/5 on MRC (Medical Research Council) scale for motor strength. Two minutes prior to this event, patient was seen ambulating in her room. She gradually became responsive over time and was loaded with Phenytoin for the suspicion of seizure. She was then transferred to the ICU care. A repeat CT scan of the head (Figure 3) showed a large right MCA territory acute nonhemorrhagic infarction with significant increase in size seen on previous MRI. The patient's hemoglobin was 6.9 g/dL during this event. Due to her history of uterine fibroma, the patient underwent a transvaginal ultrasound, which ruled out active bleeding. The patient received two units of packed red blood cells (PRBCs) and her hemoglobin stabilized throughout the remainder of the hospital course between 9-10 g/dL. She was enrolled into physical and speech therapy and was discharged on the fifteenth day with residual left arm upper weakness.

Note, all other possible confounding factors for stroke were excluded by doing additional tests, which were all normal, including hemoglobin electrophoresis, paroxysmal nocturnal hemoglobinuria marker, protein S and C, antithrombin III, factor Leiden V, erythrocyte sedimentation rate, antinuclear antibody, rapid plasma reagin, anticardiolipin antibody, Vitamin B12 levels, homocysteine levels, prothrombin and partial prothrombin times, hemoccult stool, TEE, and lupus anticoagulant antibodies.

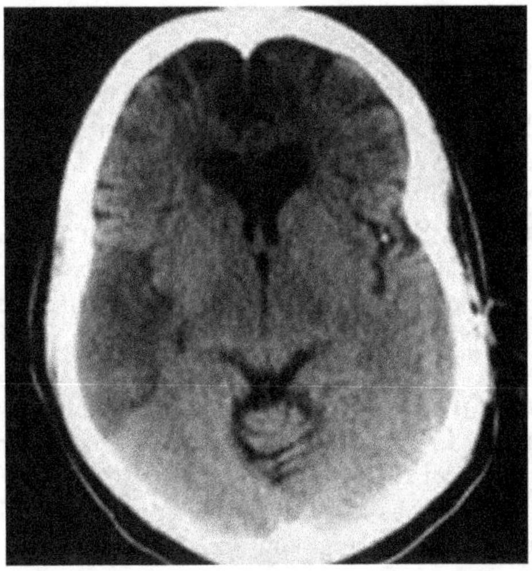

FIGURE 3: CT scan of the head without contrast showing a larger right MCA infarction compared Figure 1.

## 3. Discussion

Strokes can occur at any age and although the majority occurs over the age of 65, nearly one-fourth of strokes occur in people under the age of 65. Some common causes in this population include cardioembolism, hematologic disorders, substance abuse, trauma, dissections, oral contraceptive use, connective tissue disorders, pregnancy and postpartum states, and migraine. However, the cause of stroke in young patients remains undetermined in about 30% of cases [2]. Therefore, there needs to be a greater focus on discovering the other risk factors such as IDA in this population. IDA has been suggested to have an association with stroke, but few cases have proven it thus far.

IDA has been associated with cerebrovascular disease under three conditions. First, it has been found in patients with venous sinus thrombosis [3] or central retinal vein thrombosis [4], possibly due to secondary thrombocytosis [5]. Second, severe anemia may cause reversible focal deficits on an anemic hypoxic basis [6], sometimes in the setting of severe atherosclerotic disease. Third, IDA has been associated with cerebral infarctions, presumably on an arterial basis [7, 8] either with the evidence of thrombus formation or hypoxic basis.

Childhood ischemic strokes associated with IDA have been studied in greater depth than IDA-associated strokes in young adults. Three physiological mechanisms explaining IDA to childhood ischemic stroke include a hypercoagulable state secondary to IDA, thrombocytosis secondary to IDA, and anemic hypoxia induced by IDA [9]. Hartfield et al. reported a series of six children, between 6–18 months of age with an ischemic stroke or venous thrombosis after a viral prodrome. All patients had iron deficiency as a consistent finding among the group, and other known etiologies of childhood stroke were excluded [10]. These risk factors could possibly be a cause of stroke in the adult population as well.

Cases of carotid thrombus associated with iron deficiency anemia and thrombocytosis have been reported in adults. One reason is due to an anemic patient needing more blood flow to the brain to compensate for the lack of oxygen. Therefore, the increase in blood flow can cause endothelial vessel damage, causing a cascade of thrombus formation to occur. Akins et al. reported three case reports in which young women with severe IDA and thrombocytosis secondary to menorrhagia develop carotid artery thrombosis. The patient's profile and workup were similar to our case. The three women in these cases were 44, 20, and 39 years old, and the hemoglobin levels ranged between 6.3–7.1 g/dL [1]. Each of the case reports had evidence of thrombus by angiography due to suspicion of thrombus-induced stroke. They also ruled out other common causes for stroke by performing similar tests such as in our case.

Our paper shows an example of a hypoxia-induced stroke secondary to IDA in a young woman with menorrhagia. Thrombus formation was ruled out as the MRA showed no evidence. As all other known causes for stroke were ruled out, the patient's IDA is a reasonable cause for her stroke. Iron deficiency decreases the amount of hemoglobin, which consequently decreases the amount of oxygen in the blood resulting in low oxygen delivery to the brain. This causes hypoxic conditions in the brain, leading to death of brain tissue. Thus, we suggest a possible relationship between IDA and ischemic stroke in young adults.

Our patient had presented to the emergency department with hemoglobin of 7.6 g/dL, which was not focused on as a possible cause for stroke at that time. The patient then became unresponsive with sudden onset of left extremity weakness during her continued hospital stay with a lower hemoglobin of 6.9 g/dL. The patient was transfused with two units of PRBCs and thereafter she gradually showed improvement in motor strength and speech. After ruling out the common causes of stroke, it became clear that the low hemoglobin was most likely the culprit. It is likely that the persistent low hemoglobin and upright position of the patient may have caused hypoxia and an acute ischemic attack in her brain due to lack of oxygen delivery. This is an example of the hypoxia-induced mechanism, which was supported by the development of larger infarction in the right MCA region.

Anemia is often overlooked as an important factor in the setting of ischemic stroke, which upon correction may significantly improve the outcome. Huang et al. focused on the influence of anemia on clinical presentation and outcome of patients with first-ever atherosclerosis-related ischemic stroke. It has been shown that within three years of initial onset of first-ever atherosclerosis-related ischemic stroke, the mortality rate was significantly higher in patients who had anemia at the time of admission [11]. This topic clearly needs serious attention and further research.

If our patient had been treated for anemia on admission, this may have prevented her from progressing to a larger stroke, thus providing a more favorable outcome. Therefore, considering such risk factors like anemia is important in the prevention of such devastating and debilitating events.

## 4. Conclusion

This case has been reported because of the unique sequence of events that led to an interesting correlation between IDA and hypoxia-induced ischemic stroke. When stroke occurs in younger individuals, we need to search for other risk factors, such as dissection, AV malformations, coagulopathies, connective tissue disorders, OCP use, and now discovering that IDA should not be overlooked. IDA is a common concern predominantly in younger women, which must be addressed as a risk factor for stroke. In this case, transfusing the patient and thereby curing the anemia is what most likely saved the patient's life and prevented her from further possible ischemic strokes. If anemia was a known risk factor and our patient's anemia was corrected upon admission, the outcome may have been favorable, preventing the residual left extremity weakness. Therefore, a standard set of guidelines should be made regarding transfusions in anemic patients in the setting of stroke. IDA has been overlooked as a risk factor for ischemic stroke and needs to be further studied with greater focus.

## Abbreviations

CT: Computerized tomography
MRI: Magnetic resonance imaging
MRA: Magnetic resonance angiogram
IDA: Iron deficiency anemia
RBC: Red blood cell
MCA: Middle cerebral artery
MCV: Mean corpuscular volume
MCH: Mean corpuscular hemoglobin
HDL: High-density lipoprotein
LDL: Low-density lipoprotein
MRC: Medical research council
TEE: Transesophageal echocardiography
ICU: Intensive care unit
PRBC: Packed red blood cell
OCP: Oral contraceptive pill
AV: Arterio venous.

## Consent

Written informed consent was obtained from the patient for publication of this paper and accompanying images.

## Conflict of Interests

The authors declare that they have no competing interests.

## References

[1] P. T. Akins, S. Glenn, P. M. Nemeth, and C. P. Derdeyn, "Carotid artery thrombus associated with severe iron-deficiency anemia and thrombocytosis," *Stroke*, vol. 27, no. 5, pp. 1002–1005, 1996.

[2] M. Marcoux, "Stroke in young adults," *Colorado Neurological Institute Medical Journal*, vol. 11, no. 2, 2000.

[3] N. Aoki and T. Sakai, "Cerebral sinus thrombosis in patients with severe iron deficiency anaemia due to myoma uteri," *Acta Neurochirurgica*, vol. 97, no. 3-4, pp. 131–134, 1989.

[4] Y. Shibuya and S. Hayasaka, "Central retinal vein occlusion in a patient with anorexia nervosa," *American Journal of Ophthalmology*, vol. 119, no. 1, pp. 109–110, 1995.

[5] L. L. Schloesser, M. A. Kipp, and F. J. Wenzel, "Thrombocytosis in iron-deficiency anemia," *The Journal of Laboratory and Clinical Medicine*, vol. 66, no. 1, pp. 107–114, 1965.

[6] R. S. K. Young, D. E. Rannels, and A. Hilmo, "Severe anemia in childhood presenting as transient ischemic attacks," *Stroke*, vol. 14, no. 4, pp. 622–623, 1983.

[7] H. Knizley and W. D. Noyes, "Iron deficiency anemia, papilledema, thrombocytosis, and transient hemiparesis.," *Archives of Internal Medicine*, vol. 129, no. 3, pp. 483–486, 1972.

[8] M. B. Alexander, "Iron deficiency anemia, thrombocytosis, and cerebrovascular accident," *Southern Medical Journal*, vol. 76, no. 5, pp. 662–663, 1983.

[9] J. L. Maguire, G. Deveber, and P. C. Parkin, "Association between iron-deficiency anemia and stroke in young children," *Pediatrics*, vol. 120, no. 5, pp. 1053–1057, 2007.

[10] D. S. Hartfield, N. J. Lowry, D. L. Keene, and J. Y. Yager, "Iron deficiency: a cause of stroke in infants and children," *Pediatric Neurology*, vol. 16, no. 1, pp. 50–53, 1997.

[11] W. Y. Huang, I. C. Chen, L. Meng, W. C. Weng, and T. I. Peng, "The influence of anemia on clinical presentation and outcome of patients with first-ever atherosclerosis-related ischemic stroke," *Journal of Clinical Neuroscience*, vol. 16, no. 5, pp. 645–649, 2009.

6

# Feasibility of Functional Electrical Stimulation-Assisted Neurorehabilitation following Stroke in India: A Case Series

**Bhawna Khattar,[1] Alakananda Banerjee,[1] Rajsekhar Reddi,[2] and Anirban Dutta[3]**

[1] *Department of Physiotherapy and Rehabilitation, Max Super Speciality Hospital, Saket, New Delhi, India*
[2] *Department of Neurology, Max Super Speciality Hospital, Saket, New Delhi, India*
[3] *Department of Clinical Neurophysiology, Georg-August-University, Goettingen, Germany*

Correspondence should be addressed to Anirban Dutta, adutta@case.edu

Academic Editors: A. E. Cavanna and A. Fasano

Functional Electrical Stimulation (FES) facilitates ambulatory function after paralysis by electrically activating the muscles of the lower extremities. The Odstock Dropped Foot Stimulator (ODFS, Odstock, UK) called ODFS Pace, was used for heel-switch triggered FES-assisted walking. The ODFS is recommended as an intervention for neurologically impaired gait in the Royal College of Physicians (UK) Clinical Guidelines on Stroke. Based on the guidelines by the National Institute of Clinical Excellence (NICE, UK), we started first clinical study in India on ODFS Pace as an orthotic intervention for daily use. In this preliminary study, we also investigated improvement in volitional walking following 6 sessions (3 times per week, for 2 weeks) of 30 minutes of FES-assisted treadmill walking on 7 chronic (>6 months after stroke) stroke survivors. We found that short-duration, moderately intensive FES-assisted gait therapy improved volitional gait in 3 out of 7 stroke survivors suffering from foot drop. Even in absence of improvement in volitional walking, there were no adverse effects and the subjects found heel-switch triggered FES-assisted walking mostly "easy" (6 out of 7). Therefore FES is promising as an orthotic intervention for daily use; however, tailoring the intensity and/or frequency based on patient's ability may make it viable as a therapeutic intervention.

## 1. Introduction

The World Health Organization (WHO) defines stroke as "the rapid development of clinical signs and symptoms of a focal neurological disturbance lasting more than 24 hours or leading to death with no apparent cause other than vascular origin" [1]. Worldwide, 15 million people suffer a stroke every year, and stroke is the second leading cause of disability after dementia. India-centered studies have presented a prevalence rate of 27–34/100,000 in the 35–44 age group to 822–1116/100,000 in the 75+ age group [2–4]. The prevalence of stroke in younger individuals is higher in India as compared with high-income nations [5]. The burden of stroke on the quality of life is much greater in this younger age group of stroke survivors [5–7]. Moreover stroke drastically affects the economical productivity for that younger age group adding further to the overall disease burden [5] and therefore early rehabilitation to alleviate disability has a special significance in developing countries.

The disability due to poor ability to walk in stroke patients is frequently caused by the "foot drop" symptom that prevents the patient from being able to raise the foot during the swing phase of walking [8]. The foot slaps down on the ground after heel strike and the toe drags during the swing phase. In addition to that the patients often lack push-off power due to weakness in ankle plantar flexors (like gastrocnemius muscle), which not only reduces walking speed but also reduce ankle dorsiflexion angles during the early swing phase of gait [9]. Goldberg et al. have shown that the ankle plantar flexors are important for knee flexion velocity during push-off [10]. This leads to insufficient foot clearance that puts the patient at risk for stumbling and falling [9]. Consequently impairment of walking has been mentioned most frequently (39–90%) as the most important disabling condition in community-dwelling stroke survivors, and improving walking ability has been found to be the best way to reduce dependency [11, 12]. Almost 30% of patients who survive stroke are affected by foot drop, where the ankle dorsiflexors (e.g., tibialis anterior muscle) are functionally impaired [8, 9].

The current rehabilitation techniques following stroke are largely based on some variation of the Bobath concept which relies primarily on inhibiting spasticity and other abnormal responses through physiotherapy [13]. However there is no evidence of superiority of Bobath concept on improvements in sensorimotor control of upper and lower limb, dexterity, mobility, activities of daily living, health-related quality of life, and cost-effectiveness following stroke, and no evidence is available for the superiority of any other current approach [14]. Therefore, there is an urgent need to incorporate additional interventions based on recent findings from animal and human studies on task-specific motor learning and neuroplasticity into the framework of rehabilitation following stroke [15]. The challenge is in providing an orthotic intervention that facilitates community ambulation and in long term promotes normal recovery of gait so that the stroke survivor can wean away from the orthosis.

Functional-electrical-stimulation-(FES-) based orthosis has been shown to enhance walking abilities, increasing gait speed while lowering effort and has only recently developed into a therapeutic intervention for stroke rehabilitation [8, 16–25]. FES involves electrical stimulation of nerves and muscles with continuous short pulses of electrical current [26]. Hausdorff and Ring showed that the number of falls reduced significantly in hemiparetic patients who used FES to correct foot drop [23]. Although FES provides orthotic benefit, the "carry over" effect on volitional movement and the required dosing for long-term therapeutic benefit have not been investigated thoroughly. Daly et al. showed that gait training with FES had significant additive effect on gait coordination when compared to that without FES [24], where a treatment duration beyond 12 weeks might have shown additional gains. In this preliminary case study in India we studied (1) user response to the latest version of the Odstock Dropped Foot Stimulator (ODFS, Odstock, UK) [18] called ODFS Pace as an orthotic intervention, (2) short-duration moderate-intensity FES-assisted gait training as a therapeutic intervention at the rehabilitation clinic. We investigated changes in the volitional gait from baseline on 7 chronic (> 6 months after stroke) stroke survivors following 6 sessions (3 times a week, for 2 weeks) of 30 minutes of FES-assisted treadmill walking at their comfortable walking speed.

## 2. Case Series

The single-channel ODFS Pace (Odstock, UK) provides heel-switch triggered functional electrical stimulation (FES) to assist dorsiflexion of the ankle during walking [18]. The ODFS was recommended in the year 2000 as an intervention for neurologically impaired gait in the Clinical Guidelines on Stroke by the Royal College of Physicians (UK) and over 2000 patients have been fitted with ODFS for foot drop in UK. Based on the guidelines by the National Institute of Clinical Excellence (NICE, UK) which recommended (in July 2008) dropped foot stimulators as an intervention in stroke (http://www.nice.org.uk/Guidelines/IPG278/), we applied for ethics approval and started the first clinical study on ODFS Pace in India at the Max Super Speciality Hospitals Saket, India.

Four male and three female hemiplegic stroke survivors (age: 31–76 years) volunteered for this study. The study was approved by the Institutional Review Board of the Max Super Speciality Hospitals, Saket, India (http://www.ctri.nic.in/Clinicaltrials/pmaindet2.php?trialid=3821). Informed consent was obtained from all the subjects before their participation. The inclusion and exclusion criteria for the study are listed in Table 1. The ODFS Pace electrically stimulated the common peroneal nerve or the neuromuscular junction of the tibialis anterior (TA) muscle via self-adhesive skin electrodes which were positioned on the lower leg [18]. The placement of the stimulating electrodes is critical for balanced dorsiflexion and a trained physiotherapist fitted the stimulator to the patients. The stimulation was timed to the walking cycle by use of a switch which was placed under the heel. The stimulation was timed to begin right after or after a small delay when the heel was lifted from the ground and ended right after or after a small delay following heel strike. The electrical stimulation activated the muscles related to ankle dorsiflexion and caused the foot to lift when the user lifted the leg to step forward [18]. By extending the stimulation beyond heel strike, the stimulation stabilized the ankle when the weight was loaded on the foot (i.e., loading phase).

After the baseline assessments to verify the suitability of the prospective subjects based on our inclusion/exclusion criteria (presented in Table 1), 7 subjects were recruited for the FES-assisted gait training every alternate day for 2 weeks (i.e., thrice a week) in which 30 minutes of treadmill-walking and simultaneous "naked eye" quick observational gait analysis (OGA) [27] to adjust stimulation parameters, were performed under the supervision of a trained physiotherapist. Since interrater agreement is much higher with a binary scale [28, 29] therefore a trained physiotherapist rated gait deviations at the Ankle, Knee, Hip, Pelvis, and Trunk as "present" or "absent." The manual muscle test (MMT) on the affected ankle dorsiflexor (tibialis anterior) muscle and a measure of ankle spasticity on modified Ashworth scale (MAS) [30] were also performed before FES-assisted gait training. We investigated incremental changes (if any) in the volitional gait using pre- versus postintervention video-based OGA [27–29]. We also conducted patient survey to record their comments and subjective assessments based on Usability Rating Scale (URS) [31]. The subjective assessments was conducted on a 7-point scale with URS, of the perceived ease of use of ODFS Pace for heel switch triggered FES-assisted walking. The subject was asked to rate the ODFS Pace for FES-assisted walking as "difficult," "moderate," or "easy." After selecting one of those three choices, the subject was asked to refine his/her selection as "very," "moderately,"

Table 1: Inclusion and exclusion criteria for the stroke study.

| Inclusion criteria | Exclusion criteria |
|---|---|
| Age 21 to 80 years | Brainstem stroke |
| >6 months from a first clinical nonhemorrhagic or hemorrhagic stroke | Epilepsy |
| Medically stable | Severely impaired cognition and communication |
| Unilateral lower extremity hemiparesis | History of peroneal nerve injury |
| Able to ambulate 16 feet (5 meters) continuously with minimal assistance or less, without the use of an Ankle Foot Orthosis (AFO) | History of Parkinson's, spinal cord injury, traumatic brain injury, multiple sclerosis, and uncontrolled seizure disorder |
| AFO is clinically indicated (foot drop during ambulation) | Uncompensated hemineglect (extinguishing to double simultaneous stimulation) |
| Electrical stimulation of the paretic ankle dorsiflexors produces ankle dorsiflexion to neutral without pain | Edema of the paretic lower extremity |
| Full-voluntary dorsiflexion of the contralateral ankle | Absent sensation of lower leg and foot |
| Skin intact on hemiparetic lower extremity | History of cardiac arrhythmias with hemodynamic instability |
| | Cardiac pacemaker or other implanted electronic system |
| | Botulinum toxin injections to any lower-extremity muscle in the last 3 months |
| | Evidence of deep venous thrombosis or thromboembolism |

or "barely." The case series is described below and the diagnostic scores are summarized in Table 2.

*Case 1.* A 31-year-old young, energetic, and moderately obese gentleman suffered stroke in July 2008 (3 years, 8 months after stroke) which resulted in left hemiplegia. The subject complained of putting on weight due to sedentary lifestyle since the instability in his affected ankle led to decreased mobility. He was recommended FES-assisted gait therapy to develop confidence for community ambulation, to improve cardiovascular endurance, and possible therapeutic benefits. His preintervention video-based OGA of the affected side showed lack of dorsiflexion at heel strike resulting in foot slap, and mostly inverted foot during swing phase. Also, he had inadequate knee flexion during swing phase, and hip hiking with inadequate hip flexion during terminal swing phase. The pelvis and trunk however showed no significant deviations from normal. He underwent our two weeks of FES-assisted gait training as described earlier. His postintervention video-based OGA of the affected side during volitional walking showed improved toe off during terminal stance phase, improvement in knee flexion during swing phase, but no significant changes at the hip from preintervention. The subject graded "easy" on URS and reported less-perceived effort during FES-assisted walking.

*Case 2.* A 58-year-old, moderately obese lady with coronary artery disease leading to percutaneous transluminal coronary angioplasty (PTCA), hypertension, diabetes mellitus, and acute renal failure due to diabetic nephropathy, suffered stroke in April 2009 (3 years after stroke) resulting in right hemiplegia. The subject complained of inability to walk without support and was dependent on her caregiver for activities of daily living (ADL). She was recommended FES-assisted gait therapy to develop confidence during walking and to reduce dependence on her caregiver for ADL. Her preintervention video-based OGA of the affected side during volitional walking showed lack of dorsiflexion at heel strike resulting in foot slap, and inverted foot during swing phase. She also had inadequate knee flexion during swing phase, inadequate hip flexion during terminal swing, and significant hip hiking during swing phase. She however had no significant deviation from normal at the pelvis and trunk. She underwent our two weeks of FES-assisted gait training as described earlier. Her postintervention video-based OGA of the affected side during volitional walking showed no significant change from preintervention. The subject however perceived "the leg is lighter" and "lesser twist in the foot" during FES-assisted walking. She graded "easy" on URS.

*Case 3.* A 72-year-old outgoing lady with hypertension suffered stroke in 2006 (6 years after stroke), which resulted in left hemiparesis. The subject recently complained of falls due to ankle instability. Due to fear of falls she had low confidence in activities outside her home for ADL. She was recommended FES-assisted gait therapy to develop confidence during walking and for therapeutic benefit. Her preintervention video-based OGA of the affected side during volitional walking showed lack of heel strike (i.e., foot slap) and inadequate toe off, lack of dorsiflexion during midswing to terminal swing, and inadequate ground clearance. There was also inadequate knee extension during midstance, inadequate knee flexion during swing phase, inadequate contralateral hip extension and improper hip flexion during swing phase, and circumduction during midswing. There was a lack of pelvic rotation during midswing to terminal swing, and a forward lean of the trunk during stance phase. She underwent our two weeks of FES-assisted gait training as described earlier. Her postintervention video-based OGA of the affected side during volitional walking showed improved ground clearance of the foot, improved knee flexion during

TABLE 2: Summary of the case series (M: male, F: female, MCA: middle cerebral artery, PTCA: percutaneous transluminal coronary angioplasty, CABG: coronary artery bypass graft, TA: tibialis anterior muscle, MMT: manual muscle test, MAS: modified Ashworth scale, URS: usability rating scale, OGA: observational gait analysis, MRI: magnetic resonance imaging).

| Case | Age/gender | MRI diagnosis | Comorbidities | Year of stroke | TA MMT | Ankle MAS | URS | Pre versus postintervention OGA |
|---|---|---|---|---|---|---|---|---|
| 1 | 31/M | Right MCA stroke: infarct in right basal ganglia, fronto-temporal, and perisylvian grey and white matter. | None | 2008 | 1+ | 3 | Easy | Improvement |
| 2 | 58/F | Left MCA stroke: acute non-hemorrhagic infarct in left basal ganglia and paraventricular white matter/corona radiate with lacunar infarct in left high frontal pre-central cortex. | Diabetes, hypertension, post-PTCA | 2009 | 2− | 2 | Easy | No change |
| 3 | 72/F | Right basal ganglia infarct: gliotic area and old hemorrhagic remnant in right basal ganglia and thalamus with chronic ischemic changes in the brain. | Hypertension | 2006 | 3− | 2 | Moderately difficult | Improvement |
| 4 | 63/M | Left MCA stroke including basal ganglia: infarct in the territory supplied by left Middle Cerebral Artery (MCA) including basal ganglia. | Diabetes mellitus type II, hypertension | 2009 | 2 | 2 | Easy | No change |
| 5 | 73/M | Left MCA stroke. | Post-CABG | 2010 | 3− | 1+ | Easy | Improvement |
| 6 | 76/F | Right MCA stroke, including basal ganglia. | Post-CABG | 2009 | 3− | 1+ | Easy | No change |
| 7 | 65/F | Left MCA stroke, including basal ganglia and subcortical white matter. | None | 2009 | 1 | 3 | Easy | No change |

swing phase, and improved hip flexion during the swing phase. She commented during FES-assisted walking that "I am able to lift my foot," "I can walk more confidently," "My walking speed has increased." She graded "moderately difficult" on URS.

*Case 4.* A 63-year-old gentleman with hypertension and diabetes mellitus type II suffered stroke in August 2009 (2 years, 7 months after stroke) which resulted in left hemiplegia. He complained of labored walking. He was undergoing regular rehabilitation for last 15 months but showed no improvement. He was recommended FES-assisted gait therapy for possible therapeutic benefits. His preintervention video-based OGA of the affected side during volitional walking showed ground contact with forefoot, flat foot during the loading phase, and lack of dorsiflexion during swing phase. The knee was hyperextended during midstance and the subject suffered from reduced knee flexion during swing phase. He also suffered from hip hiking during swing phase, external rotation of the affected limb during toe off, and circumduction from preswing to terminal swing phase. The affected left pelvis hiked towards right from preswing to terminal swing, and there was no forward rotation of the pelvis during initial swing to terminal swing phase. There was also significant backward lean in the trunk from stance to preswing phase. He underwent our two weeks of FES-assisted gait training as described earlier. His postintervention video-based OGA of the affected side during volitional walking showed no significant change from preintervention. The subject liked FES-assisted treadmill walking where the foot assisted by FES could clear the ground more easily during the swing phase. However the rotation of the leg was still present during FES-assisted treadmill walking which demonstrated a weakness at the hip which couldnot be alleviated with the single-channel ODFS Pace. The subject graded "easy" on URS.

*Case 5.* A 73-year-old gentleman with coronary artery bypass graft (CABG) had a stroke in November 2010 (2 years, 3 months after stroke) which resulted in right hemiplegia. His primary concern was propensity for fall on uneven surfaces due to reduced ground clearance with foot drop. He was recommended FES-assisted gait therapy to develop confidence during walking and possible therapeutic benefits. His preintervention video-based OGA of the affected side during volitional walking showed ground contact with foot flat continuing into the loading phase, inadequate toe off, and inadequate dorsiflexion during swing phase. There was also inadequate knee flexion during terminal stance, and inadequate knee extension at the heel strike. There was inadequate hip extension from midstance to preswing, and slight circumduction from preswing to terminal swing phase. There were however no significant deviations at the pelvis or trunk. He underwent our two weeks of FES-assisted gait training as described earlier. His postintervention video-based OGA of the affected side during volitional walking showed improved toe off, improved knee flexion in swing phase, and improved hip extension. The subject remarked—"easy to lift foot with FES"—during his gait training. The subject graded "easy" on URS.

*Case 6.* A 76-year-old female with CABG had a stroke in November 2009 (2 years, 3 months after stroke) resulting in left hemiplegia. Her primary concern was weakness in the affected ankle. She was recommended FES-assisted gait therapy to develop confidence during walking and possible therapeutic benefits. Her preintervention video-based OGA of the affected side during volitional walking showed ground contact with foot flat continuing in the loading phase, inadequate knee flexion during swing phase, inadequate hip flexion during midstance, slight circumduction from preswing to terminal swing, inadequate pelvic rotation, and hip hiking from preswing to terminal swing. The trunk however showed no significant deviation from normal. She underwent our two weeks of FES-assisted gait training as described earlier. Her postintervention video-based OGA of the affected side during volitional walking showed no significant change when compared to preintervention. The subject however reported less effort during walking with FES-assistance and graded "easy" on URS.

*Case 7.* A 65-year-old physically active gentleman suffered stroke in October 2009 (2 years, 5 months after stroke) resulting in right hemiplegia. His primary concern was labored walking and foot drop which was corrected for ADL with an AFO, resulting in muscle atrophy at the ankle. He was recommended FES-assisted gait therapy to reduce muscle atrophy and possible therapeutic benefits. His preintervention video-based OGA of the affected side during volitional walking showed ground contact with forefoot or foot flat continuing in the loading phase, and lack of dorsiflexion. There was also inadequate knee flexion during swing phase, inadequate hip extension from midstance to terminal swing phase, and slight circumduction from preswing to terminal swing phase. There was a lack of pelvic rotation, significant hip hiking from initial swing to mid-swing, and lack of lateral horizontal shift of the trunk during stance phase. He underwent our two weeks of FES-assisted gait training as described earlier. His postintervention video-based OGA of the affected side during volitional walking however showed no significant change from preintervention. The subject liked FES-assistance to lift the foot during treadmill walking. He graded "easy" on URS.

## 3. Discussion

We found that our short-duration, moderately intensive FES-assisted gait therapy improved volitional gait in 3 out of 7 stroke survivors suffering from foot drop. Even though prior work [17] showed a treatment duration beyond 12 weeks necessary for reaching a plateau for therapeutic benefits, we kept the duration of the FES-assisted gait therapy short (only 2 weeks) to monitor only incremental change and didnot want the therapeutic benefits to plateau before a planned randomized controlled crossover study on electromyogram-triggered FES-assisted gait training [32]. Even in absence of improvement in volitional walking following FES-assisted gait therapy, there were no adverse effects and the subjects found heel-switch triggered FES-assisted gait with ODFS Pace mostly "easy" (6 out of 7 subjects) on URS. We postulate that the "carry over" effect that we intended to observe following short-duration, moderately intensive FES-assisted gait therapy is patient specific and we need to perform a case-by-case study with a larger cohort in future.

In published reports, the functional integrity of the corticospinal tracts (CSTs) has been associated with an individuals capacity for further functional improvement following stroke [33–35]. Moreover, stroke presents with heterogeneous patient-specific impairments in motor, sensory, tone, visual, perceptual, cognition, aphasia, apraxia, coordination, and equilibrium. Therefore the functional limitations following stroke are varied, including gait dysfunction, fall risk, limited activities of daily living, difficulties in swallowing, reduced upper extremity function, altered communication, besides others. Based on the residual function of a stroke survivor, the number of muscles that need FES assistance, intensity, frequency, and duration of the FES-assisted gait training need to be decided. The ability of a stroke survivor to undergo FES-assisted gait therapy also depends on their cardiovascular and neuromuscular capacity besides psychological factors such as motivation. We found that one channel of FES that is available with ODFS Pace was not enough to provide functional gait to some of our subjects (e.g., Cases 3, 4, 6, and 7), who needed more channels due to significant deviations in pelvis and trunk gait trajectories from normal as found from preintervention video-based OGA. Therefore in those cases, the therapeutic benefits may have been limited by the lack of gait training with multijoint coordination assisted with multichannel FES [25].

It has been shown that only 10% of stroke survivors recover limb strength and mobility rapidly enough to prevent contractures [36]. Also, 20% of stroke survivors suffer muscle atrophy which underlie worsening metabolic fitness in the chronic phase of stroke including gross muscular atrophy, altered muscle molecular phenotype, increased intramuscular area fat, elevated tissue inflammatory markers, and diminished peripheral blood flow dynamics [37]. Moreover, bone resorption begins after 30 hours of immobility which results in 17% bone loss in the paretic arm and up to 12% in the paretic leg in the chronic stages of stroke [38]. Therefore hip fracture, which is the most frequent fracture following stroke, can have incidences 2–4 times higher in stroke patients compared with the reference population [39]. FES-assisted gait training may alleviate these debilitating conditions where increased intensity and frequency of rehabilitation may help [40]. In fact recent studies in India on therapeutic benefits of FES-assisted gait training in conjunction with conventional physiotherapy have shown the additive effects of FES on reducing spasticity, improving dorsiflexor strength, improving walking ability, and improving metabolic fitness [41–43].

However lack of accessible rehabilitation facilities and high cost of rehabilitation at the well-equipped clinics are current challenges in India which usually lead to high-dropout of individuals from rehabilitation therapy following stroke. Any deconditioned chronic stroke survivor will need to recondition their cardiovascular endurance, metabolic fitness, muscle conditions, and bone strength with a gradual increase in the intensity (number of hours per day) and frequency (number of days per week) of FES-assisted gait therapy, providing a higher level as they improve their function. Also, the FES-assisted gait training should be started as soon as the patient becomes clinically stable since early intervention has shown better functional outcomes, survival rates, and reduced length of required therapy [44]. Therefore we are currently investigating a home-based rehabilitation model where stroke survivors can use a low-cost FES device (such as ODFS Pace) as an orthotic intervention for daily use during walking at home and subsequently for community ambulation after they achieve proficiency. Following a short stay in rehabilitation clinic, home-based FES-assisted treadmill-gait therapy may also be more economical and feasible, with a consulting physiotherapist in case of more affected stroke survivors. However these home-based models need to be validated with stroke survivors in India where well-equipped rehabilitation clinics are expensive, far, and few.

In closing, we would summarize our research hypothesis for stroke neurorehabilitation following Ward and Cohen [15], who have presented lessons from animal models where manipulation of environmental, behavioral, and pharmacologic contexts influenced cerebral reorganization and consequently the process of recovery of function following stroke. We propose that early task-specific FES-assisted gait therapy may drive functionally relevant neuroplastic changes in the brain. However such FES-assisted gait therapy needs to be tailored to individual health condition as identified based on WHO International Classification of Functioning (ICF). The WHO ICF model recommends intervention at multiple levels (e.g., impairment, activity, participation) where environment and personal factors can play an important role. We also need to measure at each level for example, individuals capacity for functional recovery measured with imaging techniques [26–28], metabolic fitness, and cardiovascular health measured with physiological cost index [31], and functional gait analysis to select the paretic muscles to be assisted with FES. With the WHO ICF model, we may be able to understand the response to the FES-assisted gait therapy at each level, and also understand the relationships between different levels for future planning.

## Authors' Contribution

Bhawna Khattar and Alakananda Banerjee contributed equally to this work.

## Conflict of Interests

The authors declare no existence of competing interests during the conduction of this study where the professional judgment concerning patients' welfare and the validity of the research may be influenced by financial gain or personal opinion.

## Acknowledgments

Dr. A. Dutta (Ph.D.) was supported by the Alexander von Humboldt Foundation, Germany. Drs. R. Reddi (M.D.), A. Banerjee (P.T.), and B. Khattar (P.T.) were supported by the Max Super Speciality Hospitals, Saket, New Delhi. The voluntary help received from the subjects is gratefully acknowledged.

## References

[1] World Health Organisation, *Preventing Chronic Diseases: A Vital Investment*, Geneva, Switzerland, 2005.

[2] P. Dalal, M. Bhattacharjee, J. Vairale, and P. Bhat, "UN millennium development goals: can we halt the stroke epidemic in India?" *Annals of Indian Academy of Neurology*, vol. 10, no. 3, pp. 130–136, 2007.

[3] P. M. Dalal, S. Malik, M. Bhattacharjee et al., "Population-based stroke survey in Mumbai, India: incidence and 28-day case fatality," *Neuroepidemiology*, vol. 31, no. 4, pp. 254–261, 2008.

[4] S. E. Sridharan, J. P. Unnikrishnan, S. Sukumaran et al., "Incidence, types, risk factors, and outcome of stroke in a developing country the trivandrum stroke registry," *Stroke*, vol. 40, no. 4, pp. 1212–1218, 2009.

[5] M. Tripathi and D. Vibha, "Stroke in young in India," *Stroke Research and Treatment*, vol. 2011, Article ID 368629, 2011.

[6] B. Shah, "Development of sentinel health monitoring centers for surveillance of risk factors for non-communicable disease in India," Report From the Division of Non-Communicable Diseases, Indian Council of Medical Research, New Delhi, India, 2005.

[7] B. Shah and P. Mathur, Workshop Report on Stroke Surveillance in India, Division of noncommunicable Diseases, Indian Council of Medical Research, New Delhi, India, 2006.

[8] M. H. Granat, D. J. Maxwell, A. C. B. Ferguson, K. R. Lees, and J. C. Barbenel, "Peroneal stimulator: evaluation for the correction of spastic drop foot in hemiplegia," *Archives of Physical Medicine and Rehabilitation*, vol. 77, no. 1, pp. 19–24, 1996.

[9] V. Weerdesteyn, M. De Niet, H. J. R. Van Duijnhoven, and A. C. H. Geurts, "Falls in individuals with stroke," *Journal of Rehabilitation Research and Development*, vol. 45, no. 8, pp. 1195–1213, 2008.

[10] S. R. Goldberg, F. C. Anderson, M. G. Pandy, and S. L. Delp, "Muscles that influence knee flexion velocity in double support: implications for stiff-knee gait," *Journal of Biomechanics*, vol. 37, no. 8, pp. 1189–1196, 2004.

[11] N. A. Solomon, H. A. Glick, C. J. Russo, J. Lee, and K. A. Schulman, "Patient preferences for stroke outcomes," *Stroke*, vol. 25, no. 9, pp. 1721–1725, 1994.

[12] H. Barbeau and J. Fung, "The role of rehabilitation in the recovery of walking in the neurological population," *Current Opinion in Neurology*, vol. 14, no. 6, pp. 735–740, 2001.

[13] B. Bobath, "Treatment of adult hemiplegia," *Physiotherapy*, vol. 63, no. 10, pp. 310–313, 1977.

[14] B. J. Kollen, S. Lennon, B. Lyons et al., "The effectiveness of the bobath concept in stroke rehabilitation what is the evidence?" *Stroke*, vol. 40, no. 4, pp. e89–e97, 2009.

[15] N. S. Ward and L. G. Cohen, "Mechanisms underlying recovery of motor function after stroke," *Archives of Neurology*, vol. 61, no. 12, pp. 1844–1848, 2004.

[16] R. Merletti, A. Andina, M. Galante, and I. Furlan, "Clinical experience of electronic peroneal stimulators in 50 hemiparetic patients," *Scandinavian Journal of Rehabilitation Medicine*, vol. 11, no. 3, pp. 111–121, 1979.

[17] U. Bogataj, N. Gros, M. Malezic, B. Kelih, M. Kljajic, and R. Acimovic, "Restoration of gait during two to three weeks of therapy with multichannel electrical stimulation," *Physical Therapy*, vol. 69, no. 5, pp. 319–327, 1989.

[18] P. N. Taylor, J. H. Burridge, A. L. Dunkerley et al., "Clinical use of the odstock dropped foot stimulator: its effect on the speed and effort of walking," *Archives of Physical Medicine and Rehabilitation*, vol. 80, no. 12, pp. 1577–1583, 1999.

[19] L. R. Sheffler, M. T. Hennessey, G. G. Naples, and J. Chae, "Peroneal nerve stimulation versus an ankle foot orthosis for correction of footdrop in stroke: impact on functional ambulation," *Neurorehabilitation and Neural Repair*, vol. 20, no. 3, pp. 355–360, 2006.

[20] A. I. R. Kottink, H. J. Hermens, A. V. Nene, M. J. Tenniglo, C. G. Groothuis-Oudshoorn, and M. J. Ijzerman, "Therapeutic effect of an implantable peroneal nerve stimulator in subjects with chronic stroke and footdrop: a randomized controlled trial," *Physical Therapy*, vol. 88, no. 4, pp. 437–448, 2008.

[21] J. H. Burridge, P. N. Taylor, S. A. Hagan, D. E. Wood, and I. D. Swain, "The effects of common peroneal stimulation on the effort and speed of walking: a randomized controlled trial with chronic hemiplegic patients," *Clinical Rehabilitation*, vol. 11, no. 3, pp. 201–210, 1997.

[22] J. H. Burridge and M. Ladouceur, "Clinical and therapeutic applications of neuromuscular stimulation: a review of current use and speculation into future developments," *Neuromodulation*, vol. 4, no. 4, pp. 147–154, 2001.

[23] J. M. Hausdorff and H. Ring, "Effects of a new radio frequency-controlled neuroprosthesis on gait symmetry and rhythmicity in patients with chronic hemiparesis," *American Journal of Physical Medicine and Rehabilitation*, vol. 87, no. 1, pp. 4–13, 2008.

[24] J. J. Daly, J. Zimbelman, K. L. Roenigk et al., "Recovery of coordinated gait: randomized controlled stroke trial of functional electrical stimulation (FES) versus no FES, with weight-supported treadmill and over-ground training," *Neurorehabilitation and Neural Repair*, vol. 25, no. 7, pp. 588–596, 2011.

[25] J. J. Daly and R. L. Ruff, "Feasibility of combining multichannel functional neuromuscular stimulation with weight-supported treadmill training," *Journal of the Neurological Sciences*, vol. 225, no. 1-2, pp. 105–115, 2004.

[26] R. Kobetic, R. J. Triolo, and E. B. Marsolais, "Muscle selection and walking performance of multichannel FES systems for ambulation in paraplegia," *IEEE Transactions on Rehabilitation Engineering*, vol. 5, no. 1, pp. 23–29, 1997.

[27] *Observational gait analysis handbook*, Professional Staff Association of Rancho Los Amigos Medical Center, Downey, Calif, USA, 1989.

[28] M. E. Eastlack, J. Arvidson, L. Snyder-Mackler, J. V. Danoff, and C. L. McGarvey, "Interrater reliability of videotaped observational gait-analysis assessments," *Physical Therapy*, vol. 71, no. 6, pp. 465–472, 1991.

[29] D. E. Krebs, J. E. Edelstein, and S. Fishman, "Reliability of observational kinematic gait analysis," *Physical Therapy*, vol. 65, no. 7, pp. 1027–1033, 1985.

[30] R. W. Bohannon and M. B. Smith, "Interrater reliability of a modified Ashworth scale of muscle spasticity," *Physical Therapy*, vol. 67, no. 2, pp. 206–207, 1987.

[31] E. Steinfeld and G. Danford, Eds., *Enabling Environments: Measuring the Impact of Environment on Disability and Rehabilitation*, Kluwer/Plenum, 1999.

[32] A. Dutta, R. Kobetic, and R. J. Triolo, "Gait initiation with electromyographically triggered electrical stimulation in people with partial paralysis," *Journal of Biomechanical Engineering*, vol. 131, no. 8, Article ID 081002, 2009.

[33] C. M. Stinear, P. A. Barber, P. R. Smale, J. P. Coxon, M. K. Fleming, and W. D. Byblow, "Functional potential in chronic stroke patients depends on corticospinal tract integrity," *Brain*, vol. 130, no. 1, pp. 170–180, 2007.

[34] R. Lindenberg, V. Renga, L. L. Zhu, F. Betzler, D. Alsop, and G. Schlaug, "Structural integrity of corticospinal motor fibers predicts motor impairment in chronic stroke," *Neurology*, vol. 74, no. 4, pp. 280–287, 2010.

[35] A. Sterr, Shan Shen, A. J. Szameitat, and K. A. Herron, "The role of corticospinal tract damage in chronic motor recovery and neurorehabilitation: a pilot study," *Neurorehabilitation and Neural Repair*, vol. 24, no. 5, pp. 413–419, 2010.

[36] V. A. Hachinski and J. W, Norris, *The Acute Stroke*, FA Davis, Philadelphia, Pa, USA, 1985.

[37] F. M. Ivey, R. F. Macko, A. S. Ryan, and C. E. Hafer-Macko, "Cardiovascular health and fitness after stroke," *Topics in Stroke Rehabilitation*, vol. 12, no. 1, pp. 1–16, 2005.

[38] G. S. Beaupre and H. L. Lew, "Bone-density changes after stroke," *American Journal of Physical Medicine and Rehabilitation*, vol. 85, no. 5, pp. 464–472, 2006.

[39] A. Ramnemark, L. Nyberg, B. Borssén, T. Olsson, and Y. Gustafson, "Fractures after stroke," *Osteoporosis International*, vol. 8, no. 1, pp. 92–95, 1998.

[40] G. Kwakkel, R. C. Wagenaar, T. W. Koelman, G. J. Lankhorst, and J. C. Koetsier, "Effects of intensity of rehabilitation after stroke: a research synthesis," *Stroke*, vol. 28, no. 8, pp. 1550–1556, 1997.

[41] S. K. Sabut, P. K. Lenka, R. Kumar, and M. Mahadevappa, "Effect of functional electrical stimulation on the effort and walking speed, surface electromyography activity, and metabolic responses in stroke subjects," *Journal of Electromyography and Kinesiology*, vol. 20, no. 6, pp. 1170–1177, 2010.

[42] S. K. Sabut, C. Sikdar, R. Kumar, and M. Mahadevappa, "Functional electrical stimulation of dorsiflexor muscle: effects on dorsiflexor strength, plantarflexor spasticity, and motor recovery in stroke patients," *NeuroRehabilitation*, vol. 29, no. 4, pp. 393–400, 2011.

[43] A. Dutta, B. Khattar, and A. Banerjee, "Nonlinear analysis of electromyogram following gait training with myoelectrically triggered neuromuscular electrical stimulation in stroke survivors," *EURASIP Journal on Advances in Signal Processing*, vol. 2012, no. 153, 2012.

[44] M. Musicco, L. Emberti, G. Nappi, and C. Caltagirone, "Early and long-term outcome of rehabilitation in stroke patients: the role of patient characteristics, time of initiation, and duration of interventions," *Archives of Physical Medicine and Rehabilitation*, vol. 84, no. 4, pp. 551–558, 2003.

7

# A Case of Progressive Stroke on Posterior Circulation with Transient Bilateral Oculomotor Palsy

**Chiaki Takahashi**

*Department of Neurosurgery, Takaoka City Hospital, 4-1, Takara-machi, Takaoka, Toyama, Japan*

Correspondence should be addressed to Chiaki Takahashi; chiakit429@image.ocn.ne.jp

Academic Editor: Mehmet Turgut

Infarction located in the midbrain and pons presents various ophthalmic symptoms, because of the damage of the nuclei that control the movement of internal and external ocular and palpebral muscles. We experienced a case which presented with rare ocular symptoms and course. A 61-year-old man presented with left hemiparesis and dysarthria, bilateral ptosis, and bilateral impaired eyeball movement: right eyeball movement was totally impaired and left could only perform slight adduction. MRI showed fresh stroke in the right thalamus, cerebral crus, and posterior lobe and cuneate lesion on bilateral paramedian portion of the midbrain. MRA showed occlusion in the P1 area of the posterior cerebral artery (PCA). Transesophageal echocardiography (TEE) showed findings of a patent foramen ovale (PFO). These findings suggested cardioembolic stroke as a cause of PCA occlusion and we prescribed rivaroxaban. The patient's eyeball and eyelid movement, only on the left side, was improved imperfectly 2 weeks later. We thought that neurological findings and course of this case may have arisen from dysfunction of the oculomotor nucleus and oculomotor fascicles, and MLF results from the presence of the lesion in paramedian midbrain and pons.

## 1. Introduction

We sometimes encounter patients with cerebral infarction in whom the main lesion is located in the posterior circulation. In such patients, especially in a case where the lesion is in the midbrain, the severity and symptoms show great variety depending on the location and range. In particular, the vascular supply in the midbrain is much more complex than in the pons and medulla. The vasculature is supplied by branches of three arteries: the posterior cerebral artery (PCA) and the basilar and the superior cerebellar artery (SCA), depending on the level [1]. The eponymic symptoms which represent oculomotor paresis with the paramedian midbrain lesion have been named Claude syndrome [2] and Benedict syndrome [3], and these definitions are also complex. In addition, Nothnagel reported symptoms of ipsilateral or bilateral oculomotor paresis and contralateral cerebellar ataxia due to a lesion in ventral side of the midbrain including the superior colliculus [4]. We think the present case is a rare case that presented transient bilateral oculomotor paresis with ptosis and contralateral ataxia and hemiparesis. The clinical symptoms suggested Nothnagel syndrome; however, we were not able to explain some points.

## 2. Case Presentation

A 61-year-old man with no remarkable history had never had a regular medical examination. He has been smoking about forty cigarettes per day for more than forty years. On the morning of the day before admission, he found that he was not able to read a book as his vision became suddenly distorted. He had additionally noticed weakness in his left leg during the daytime but went to bed without going to the hospital. The next morning, his weakness grew worse and he visited our hospital in a wheelchair due to gait disturbance. At this first admission, his NIH Stroke Scale (NIHSS) score was 4 points: hemiparesis 2, sensory disturbance 1, and dysarthria 1. He complained of diplopia when he looked to the right, but we could not observe his ocular deviation. His head MRI-DWI showed a scattered fresh infarction including the right occipital lobe, cerebral crus, and thalamus, and MRA showed occlusion of the P2 area of the right PCA and left

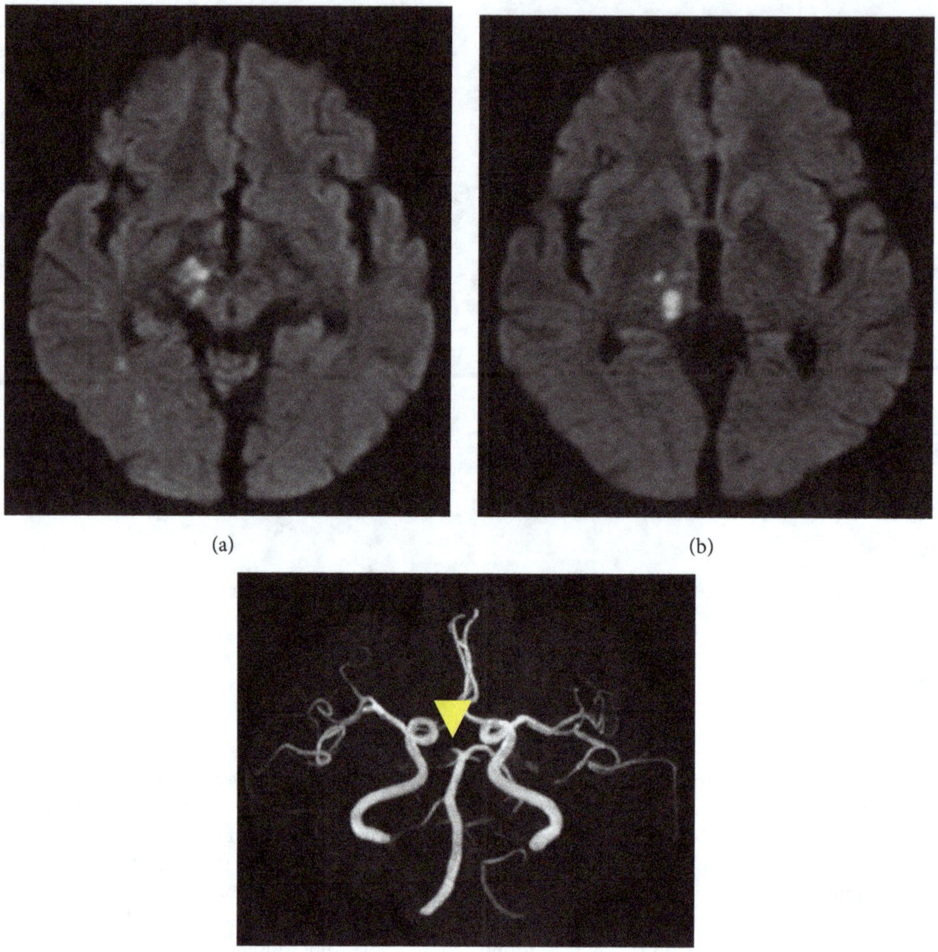

(a) (b) (c)

Figure 1: Head MRI performed about 24 hours after onset showed right occipital lobe, thalamus, cerebral crus, and midbrain fresh infarction (a, b). MRA showed right P2 (arrow head) and left SCA (superior cerebellar artery) occlusion (c).

SCA (Figure 1). Carotid ultrasound (CUS) showed findings of moderate arteriosclerosis, and plaque accumulation in the carotid bifurcation was not observed. He was admitted to our hospital. Electrocardiogram (ECG) and monitoring data showed no findings of arrhythmia. We speculated that the cause of this stroke might be atherosclerotic change at first. We decided to begin injection of argatroban hydrate and edaravone, and administered oral aspirin 100 mg.

Early the next morning, a drop in consciousness level and aggravation of left hemiparesis presented. Emergency MRI was performed and showed enlargement of the lesion in the thalamus and additional cuneate fresh stroke on the right paramedian portion of the midbrain and small spotty fresh stroke on the left paramedian portion. MRA showed the extension of the occlusion of the PCA to the P1 portion (Figure 2). At this point, we thought perforators branching from proximal part of PCA were occluded due to the progression of thrombosis in the PCA. We added cilostazol to avoid extra thrombosis. After half a day, his consciousness level began to improve, and we performed a detailed neurological examination. At this time, we observed bilateral ptosis. He could not open his eyelids on his own and showed compensated contraction of the frontal muscle. His ocular position was median; right eyeball movement was totally impaired and left could only perform slight adduction with ocular nystagmus. The right and left pupil diameters were 6.0 mm and 5.0 mm. Light reflex was not observed on the right and was observed only slightly on the left.

During the course of treatment, transesophageal echocardiography (TEE) was performed to detect the cause of the stroke. It showed a patent foramen ovale (PFO) and noncompaction of the ventricular myocardium, which could have caused the stroke. According to the findings on TEE, we were convinced that the cause of the stroke was cardioembolic and changed his prescription from aspirin to rivaroxaban 20 mg.

His consciousness level improved gradually, and oculomotor paresis including ptosis only on the left side was also improved imperfectly 2 weeks later. Finally, disturbance of upward and downward abduction remained on the left side

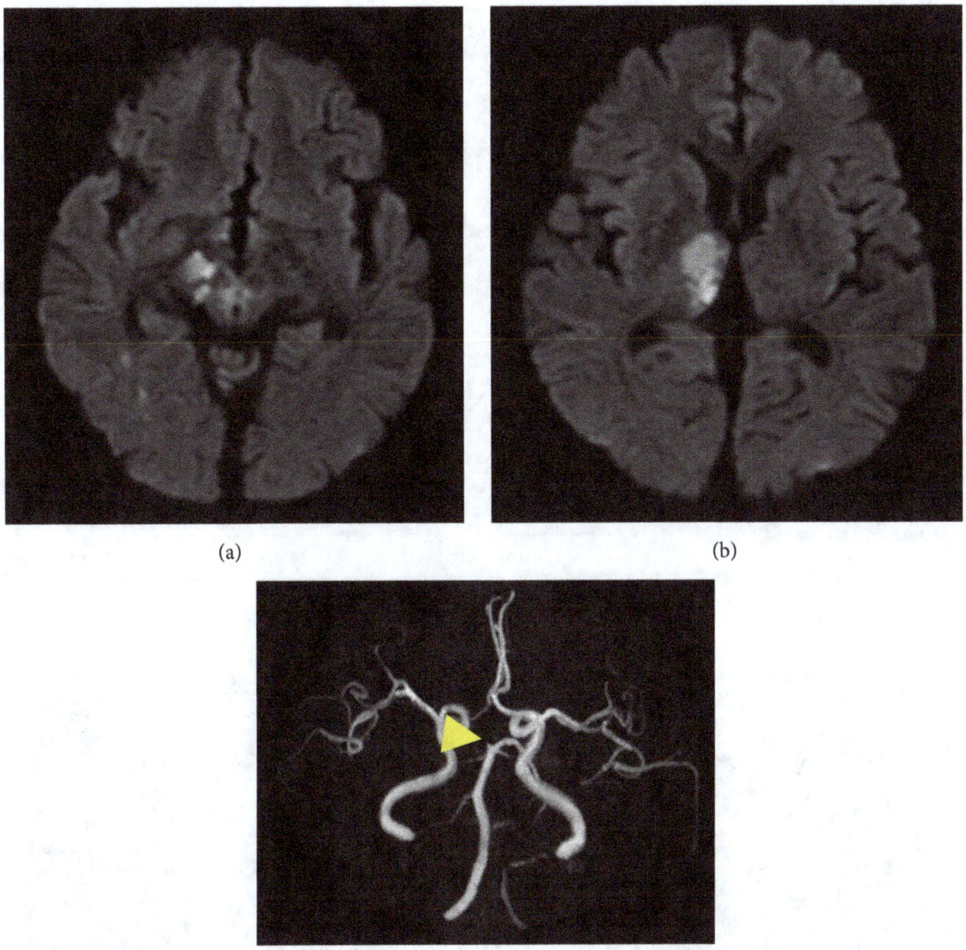

(a) (b) (c)

Figure 2: Head MRI performed after aggravation of neurological symptoms showed enlargement of infarction (a, b). MRA showed extension of occlusion (arrow head) to the P1 (c).

and severe oculomotor palsy also remained in the right side (Figure 3). He could not achieve ocular convergence and Bell phenomenon in both eyes.

In addition, with regard to the motor paresis, we observed complete hemiplegia in the left upper extremity in the flexed position and mild hemiparesis in the left lower extremity. With the improvement of his consciousness level, he started standing and walking training with physical therapists. Although his muscle strength on the left lower extremity was sufficient, he had difficulty with those types of training due to ataxia of bilateral body trunk and lower extremities and attentional deficit as a higher brain dysfunction. Ultimately, he acquired walking ability with a cane, but he risked losing his balance and falling down when he had a lapse of concentration. With regard to higher brain dysfunction, mild cognitive dysfunction and memory deficit were present. At 12 weeks after initial presentation, he could leave our hospital and go home in relatively good condition.

## 3. Discussion

At first, neurological deficits in this case due to the occlusion of the P2 area of the PCA were not severe; they later became severe as a consequence of the enlargement of infarction due to the progressive thrombosis of the PCA and occlusion of the perforators branching from the P1 area. MRI showed a thalamic, cerebral crus and cuneate fresh stroke on the right paramedian portion of the midbrain and a very small spotty fresh stroke on the left paramedian portion. At first, we did not detect the left spotty infarction, but his clinical findings could not be explained; hence, we carefully reexamined his MRI referring to his apparent diffusion coefficient (ADC) map (Figure 4). The vasculature of the paramedian midbrain tegmentum was supplied by perforators branching like a fan from the P1 area up and down. These perforators are divided into 4 groups [5]. The first branch is called the thalamoperforating artery, and the second and third branches are the median mesencephalic arteries which supply the midbrain and the fourth branch is the superior pontine tegmental branch which supplies the pons [5]. Of these, the first and second branches bifurcate to the bilateral side with a probability of 10% [6]. In that case, the symptoms of the patient become potentially severe when the first or second branches are occluded by thrombus. It will bring the bilateral mesencephalic lesion. We detected the bilateral

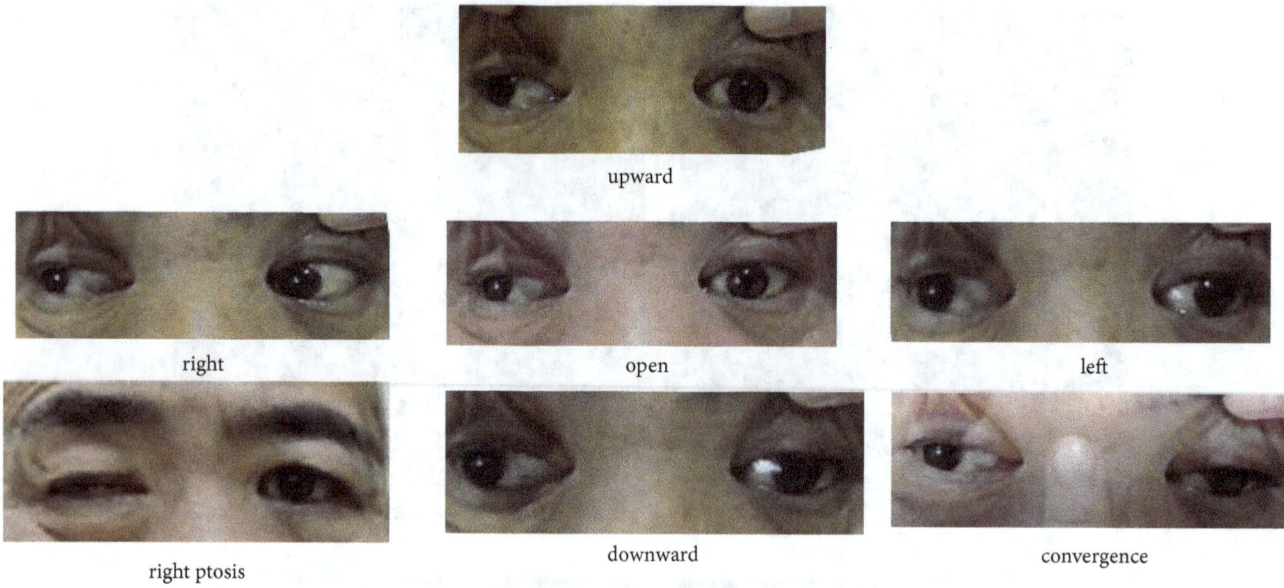


FIGURE 3: Findings of ptosis and oculomotor palsy one month after onset.

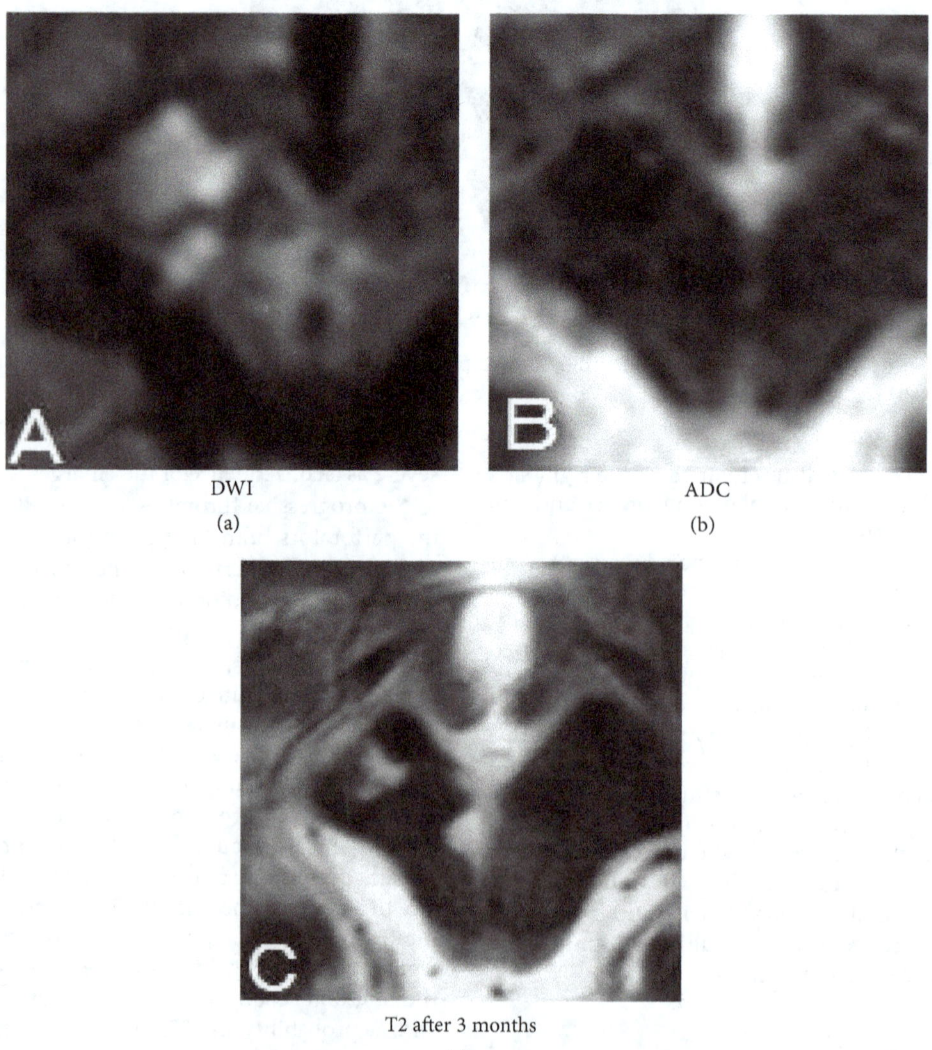


FIGURE 4: Head MRI on midbrain performed after aggravation of neurological symptoms. ADC map indicates the left paramedian lesion as stroke (a, b). Bilateral paramedian lesions three months after onset (c).

mesencephalic lesions in our case and considered that the second branch might be occluded.

When the patient's condition showed abrupt change at first, we observed these neurological symptoms: (1) bilateral total ophthalmoplegia with bilateral ptosis (the left eye could only perform slight adduction with ocular nystagmus), (2) contralateral hemiparesis and ataxia, and (3) consciousness disturbance. One month later, his neurological symptoms had improved: (1) right oculomotor palsy with ptosis, (2) contralateral abducens palsy with ocular nystagmus, (3) disturbance of bilateral suprainfraduction, (4) contralateral hemiparesis and ataxia, and (5) cognitive dysfunction and attentional deficit.

We considered the mechanism of the change of the symptoms and the affected region. At first, we could posit that the bilateral oculomotor palsy affected his symptoms because of the existence of the distinctive symptoms, bilateral ptosis, pupillary abnormality, and so on, and the lesion on paramedian midbrain lesion in MRI.

The nucleus of the oculomotor nerve is placed in the midline region of the midbrain. It exists in complex with multiple independent subnuclei, controlling the superior, inferior, and medial rectus muscle, inferior oblique muscle, levator palpebrae superioris muscle, and sphincter pupillae, respectively. Of all others, the caudal central subnucleus (CCN), which controls the levator palpebrae superioris muscle, exists in the center area of the midbrain and dominates the bilateral elevation of the eyelids [7, 8] (Figure 5). The nerve fibers which arise from the oculomotor subnucleus form the oculomotor fascicles near the red nucleus and make a transition to the extramedullary oculomotor nerve [9, 10].

At first, we inferred from his MRI and clinical symptoms that his partial neurological findings were due to nuclear damage of the whole oculomotor complex including the CCN. At that time, the severity of bilateral ptosis was almost the same between right and left eyelid. In addition, his pupil showed bilateral mydriasis. We thought that these findings are not likely with the damage of the oculomotor fascicles. However, left ptosis and oculomotor palsy were improved one month later. As a damaged CCN cannot later show unilateral improvement of ptosis [10], we determined that the CCN was not damaged and that part of the fascicles was damaged bilaterally and then showed mild or incomplete improvement on the left side. Indeed, a case of oculomotor palsy without ptosis was reported as a result of the sparing of the CCN from the damage of stroke [10]. Besides, it is said that the subnuclei of the superior rectus muscle control the contralateral side [11]. In our case strong disturbance of the supra and infraduction of the bilateral side persisted one month later. We speculated about the two possibilities to be able to evoke it. At first, according to the figure of the oculomotor complex by Warwick (Figure 5), we thought that the subnuclei of the supra- and infraduction were damaged bilaterally due to the involvement of the dorsal side of the upper to lower oculomotor complex in the infarction lesion. We thought that the bilateral nerve fibers of the levator palpebrae superioris muscle were damaged in the oculomotor fascicles and that of the other external and internal muscles controlled by the oculomotor nerve were damaged supranuclearly.

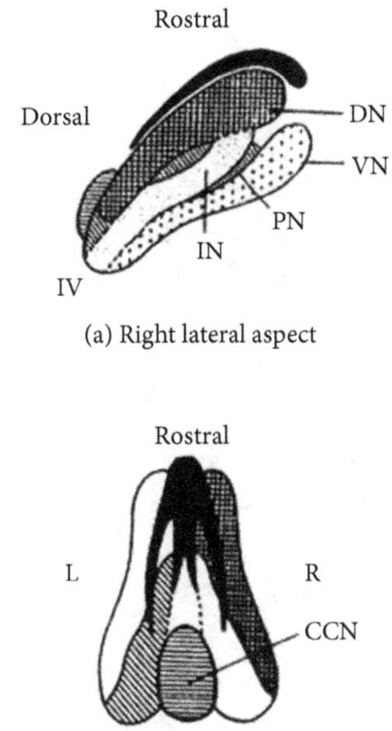


(a) Right lateral aspect

(b) Dorsal aspect

Rectus inferior
Rectus medialis
Rectus superior
Obliquus inferior
Levator palpebrae superioris
Visceral nuclei
CCN: central caudal nucleus
DN: dorsal nucleus
VN: ventral nucleus
PN: paramedial nucleus
IN: intermediate nucleus

FIGURE 5: Structure of the oculomotor complex indicated by Warwick [7].

Secondly, ischemic lesion extended to the rostral interstitial nucleus of the medial longitudinal fascicles (riMLF) or interstitial nucleus of Cajal placed in rostral-medial side of the red nucleus might bring Parinaud's syndrome [12].

Then, we considered the behaviors which are impossible to explain only with the dysfunction around the level of the oculomotor nucleus.

The positions of the bilateral eyes were almost neutral at first and he could abduct only his left eyeball slightly with ocular nystagmus. One month later, his right eyeball was fixed completely to the abducted position and he could abduct his left eyeball incompletely with ocular nystagmus.

Granted that the stroke lesion in the upper pons which was impossible to detect by MRI existed, we considered several possibilities. One-and-a-half syndrome and medial longitudinal fascicles (MLF) syndrome are caused by the damage of paramedian area of the pons. The former does not fit into the behaviors of his eye movement, because he could adduct his left eye. Besides, we also considered WEBINO syndrome which is caused by the bilateral MLF syndrome. In such a case, we could observe the alternative exotropia when

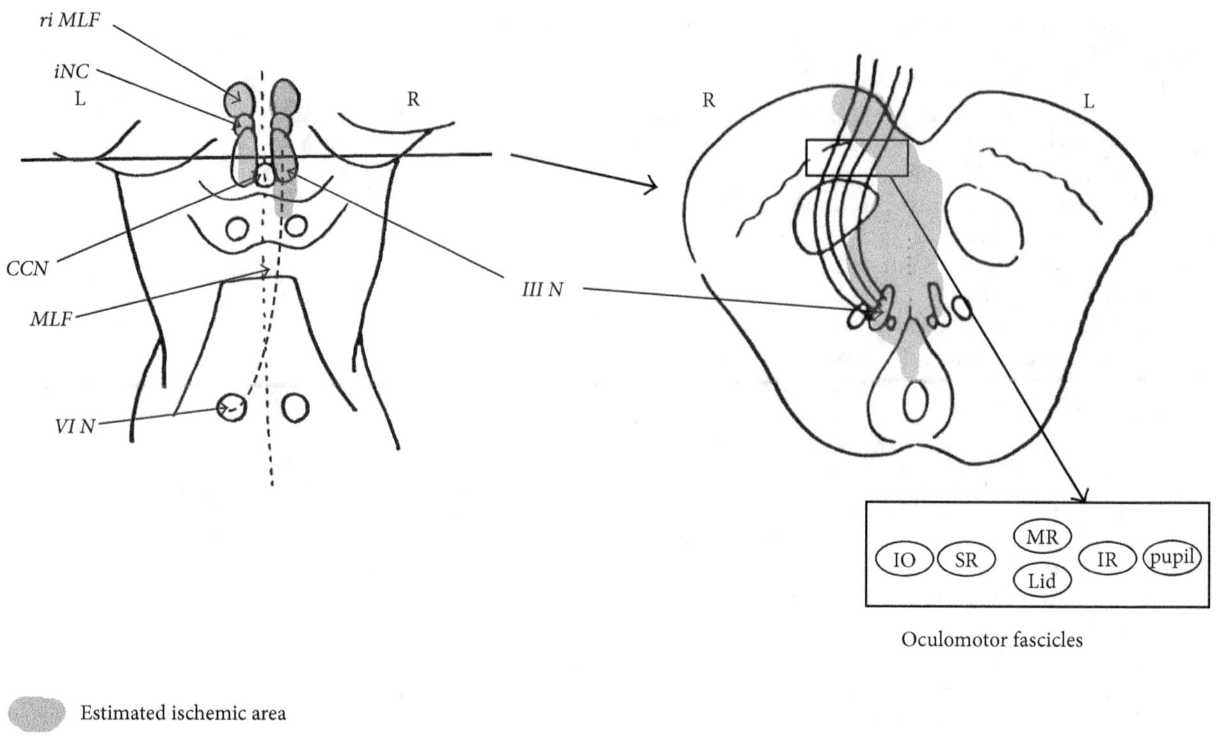


FIGURE 6: Picture in the left shows dorsal side of the midbrain and pons and in the right shows cross-sectional view of the midbrain along the line. Gray areas mark the ischemic area. riMLF: rostral interstitial nucleus of medial longitudinal fasciculus, iNC: interstitial nucleus of Cajal, CCN: caudal central subnucleus, MLF: medial longitudinal fasciculus, III N: oculomotor nucleus, VI N: abducens nucleus, IO: intraocular muscles, SR: superior rectus muscle, MR: medial rectus muscle, Lid: Levator palpebrae superioris muscle, IR: inferior rectus muscle, and pupil: sphincter pupillae muscles.

the patient holds fixation with a single eye. However his right eye always fixed into the abducted position regardless of the behavior of right eye; it also does not fit. Besides, it is reported that WEBINO syndrome due to pontine lesion often shows convergence impairment [13].

So, we speculated about it as follows.

At first, both bilateral oculomotor palsy which was stronger in the right eye and the right MLF syndrome existed, and then the left oculomotor palsy improved, and the right strong oculomotor palsy and the right MLF syndrome might remain finally. The left abducens palsy might be a movement of the intact side with nystagmus. Besides, his convergence palsy is explainable by coexisting dysfunction of the oculomotor nucleus.

We described the final estimated ischemic area in his brain stem (Figure 6). The figure in the left side shows the dorsal side of the brainstem and it describes ischemic area including the bilateral oculomotor nucleus without CCN and right MLF. The figure in the right side shows cross-sectional view of the midbrain along the line. It describes the ischemic part of the oculomotor fascicles pointed by the MRI image. Castro et al. reported these fascicles lines like the schema in the lower right side [14].

In addition, cognitive dysfunction and attentional deficit were presented and may have arisen from the inclusion of the thalamus [15]. Contralateral hemiparesis may have arisen from the stroke of the cerebral crus, and ataxia may have arisen from the thalamic stroke.

We obtained informed consent from the patient to use personal information and data including photographs of eyes, images of MRI, and health records.

## Conflicts of Interest

The authors declare no conflicts of interest concerning this manuscript.

## References

[1] E. Kumral, G. Bayulkem, A. Akyol, N. Yunten, H. Sirin, and A. Sagduyu, "Mesencephalic and associated posterior circulation infarcts," *Stroke*, vol. 33, no. 9, pp. 2224–2231, 2002.

[2] H. Claude, "Syndrome pedonculaire de la region du noyau rouge," *Revue Neurologique*, vol. 23, pp. 311–313, 1912.

[3] M. Benedikt, "Tremblement avec paralysie croisee du moteur oculaire commun," *Bulletin Medical (Paris)*, vol. 3, pp. 547-548, 1889.

[4] H. Nothnagel, "On the diagnosis of diseases of the corpora quadrigemina," *Brain*, vol. 12, no. 1-2, pp. 21–35, 1889.

[5] N. Goto, "Microanatomy of brainstem blood supply for clinical diagnosis," *Neurosurgeons*, vol. 5, pp. 127–138, 1985 (Japanese).

[6] A. Pedroza, M. Dujovny, J. I. Ausman et al., "Microvascular anatomy of the interpeduncular fossa," *Journal of Neurosurgery*, vol. 64, no. 3, pp. 484–493, 1986.

[7] R. Warwick, "Oculomotor organization," *Annals of the Royal College of Surgeons of England*, vol. 19, pp. 36–52, 1956.

[8] K. Ruchalski and G. M. Hathout, "A medley of midbrain maladies: a brief review of midbrain anatomy and syndromology for radiologists," *Radiology Research and Practice*, vol. 2012, Article ID 258524, 11 pages, 2012.

[9] N. Saeki, A. Yamaura, and K. Sunami, "Bilateral ptosis with pupil sparing because of a discrete midbrain lesion: magnetic resonance imaging evidence of topographic arrangement within the oculomotor nerve," *Journal of Neuro-Ophthalmology*, vol. 20, no. 2, pp. 130–134, 2000.

[10] J. Sargent, "Nuclear and infranuclear ocular motility disarders," in *Clinical Neuro-Ophthalmology*, N. R. Miller, P. S. Subramanian, and V. R. Patel, Eds., pp. 341–371, Wolters Kluwer, 2016.

[11] L. R. Caplan, "'Top of basilar' syndrome," *Neurology*, vol. 55, pp. 72–79, 1980.

[12] M. B. Bender, "Brain control of conjugate horjzontal and vertical eye movements: A survey of the stductural and functional correlates," *Brain*, vol. 103, no. 1, pp. 23–69, 1980.

[13] T. Yoshinaga, K. Nakamura, K. Kaneko, and A. Nakamura, "A case report of WEBINO syndrome with convergence impairment," *Journal of Neurology and Neurophysiology*, vol. 6, article 270, 2005.

[14] O. Castro, L. N. Johnson, and A. C. Mamourian, "Isolated inferior oblique paresis from brainstem infarction: perspective on oculomotor fascicular organization in the ventral midbrain tegmentum," *Archives of Neurology*, vol. 47, no. 2, pp. 235–237, 1990.

[15] R. P. Mills and P. D. Swanson, "Vertical oculomotor apraxia and memory loss," *Annals of Neurology*, vol. 4, no. 2, pp. 149–153, 1978.

# Cervical Spine Ischemic Stroke Complicated by Spastic Quadriparesis and Ogilvie Syndrome: A Case Report and Literature Review

**Salman Assad, Justin Nolte, Dharampreet Singh, Samrina Hanif, and Paul Ferguson**

*Department of Neurology, Marshall University School of Medicine, Huntington, WV, USA*

Correspondence should be addressed to Salman Assad; salmanassad91@gmail.com

Academic Editor: Peter Berlit

Infarction or ischemia of the spinal cord is a rare entity and is often misdiagnosed as inflammatory myelopathy in acute settings. Atherosclerotic disease can affect spinal arteries, leading to cord ischemia with clinical presentation mixed with myelopathy. We present a case of a 66-year-old male who came to the hospital with unsteady gait and numbness of all extremities without associated pain for the past 48 hours. The neurological examination on admission directed the diagnosis towards myelopathy of the cervical spine. However, the initial magnetic resonance imaging (MRI) of the cervical spine demonstrated gliosis and restricted diffusion of the cord with multilevel neuroforaminal stenosis but without central canal stenosis or cord compression. The MRI brain, cerebrospinal fluid analysis, and rheumatologic evaluation were unremarkable. Four days into the clinical course, the patient developed weakness and spasticity of all extremities prompting further evaluation. Computed tomography angiography (CTA) scan of the head and neck revealed right vertebral artery occlusion and intracranial atherosclerotic disease. He was started on aspirin and clopidogrel for secondary risk reduction. The hospital course was further complicated by Ogilvie syndrome (OS), and the patient underwent uncomplicated cecostomy.

## 1. Introduction

Spinal cord ischemia is caused by a vascular interruption that can lead to cord dysfunction, ischemia, and infarction [1]. The blood supply of the spinal cord consists of anterior and posterior spinal arteries. The cervical cord lesions can typically present with either acute quadriparesis or paraparesis. Three vessels arising from vertebral arteries supply the spinal cord in the neck consisting of anterior and two posterior spinal arteries [2]. The manifestation of cord infarction is spontaneous with unknown etiology. Vascular aneurysm, dissection, and post-surgical complications should be ruled out when suspecting a cord ischemic stroke [3]. We present a unique and first-ever report of cryptogenic cervical cord acute ischemic infarction with late-onset development of Ogilvie syndrome.

## 2. Case Presentation

A 66-year-old male with a past medical history of hypertension, hyperlipidemia, coronary artery disease, prostate cancer, and gastroesophageal reflux disease presented to the emergency department with intermittent symptoms of disequilibrium, gait instability, and progressive numbness of all extremities. The patient also developed hypotension and required vasopressors and intravenous fluid support after his neurologic symptomatology further evolved into weakness and spasticity. Laboratory investigation revealed hypercholesterolemia with normal thyroid-stimulating hormone, vitamin B12, and folate levels. Transthoracic echocardiography showed ejection fraction >55%, no wall abnormalities, and no patent foramen ovale. The MRI of the brain was unremarkable. The computed tomography angiography (CTA) of the head and neck showed right vertebral artery occlusion with moderate diffuse intracranial atherosclerosis (Figure 1). On day 2 of admission, the patient's weakness of all four extremities worsened and became acutely myelopathic with Babinski and Hoffman's sign in the setting of diffuse hyperreflexia and quadriparesis. An MRI of the cervical spine with and without gadolinium demonstrated a restriction on diffusion-weighted imaging (DWI)

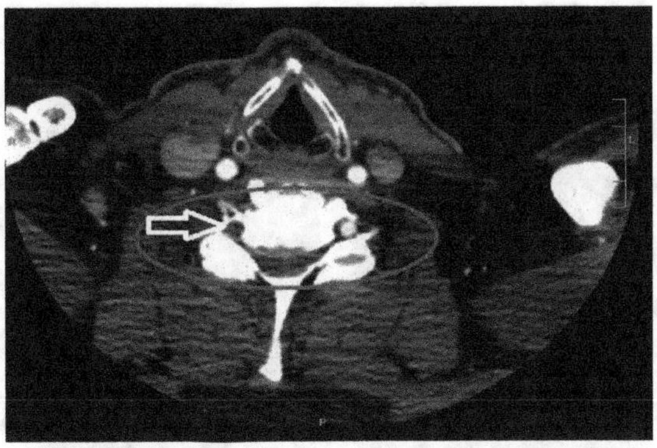

FIGURE 1: The computed tomography angiography (CTA) of the the head and neck showed right vertebral artery occlusion with moderate diffuse intracranial atherosclerosis.

corresponding to the signal abnormality foci seen on short-TI inversion recovery (STIR) images (Figure 2).

He further developed urinary retention and Ogilvie's (acute colonic pseudo-obstruction) syndrome. The MRI of the thoracolumbar region did not reveal any abnormality. For spasticity, the patient was given baclofen 20 mg three times per day and tizanidine 2 mg every 8 hours. For Ogilvie's syndrome, cecostomy was performed by the surgery team. The lumbar puncture and cerebrospinal fluid analysis showed normal IgG index 0.6 (normal range 0.0–0.7), high myelin basic protein 12 (normal range 0–1.2 nanograms/milliliter (ng/ml)), no oligo clonal bands, negative neuromyelitis optica spectrum disorders (NMOSD) antibody, and negative myelin oligodendrocyte glycoprotein (MOG) antibody. The blood cultures, urine cultures, and CSF diagnostic workup for viral, bacterial, or fungal infections were noncontributory. The patient was started on subcutaneous heparin for deep venous thrombosis prophylaxis, aspirin 81 mg daily, clopidogrel 75 mg daily, and atorvastatin 40 mg daily for secondary risk reduction. The patient was discharged to a rehabilitation facility.

## 3. Discussion

The onset of spinal cord ischemia or infarction symptomatology is usually abrupt like that noted in cerebral ischemia. A diffuse atherosclerotic process can affect spinal arteries and can lead to focal or nonfocal neurological deficits [3]. Cigarette smoking, uncontrolled hypertension, diabetes, positive family history of vascular insults, and hyperlipidemia are the major risk factors for spinal cord infarction [4]. The vertebrobasilar insufficiency can present with a multitude of symptoms such as bilateral body weakness, headaches, vomiting, diplopia, blindness, dizziness, and gait instability [5]. The symptoms of bladder dysfunction, quadriparesis, bilateral loss of pain, temperature sensation with intact proprioception, and vibration sensation are indicative of anterior spinal artery (ASA) syndrome [5]. The patient in our case has occluded right nondominant vertebral artery indicative of vertebrobasilar insufficiency. The functional outcome with spinal cord infarction is promising due to the noninvolvement of cognitive deficits [6]. Elzamly et al. reported a case of posterior cervical cord infarction after the neuro-endovascular intervention for vertebrobasilar insufficiency [7]. It is imperative to mention that we did not consider thrombolysis in our case as cord infarction might have happened due to hypotensive episode. The patient in our report also developed neurogenic bladder and Ogilvie syndrome (colonic pseudo-obstruction), which is usually common with lesions below thoracic spine vertebra level 10 (T10) as reported by Korsten et al. [8].

Davda and Osman also mentioned a similar anterior spinal cord infarct with an affected spinothalamic tract involving the pain and temperature sensation [9]. This finding is in contrast to our report where both vibration and fine touch with pain and temperature sensations were affected, highlighting the involvement of both anterior and posterior spinal arteries. Ota et al. mentioned a patient who initially presented with sudden onset quadriplegia with an MRI cervical spine indicative of myelopathy [10]. After almost one week of the worsening of neurological symptoms, DWI and ADC images of the MRI cervical spine were obtained that showed acute cord infarction [10]. On the other hand, our patient developed spastic quadriplegia almost after 10 days of onset with intermittent episodes of unsteady gait. Müller et al. and Restrepo et al. mentioned the prompt recovery within few days of ASA syndrome in patients presented within 3 hours of symptoms and treated with intravenous recombinant tissue plasminogen activator (tPA) [4, 11]. It is also necessary to look for vascular dissection, aneurysm, or malformations before giving tPA [11]. The fluid resuscitation and use of dual antiplatelet therapy (DAPT) with statins were found to be associated with good outcomes in ASA syndrome patients [4]. The role of a mechanical thrombectomy or neuroendovascular procedures in such cases is still debatable and will require future studies.

The first limitation of our case presentation was not taking into consideration the magnetic resonance angiography (MRA) or conventional angiogram of the cervical spine in the beginning. The second limitation was not ordering a repeat MRI or MRA of the thoracolumbar spine on day 14 of hospitalization after the patient developed Ogilvie syndrome to rule out thoracolumbar infarction. However,

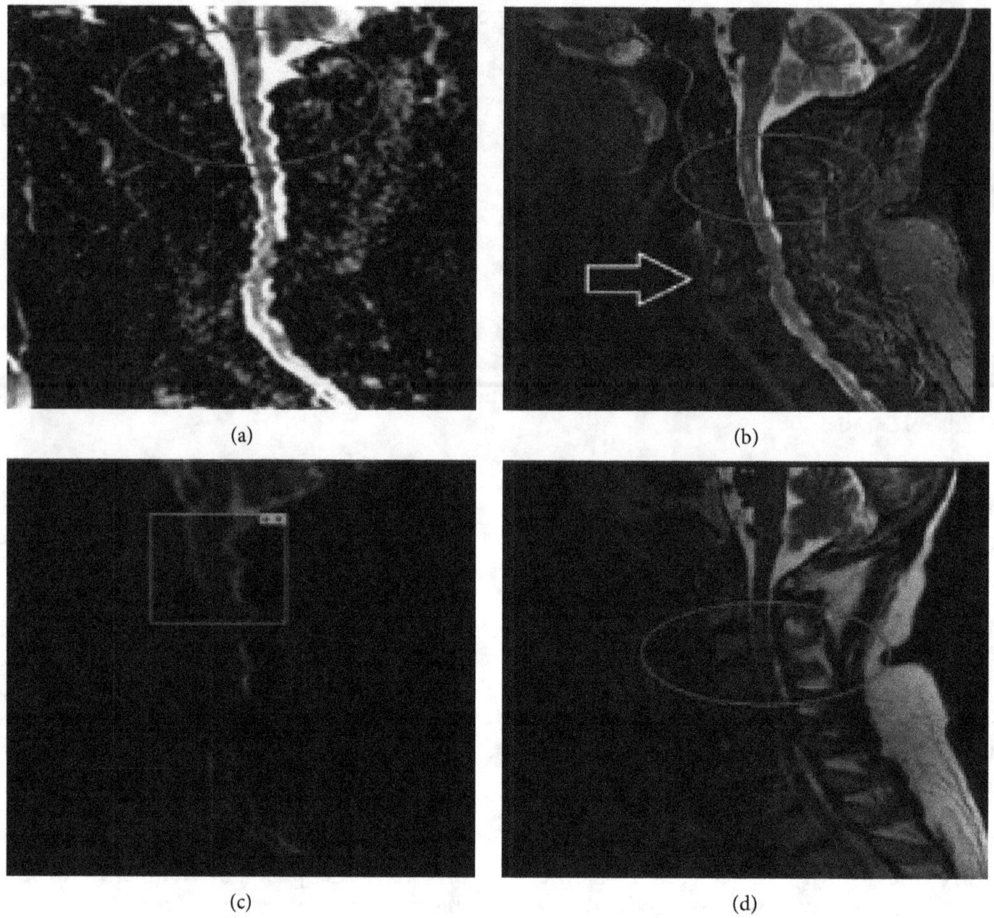


FIGURE 2: (a–d) MRI of the cervical spine with and without gadolinium demonstrated a restriction on diffusion-weighted imaging (DWI) (a) corresponding to the signal abnormality foci seen on short-TI inversion recovery (STIR) images (red circles in (b) and (d) and white marker image in (c)) and anterior compression from displaced cervical discs (white arrow in (b)).

the CTA of the head and neck was done and vascular dissection or aneurysm was not reported which in the past has been associated with spinal cord vascular syndromes. We conclude that the timely diagnosis of cord ischemia is important and MRI with DWI/ADC, MRA, or conventional angiogram should be considered in such cases. If within the window, tPA can be considered followed by DAPT for 3–6 months based on clinical discretion until clinical trials are available in the literature.

## Conflicts of Interest

The authors declare no conflicts of interest.

## References

[1] M.-Y. Cheng, R.-K. Lyu, Y.-J. Chang et al., “Spinal cord infarction in Chinese patients. Clinical features, risk factors, imaging and prognosis,” *Cerebrovascular Diseases*, vol. 26, no. 5, pp. 502–508, 2008.

[2] S. Prasad, R. S. Price, S. M. Kranick, J. H. Woo, R. W. Hurst, and S. Galetta, “Clinical reasoning: a 59-year-old woman with acute paraplegia,” *Neurology*, vol. 69, no. 24, pp. E41–E47, 2007.

[3] T. A. Bley, C. C. Duffek, C. J. François et al., “Presurgical localization of the artery of adamkiewicz with time-resolved 3.0-T MR angiography,” *Radiology*, vol. 255, no. 3, pp. 873–881, 2010.

[4] K. I. Müller, L. H. Steffensen, and S. H. Johnsen, “Thrombolysis in anterior spinal artery syndrome,” *BMJ Case Reports*, vol. 2012, no. 2, 2012.

[5] A. Lima Neto, R. Bittar, G. Gattas et al., “Pathophysiology and diagnosis of vertebrobasilar insufficiency: a review of the literature,” *International Archives of Otorhinolaryngology*, vol. 21, no. 3, pp. 302–307, 2017.

[6] K. Nedeltchev, T. J. Loher, F. Stepper et al., “Long-term outcome of acute spinal cord ischemia syndrome,” *Stroke*, vol. 35, no. 2, pp. 560–565, 2004.

[7] K. Elzamly, C. Nobleza, E. Parker, and R. Sugg, “Unilateral upper cervical posterior spinal cord infarction after a neuroendovascular intervention: a case report,” *Case Reports in Neurological Medicine*, vol. 2018, Article ID 5070712, 3 pages, 2018.

[8] M. A. Korsten, A. S. Rosman, A. Ng et al., “Infusion of neostigmine-glycopyrrolate for bowel evacuation in persons with spinal cord injury,” *The American Journal of Gastroenterology*, vol. 100, no. 7, pp. 1560–1565, 2005.

[9] N. Davda and C. Osman, “Anterior spinal cord infarct: a rare yet disabling stroke,” *BMJ Case Reports*, vol. 7, pp. 22017–221655, 2018.

[10] K. Ota, R. Iida, K. Ota et al., "Atypical spinal cord infarction: a case report," *Medicine (Baltimore)*, vol. 97, no. 23, Article ID e11058, 2018.

[11] L. Restrepo and J. F. Guttin, "Acute spinal cord ischemia during aortography treated with intravenous thrombolytic therapy," *Texas Heart Institute Journal*, vol. 33, no. 1, pp. 74–77, 2006.

# 9

# Papillary Fibroelastoma as a Cause of Cardiogenic Embolic Stroke in a β-Thalassemia Patient: Case Report and Literature Review

**Re-I Chin,[1] John J. Monda,[1] Maulik Sheth,[2] William Ogle,[3] Gloria Merenda,[4] and Debapriya De[2]**

[1]*Saint Louis University School of Medicine, 1402 S Grand Blvd, Saint Louis, MO 63104, USA*
[2]*Department of Internal Medicine, SSM St. Mary's Health Center, 6420 Clayton Rd, Richmond Heights, MO 63117, USA*
[3]*Department of Cardiothoracic Surgery, SSM St. Mary's Health Center, 6420 Clayton Rd, Richmond Heights, MO 63117, USA*
[4]*Department of Pathology, SSM St. Mary's Health Center, 6420 Clayton Rd, Richmond Heights, MO 63117, USA*

Correspondence should be addressed to Re-I Chin; chinr@slu.edu

Academic Editor: Aiden Abidov

We describe a case of a young male without stroke risk factors who presented with a sudden onset of left-sided weakness, left hand numbness, and left eye blurriness. CT scan of the head without contrast and diffusion-weighted MRI of the brain with contrast revealed an ischemic stroke in the right middle cerebral artery distribution. Transesophageal echocardiography (TEE) revealed a mobile pedunculated mass on the posterior surface of the mitral valve. This mass was resected and pathology showed a cardiac papillary fibroelastoma (CPFE), which was determined to be the cause of the patient's cardioembolic stroke. Further workup also found that patient had microcytic anemia secondary to β-thalassemia intermedia, a rare hematologic disorder due to defective hemoglobin synthesis. Recently, another case report suggested β-thalassemia major may underlie the pathogenesis of CPFE. β-Thalassemia major causes a state of chronic inflammation and endothelial damage, which can mediate CPFE formation. Based on literature review, this is the first case report of a CPFE in a patient with β-thalassemia intermedia. This hypothesis-generating case report calls attention to the need for elucidating the relationship between CPFE and β-thalassemia in future studies to better understand the diagnosis and management of a rare cardiac tumor.

## 1. Introduction

Primary tumors of the heart are rare, occurring at a frequency of 0.001–0.03% based on autopsy studies [1, 2]. Cardiac papillary fibroelastomas (CPFEs) are historically known as the second most common primary cardiac tumors after cardiac myxomas. However, more recent studies suggest that CPFEs may be the most common cardiac tumor due to increasing diagnosis with echocardiography [3]. CPFEs consist of a small, papillary, pedunculated, and avascular tumor covered by endothelium surrounded by a hyaline stroma [4], though some authors believe that CPFEs are hamartomatous instead of neoplastic [5, 6]. Most of CPFEs are found on the valvular endocardium of the aortic and mitral valves, followed by the tricuspid and pulmonary valves and nonvalvular sites scattered in the atria and ventricles [7]. Multiple CPFEs can also form at the same location [3].

Although CPFEs are histologically benign and are usually asymptomatic, symptoms can occur when either the tumor itself or a thrombus embolizes. The most common clinical presentation is stroke or transient ischemic attack, followed by angina, myocardial infarction, sudden death, heart failure, syncope or presyncope, and systemic or pulmonary embolic events [7, 8]. Both transthoracic echocardiogram (TTE) and transesophageal echocardiogram (TEE) can be used to diagnose CPFE with high sensitivity and specificity [9]. On echocardiography, the tumor appears as a well-demarcated homogeneous round or oval structure and can appear "speckled" with stippling around the perimeter if the image quality is high [8, 9]. This report describes a case of a young male who

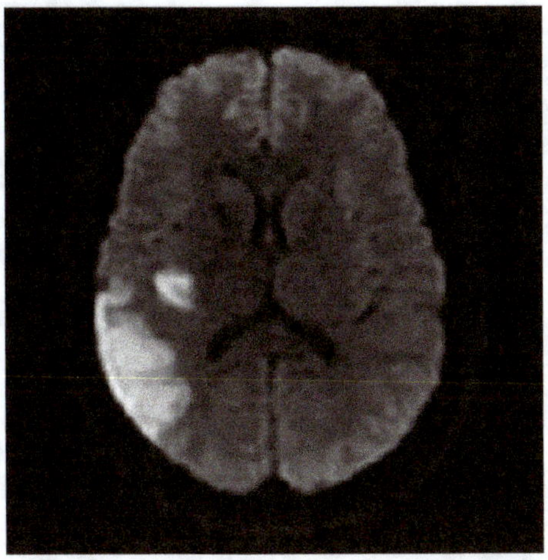

FIGURE 1: Axial images of diffusion-weighted MRI of the brain with contrast showing hyperintensity in the temporal and occipital lobes.

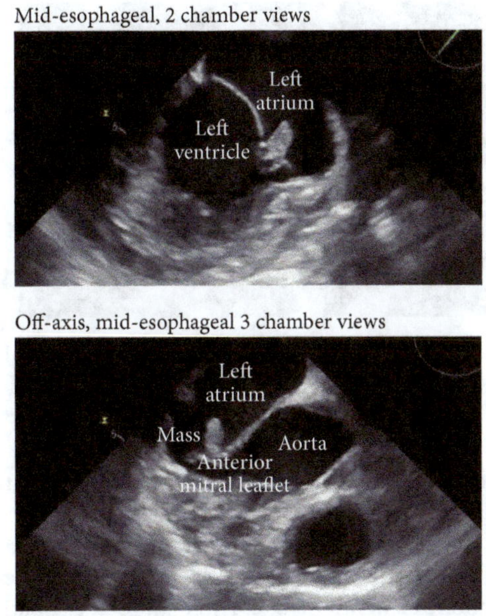


FIGURE 2: Transesophageal echocardiogram (TEE) image showing a pedunculated mass on the atrial aspect of the posterior leaflet of the mitral valve before surgical resection of the CPFE.

presented with a cardioembolic stroke secondary to a CPFE diagnosed on TEE who was found to have $\beta$-thalassemia intermedia.

## 2. Case Presentation

The patient was a 29-year-old African American male without significant past medical history who presented to the emergency room with sudden weakness in his left lower extremity. While at work he suddenly felt lightheaded dizziness. Then, his left leg "gave out" while walking. Two days priorly, patient also had noted that his vision in his left eye suddenly became blurry, and his left hand clenched together uncontrollably and felt numb. Physical examination was normal except for mild loss of sensation in his left forearm. Troponin I was 0.196 and hemoglobin and MCV were 10.7 gm/dL and 70.8 fL, respectively. Urine drug screen was positive for cannabinoids. EKG revealed normal sinus rhythm with early repolarization changes. CT scan of the head without contrast showed loss of grey-white matter differentiation in the right insular cortex signifying a subacute ischemic stroke in the right middle cerebral artery distribution. He was started on aspirin, clopidogrel, and statin and was admitted for further workup.

The patient lacked significant cardiovascular risk factors that often cause ischemic stroke. He was young and normotensive and denied a family history of early cardiovascular disease. He smoked less than half a pack of cigarettes per day and used marijuana recreationally. He denied any IV drug use. He was generally active, with his most recent episode of prolonged immobilization being a six-hour car ride two weeks prior to presentation. He denied any past DVTs or a family history of hypercoagulability. The patient's neurological exam returned to normal within 48 hours of hospital admission.

For stroke workup, patient underwent CT angiogram of the head and neck, which was normal. MRI of the brain with contrast showed abnormal signal in the right parietal lobe and other areas of small bright signals in the temporal lobe, occipital white matter, and right cerebellum consistent with multiple subacute infarcts (Figure 1). Transesophageal echocardiogram showed an 8 × 5 mm pedunculated mass on the atrial aspect of the posterior leaflet of the mitral valve (Figure 2), suggesting either a cardiac tumor or a vegetation of infectious or noninfectious etiology. Endocarditis was considered less likely due to lack of fever, along with four sets of negative blood cultures. In terms of the risk for endocarditis, the patient only met one minor Duke criterion, which was having a vascular phenomenon such as thromboembolic event.

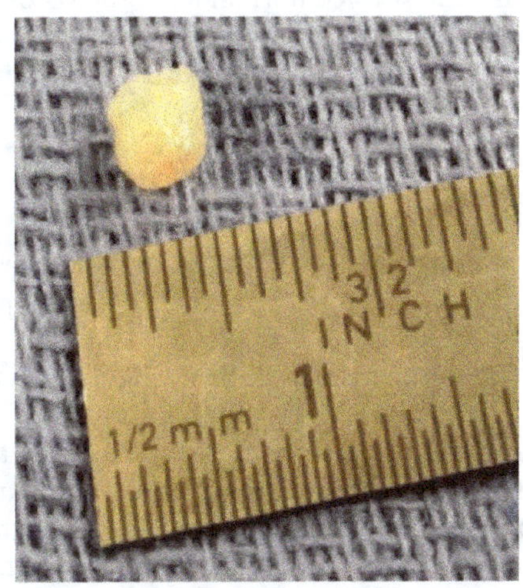

FIGURE 3: Surgical resection of the cardiac mass.

The patient was evaluated by cardiothoracic surgery and the lesion was resected three weeks later (Figure 3). Repeat TEE demonstrated the complete removal of the pedunculated mass (Figure 4). Pathology showed papillary structures lined

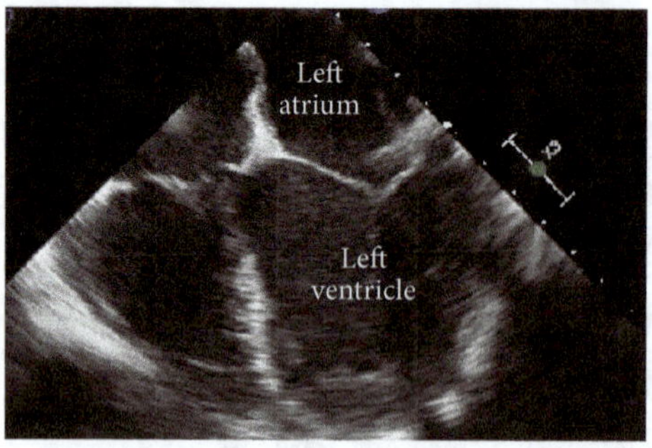


FIGURE 4: Transesophageal echocardiogram (TEE) image showing a preserved mitral valve after surgery resection of the CPFE.

by endothelium consisting of fibromyxoid stroma with dense areas of hyalinized stroma, confirming the diagnosis of a papillary fibroelastoma of the mitral valve (Figure 5). Fragments of this cardiac tumor were deemed the source of his cardioembolic ischemic stroke. After surgery, the patient was stable without further thromboembolic events or neurologic deficits. Hypercoagulable workup, including lupus anticoagulant, PT/PTT, anticardiolipin, homocysteine, and ANA, was negative. HIV serology was negative. Further workup of his microcytic anemia showed normal ferritin level of 197. Notably, on hemoglobin electrophoresis, Hgb A1 was decreased at 83.8% and Hgb F was increased at 13.2%, consistent with beta-thalassemia intermedia that was newly diagnosed.

## 3. Discussion

A stroke in a young and otherwise healthy individual without traditional risk factors presents an intriguing opportunity to investigate the cause of this clinical condition. Although CPFEs are rare and histologically benign, they should be managed with caution because they are a source of cardioembolic stroke [10]. Embolic strokes caused by arrhythmias and valvular diseases often require anticoagulation, but embolic strokes from CPFEs can be prevented through surgical resection of the tumor alone [8]. Surgical resection is the mainstay treatment and should be considered especially for CPFEs that are more than 10 mm in diameter, highly mobile, and associated with systemic embolization [11]. The outcomes following surgery are excellent: most valves retain their functionality and the tumors rarely recur [3]. Since CPFE has a curative management, understanding the pathogenesis of CPFE can guide disease diagnosis and prevent devastating neurological complications.

While CPFE is classified as a cardiac tumor, its pathogenesis differs significantly from that of other solid tumors and remains controversial. Instead of being driven by mutational changes and genomic instability, CPFEs are thought to arise from a combination of nongenetic causes: endothelial damage, viral-induced growth, microthrombi aggregation, and hamartomatous origin [7]. One of the more widely discussed theories suggests hemodynamic stress of blood flow causes damage to the endocardium, and continued hemodynamic stress over time leads to the accumulation of successive fibrin layers within the tumor [9]. Clinical studies support

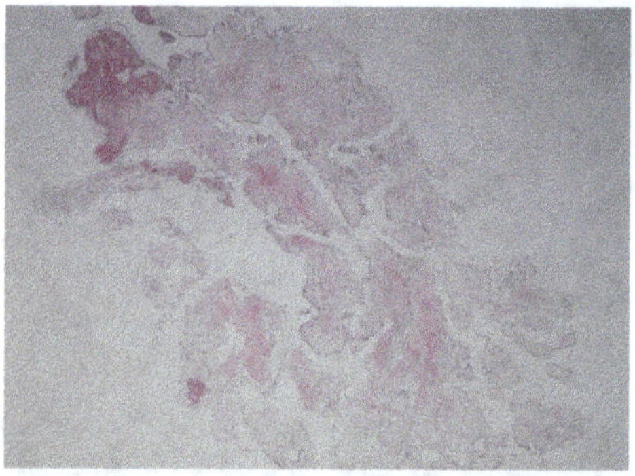

(a)

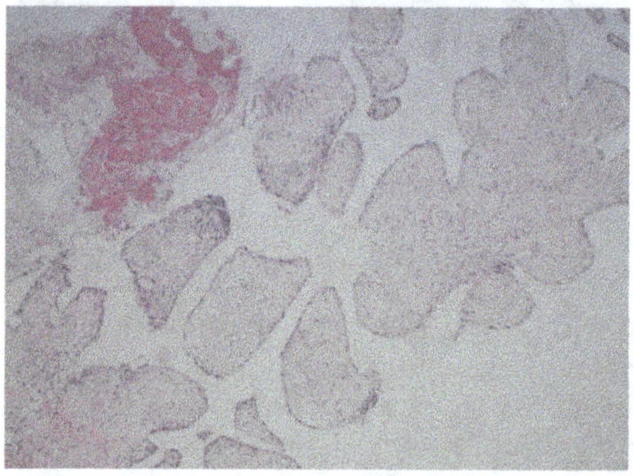

(b)

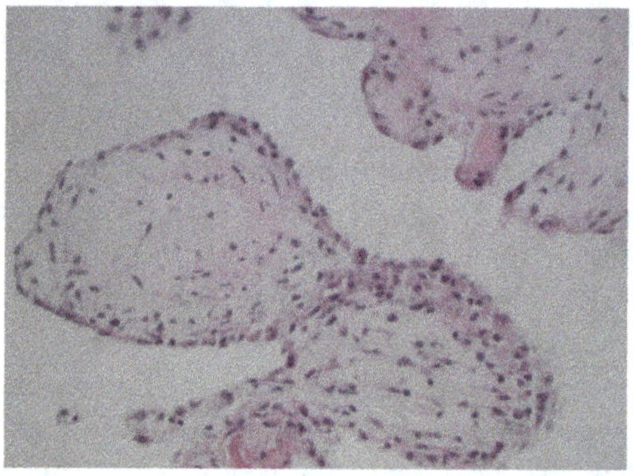

(c)

FIGURE 5: (a) H&E 40x reveals multiple papillary structures lined by endothelial cells; (b) H&E 100x reveals the papillary structures are avascular and contain fibromyxoid stroma; (c) H&E 400x reveals the papillary structures are lined by bland endothelial cells.

this hypothesis, showing that a large proportion of patients with CPFEs have associated cardiac and valvular conditions that increase hemodynamic stress [9]. The observation that CPFEs developed after iatrogenic stress to the endocardium through cardiac surgery and thoracic irradiation further supports this hypothesis [12].

More recently, a case report suggested a novel cause of damage to the endocardium in association with CPFEs in patient with $\beta$-thalassemia major [13]. $\beta$-Thalassemia, an inherited hemolytic disorder caused by the partial or complete inability to synthesize the $\beta$-chain in hemoglobin, is categorized into three groups based on the genetic alterations and clinical severity: major, intermedia, and minor. In the serum and plasma of patients with thalassemia, in vitro studies showed that there are elevated levels of endothelial adhesion proteins (intercellular adhesion molecule-1 [ICAM-1], E-selectin [ELAM-1], vascular cell adhesion molecule-1 [VCAM-1], von Willebrand factor [VWF], and thrombomodulin) [14, 15]. These endothelial adhesion proteins are elevated in the setting of endothelial activation and damage as well as chronic inflammation, suggesting these two processes underlie the pathophysiology of $\beta$-thalassemia [16]. These same processes, like hemodynamic stress, can also contribute to the formation of CPFEs.

In this case, this otherwise healthy patient did not have any cardiac or iatrogenic causes of increased hemodynamic stress. Based on literature review, this case is the second report that associates $\beta$-thalassemia with CPFE and is the first report specifically for $\beta$-thalassemia intermedia. While there is insufficient evidence to conclude whether his $\beta$-thalassemia contributed to the formation of the CPFE, this hypothesis-generating case calls attention to the need for elucidating the relationship between these two conditions in future studies.

## Conflicts of Interest

The authors declare no conflicts of interest.

## References

[1] K. Reynen, "Frequency of primary tumors of the heart," *The American Journal of Cardiology*, vol. 77, no. 1, p. 107, 1996.

[2] P. Centofanti, E. Di Rosa, L. Deorsola et al., "Primary cardiac tumors: early and late results of surgical treatment in 91 patients," *Annals of Thoracic Surgery*, vol. 68, no. 4, pp. 1236–1241, 1999.

[3] S. S. Tamin, J. J. Maleszewski, C. G. Scott et al., "Prognostic and bioepidemiologic implications of papillary fibroelastomas," *Journal of the American College of Cardiology*, vol. 65, no. 22, pp. 2420–2429, 2015.

[4] J. Butany, V. Nair, A. Naseemuddin, G. M. Nair, C. Catton, and T. Yau, "Cardiac tumours: diagnosis and management," *Lancet Oncology*, vol. 6, no. 4, pp. 219–228, 2005.

[5] H. R. Dudley, F. Goodale, and R. M. O'Neal, "Fibro-elastic hamartomas of heart valves," *The American Journal of Pathology*, vol. 32, no. 1, pp. 35–39, 1956.

[6] C. Raeburn, "Papillary fibro-elastic hamartomas of the heart valves," *The Journal of Pathology and Bacteriology*, vol. 65, no. 2, pp. 371–373, 1953.

[7] R. M. Gowda, I. A. Khan, C. K. Nair, N. J. Mehta, B. C. Vasavada, and T. J. Sacchi, "Cardiac papillary fibroelastoma: a comprehensive analysis of 725 cases," *American Heart Journal*, vol. 146, no. 3, pp. 404–410, 2003.

[8] J. P. Sun, C. R. Asher, X. S. Yang et al., "Clinical and echocardiographic characteristics of papillary fibroelastomas: a retrospective and prospective study in 162 patients," *Circulation*, vol. 103, no. 22, pp. 2687–2693, 2001.

[9] K. W. Klarich, M. Enriquez-Sarano, G. M. Gura, W. D. Edwards, A. J. Tajik, and J. B. Seward, "Papillary fibroelastoma: echocardiographic characteristics for diagnosis and pathologic correlation," *Journal of the American College of Cardiology*, vol. 30, no. 3, pp. 784–790, 1997.

[10] E. J. Kasarskis, O. William, and G. Earle, "Embolic stroke from cardiac papillary fibroelastomas," *Stroke*, vol. 19, no. 9, pp. 1171–1173, 1988.

[11] M. M. Anastacio, M. R. Moon, R. J. Damiano Jr., M. K. Pasque, H. S. Maniar, and J. S. Lawton, "Surgical experience with cardiac papillary fibroelastoma over a 15-year period," *Annals of Thoracic Surgery*, vol. 94, no. 2, pp. 537–541, 2012.

[12] A. N. Kurup, H. D. Tazelaar, W. D. Edwards et al., "Iatrogenic cardiac papillary fibroelastoma: a study of 12 cases (1990 to 2000)," *Human Pathology*, vol. 33, no. 12, pp. 1165–1169, 2002.

[13] J. Kokotsakis, I. Nenekidis, V. Anagnostakou et al., "Papillary fibroelastoma of the aortic valve in a $\beta$-thalassemia patient," *General Thoracic and Cardiovascular Surgery*, vol. 59, no. 10, pp. 712–714, 2011.

[14] P. Butthep, A. Bunyaratvej, Y. Funahara et al., "Alterations in vascular endothelial cell-related plasma proteins in thalassaemic patients and their correlation with clinical symptoms," *Thrombosis and Haemostasis*, vol. 74, no. 4, pp. 1045–1049, 1995.

[15] P. Butthep, A. Bunyaratvej, Y. Funahara et al., "Possible evidence of endothelial cellactivation and disturbance in thalassemia: an in vitro study," *Southeast Asian Journal of Tropical Medicine and Public Health*, vol. 28, supplement 3, pp. 141–148, 1997.

[16] I. Kanavaki, P. Makrythanasis, C. Lazaropoulou et al., "Soluble endothelial adhesion molecules and inflammation markers in patients with $\beta$-thalassemia intermedia," *Blood Cells, Molecules, and Diseases*, vol. 43, no. 3, pp. 230–234, 2009.

# 10

# Bilateral Medial Medullary Stroke: A Challenge in Early Diagnosis

**Amir M. Torabi**

*East Dallas Neurological Services Baylor Medical Center, Garland, TX, USA*

Correspondence should be addressed to Amir M. Torabi; amir_torabi@yahoo.com

Academic Editors: T. K. Banerjee, S. T. Gontkovsky, and J. C. Kattah

Bilateral medial medullary stroke is a very rare type of stroke, with catastrophic consequences. Early diagnosis is crucial. Here, I present a young patient with acute vertigo, progressive generalized weakness, dysarthria, and respiratory failure, who initially was misdiagnosed with acute vestibular syndrome. Initial brain magnetic resonance imaging (MRI) that was done in the acute phase was read as normal. Other possibilities were excluded by lumbar puncture and MRI of cervical spine. MR of C-spine showed lesion at medial medulla; therefore a second MRI of brain was requested, showed characteristic "heart appearance" shape at diffusion weighted (DWI), and confirmed bilateral medial medullary stroke. Retrospectively, a vague-defined hyperintense linear DWI signal at midline was noted in the first brain MRI. Because of the symmetric and midline pattern of this abnormal signal and similarity to an artifact, some radiologists or neurologists may miss this type of stroke. Radiologists and neurologists must recognize clinical and MRI findings of this rare type of stroke, which early treatment could make a difference in patient outcome. The abnormal DWI signal in early stages of this type of stroke may not be a typical "heart appearance" shape, and other variants such as small dot or linear DWI signal at midline must be recognized as early signs of stroke. Also, MRI of cervical spine may be helpful if there is attention to brainstem as well.

## 1. Introduction

Bilateral medial medullary stroke is very rare, and clinical diagnosis without neuroimaging is very difficult [1]. Brainstem encephalitis and Guillain-Barre's syndrome (GBS) can present similarly [2]. Despite a huge progress in MRI technology, still human factor and experience can determine correct interpretation. Here, I discuss a clinical case and MRI findings of a patient with this diagnosis.

## 2. Case Presentation

A 59-year-old white male patient, right-handed, presented with acute vertigo, nausea, and vomiting to a University Hospital in Dallas, TX, USA, on April 17, 2013. Past medical history was remarkable for untreated hypertension and moderate alcohol consumption. He was not taking any medication at home. Initial examiner (an internist) in that hospital noted bilateral nystagmus, although he did not specify direction or other characteristics of the nystagmus.

MRI of brain was done and read as normal (Figure 1), although a faint linear signal at DWI at midline medulla could be seen retrospectively. MR angiography of head (Figure 2) and neck was normal. Patient was told may have acute labyrinthitis and was discharged home two days later. After discharge his condition slowly deteriorated, and he presented to our hospital, Baylor Medical Center at Garland, TX, USA, three days later with generalized weakness, falls, slurred speech, respiratory failure, and dysphagia. Initially he was intubated due to risk of aspiration. His evaluation after extubation showed severe dysarthria with normal comprehension. His cranial nerves revealed direction changing gaze evoked horizontal nystagmus. No facial palsy noted, and extraocular movement still was full. Hypoglossal diplegia as well as decreased gag reflex was noted. Motor exam showed diffuse bilateral weakness of both upper and lower extremities at the range of 2-3/5, along with decreased tone and absent deep tendon reflexes everywhere, similar to an acute spinal cord shock state. He had mute Babinski response bilaterally.

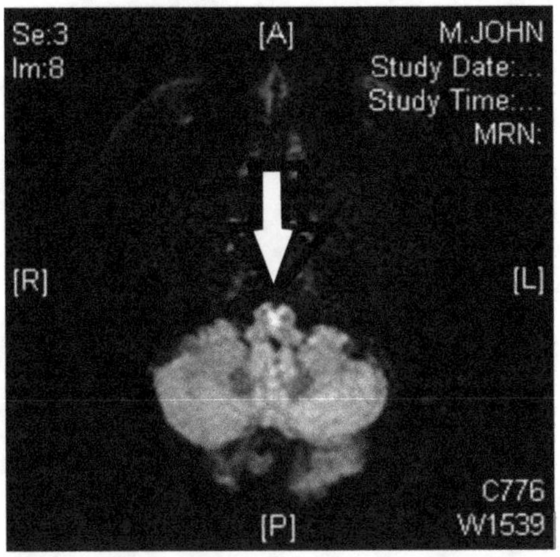


FIGURE 1: MRI of brain and DWI at presentation. Abnormal signal at DWI, a midline dot-linear signal, was similar to an artifact.

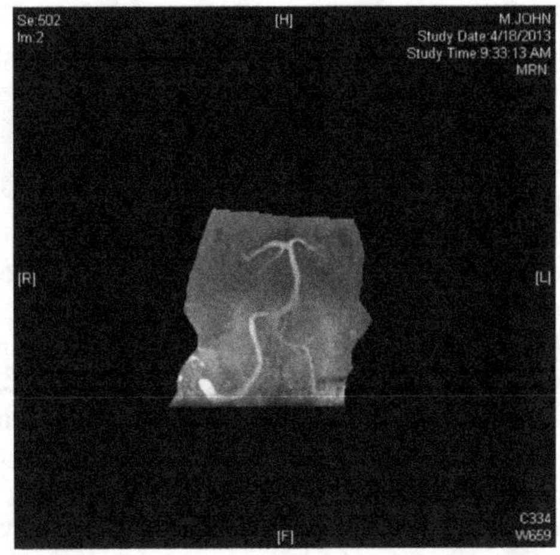


FIGURE 2: MRA of brain does not show any abnormality of vertebral arteries.

Shortly after examination, he developed respiratory failure and was reintubated.

For the possibility of GBS and brainstem encephalitis, lumbar puncture was performed which showed normal cell, protein, and glucose. Blood and CSF cultures were negative. Since GBS still could not be excluded, he was started on empiric intravenous immunoglobulin (IVIG). Thiamine 100 mg intravenous was given for the possibility of Wernicke's encephalopathy, and Aspirin 325 mg per day was added for the possibility of stroke. MRI of cervical spine (Figure 3) was ordered to make sure that there was no high cervical cord lesion. Cervical cord was unremarkable, but interestingly, a T2-hyperintense lesion was noted at midanterior medulla (Figure 3). Because of this finding, a repeat MRI of brain was requested (Figure 4), which confirmed bilateral anterior medial medullary stroke, typical "heart appearance sign." IVIG was stopped, and he was put on full dose enoxaparin 1 mg/kg twice a day, but there was progressive weakness to the point of quadriplegic state in less than two days. Still he was able to communicate with eye movements and blinking. He had tracheostomy and remained ventilator dependent for another five days, then he decided to stop his ventilator, and shortly after he died of respiratory failure.

## 3. Discussion

Bilateral medial medullary stroke is a very rare type of stroke. The most common symptoms are weakness, dysarthria, hypoglossal palsy, flaccid, or spastic quadriplegia. It has generally a poor prognosis [1, 3, 4]. The characteristic brain MRI finding of "heart appearance" at DWI has been described in multiple case reports [1, 3, 4]. In this case, the first MRI (Figure 1) done in acute phase did show a small linear abnormal DWI signal at midline but was missed by radiologist and clinician.

There have been other case reports of this type of stroke, missed by radiologists. Considering interventions such as thrombolytic in the acute phase, it is important to diagnose any stroke as early as possible, and such subtle finding needs

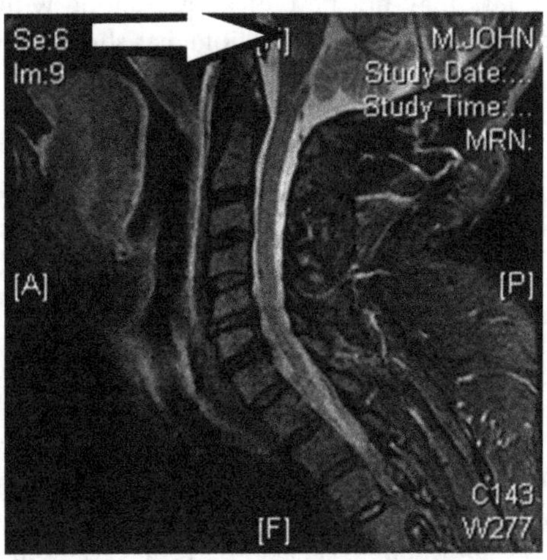


FIGURE 3: MRI of cervical spine, sagittal, shows abnormal T2 hyperintense lesion at mid-upper medulla.

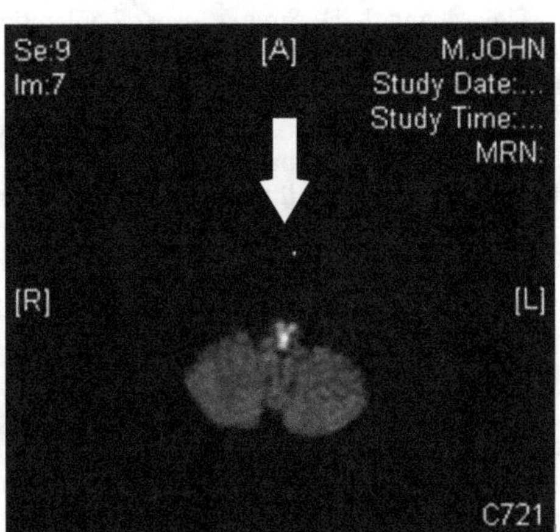


FIGURE 4: Second brain MRI, DWI shows characteristic "heart appearance" sign suggestive of bilateral medial medullary infarct.

to be picked up by radiologist or neurologist for an effective treatment. Normal MRA of brain may suggest small vessel disease of one of the paramedian perforatings (from vertebral or anterior spinal arteries). It is possible if one paramedian artery is supplying both pyramids in rare cases.

Brainstem encephalitis is also very rare and has a broad range of differential diagnosis including infectious and autoimmune causes. It has features such as ophthalmoparesis, ataxia, weakness, and upper motor neuron signs. In this case, negative CSF, absence of ophthalmoplegia, and MRI findings are all against brainstem encephalitis. GBS similarly can mimic the presentation, particularly with diffuse areflexia and progressive weakness, and was excluded by MRI findings [2]. MRI of cervical spine was helpful to view abnormal signal at upper medulla. Sagittal FLAIR brain MRI is equally helpful but may not be done routinely.

Overall outcome of this type of stroke is not good with severe morbidity and mortality, and early diagnosis based on combination of clinical and MRI findings by both neurologist and radiologist is critical. MRI findings particularly in the first few hours may not be typical, and along with clinical presentation neurologists and radiologists should have a high index of suspicion.

## Conflict of Interests

The author declare that there is no conflict of interest.

## References

[1] E. Kumral, N. Afsar, D. KIrbas, K. BalkIr, and T. ÖzdemirkIran, "Spectrum of medial medullary infarction: clinical and magnetic resonance imaging findings," *Journal of Neurology*, vol. 249, no. 1, pp. 85–93, 2002.

[2] L. Ma, Y. Deng, J. Wang et al., "Bilateral medial medullary infarction presenting as Guillain-Barré- like syndrome," *Clinical Neurology and Neurosurgery*, vol. 113, no. 7, pp. 589–591, 2011.

[3] G. Kleinert, F. Fazekas, R. Kleinert et al., "Bilateral medial medullary infarction: magnetic resonance imaging and correlative histopathologic findings," *European Neurology*, vol. 33, no. 1, pp. 74–76, 1993.

[4] W. M. Jagiella and J. H. Sung, "Bilateral infarction of the medullary pyramids in humans," *Neurology*, vol. 39, no. 1, pp. 21–24, 1989.

[5] M. Maeda, T. Shimono, H. Tsukahara, S. E. Maier, and K. Takeda, "Acute bilateral medial medullary infarction: a unique "heart appearance" sign by diffusion-weighted imaging," *European Neurology*, vol. 51, no. 4, pp. 236–237, 2004.

[6] K. Tokuoka, N. Yuasa, T. Ishikawa et al., "A case of bilateral medial medullary infarction presenting with "heart appearance" sign," *Tokai Journal of Experimental and Clinical Medicine*, vol. 32, no. 3, pp. 99–102, 2007.

[7] K. Parsi, R. K. Itgampalli, A. Suryanarayana, and K. R. Kumar, "Bilateral medial medullary infarction: heart appearance," *Neurology India*, vol. 61, pp. 84–85, 2013.

# 11

# A Case Report Exploring Activity Intensity in Inpatient Rehabilitation after Stroke

**Kathryn Zalewski,[1] Julie Kerk,[2] Kristina Laundre,[1] Amber Wacek,[1] and Melissa Wiedmeyer[1]**

[1] *College of Health Sciences, Department of Human Movement Science, Doctor of Physical Therapy Program, University of Wisconsin-Milwaukee, P.O. Box 413 Pavilion 360, Milwaukee, WI 53201, USA*
[2] *Neurorehabilitation Unit, Department of Physical Therapy, Froedtert Memorial Lutheran Hospital, 9200 West Wisconsin Avenue, Milwaukee, WI 53226, USA*

Correspondence should be addressed to Kathryn Zalewski, zalewski@uwm.edu

Academic Editor: Nam-Jong Paik

*Background and Purpose.* Inpatient rehabilitation in countries other than the United States (US) has been described as a time where patients are often not engaged in intensive physical activity. The purpose of this case report is to explore the amount and intensity of physical activity provided in inpatient rehabilitation after stroke in the US. *Methods.* This study presents a case report of a person admitted to an inpatient rehabilitation unit after sustaining a first stroke. A customized data collection tracked type of activity, activity intensity and social interaction every 5 minutes during the rehabilitation day. *Results.* 74 percent of the day was spent in low intensity, often seated, physical activity; 14% of the day was spent resting or sleeping. Only 2.91% the day was spent in moderate or high intensity activity with a mobility focus. *Conclusions.* Consistent with other studies, this case report suggests a relatively low physical demand to rehabilitation delivered in inpatient stroke rehabilitation. This case begins to raise questions about optimized rehabilitation parameters for acute stroke rehabilitation.

## 1. Introduction

Amount and duration of rehabilitation therapy delivered after stroke is largely influenced by regulations guiding reimbursement from federal funding programs. Inpatient rehabilitation is viewed as being beneficial to people in the early stages of stroke recovery [1]. The combined impact of physical therapy (PT), occupational therapy (OT), and speech therapy (ST) for individuals recovering from first stroke (CVA) is estimated at 20 points on the Functional Independence Measure (FIM) [2]. The functional impact of therapy is in part a function of dosage calculated by exploring daily physical activity (physical therapy sessions or nontherapeutic physical activity), total length of stay, and intensity of the sessions. Functional recovery, including the recovery of ambulation is tied to the total time spent practicing walking, and in particular time spend in high-intensity repetitive and task-specific practice [3]. Total activity dosage in inpatient rehabilitation, including therapeutic activity delivered in PT and nontherapeutic ambulation is not well described.

On average, rehabilitation units in the United States provide 1.5–1.6 thirty minute sessions of physical, occupational and speech therapy daily [2, 4]. Physical therapy sessions are described to last 38 minutes. A majority of the sessions (81.1%) include some type of pregait or gait activities [4]. These observations suggest that most patients receive approximately 60 minutes of structured physical therapy daily. Nonstructured physical activity is harder to quantify; there are no known descriptions of the nontherapeutic activity in inpatient rehabilitation.

An emerging body of evidence from stroke centers in other countries characterizes the acute rehabilitation window as lacking in activity intensity. A small study comparing the time use of people recovering from stroke in Belgium and Switzerland found discrepancies between hours spent in therapeutic activities (2.5 versus 4 hours), with PT the predominant therapy provided by both countries. In both countries, the bulk of the care was provided in the patient's room. The intensity of the PT services was not documented [5]. Bernhardt et al. documented stroke rehabilitation intensity in a hospital in Melbourne, Australia. Their findings suggest that people in the early stages of stroke recovery engage in moderate or high intensity activities less than 13 percent of the therapeutic day. Over 50% of the time, people in rehabilitation were resting in bed. This pattern of inactivity seemed to be independent of the frailty of the individual, as when the data were analyzed to remove those who were restricted to bed rest, the data were not significantly changed. In addition, people engaged in stroke rehabilitation were alone over 60% of the time. The authors conclude the inpatient rehabilitation stay is characterized by people being "inactive and alone" [6]. The finding of relative inactivity and social isolation was replicated in a case series exploring subacute rehabilitation [7]. While there is no known description of the comprehensive inpatient rehabilitation stay in the United States that examines both services delivered and intensity of those services delivered, if the rehabilitation environment parallels that of other countries, it is possible that the rehabilitation day is characterized by underactivity.

The prospective payment system (PPS) used by the Centers for Medicare and Medicaid to reimburse care in inpatient rehabilitation facilities (IRFs) was passed as part of the Balance Budget Act in 1997 and implemented in 2002 [8]. While the full impact of the restructuring of rehabilitation payment is not known, trends towards shorter lengths of stay seem to be consistent [9], with lengths of stay for people recovering from stroke approximately 15 days (±12) [2]. O'Brien's recent review of trends in rehabilitation outcomes based on FIM score, discharge destination, and lengths of stay before and after introduction of PPS begin to suggest that while functional outcomes may not be changed with shorter lengths of stay, fewer individuals may be returning home [9]. A shorter length of stay, coupled with a rehabilitation environment characterized by underactivity creates the possibility that physical activity dosage in acute rehabilitation may be inadequate to meet the functional challenges of the patient and his/her family in the transition to a home environment.

Undertreatment may have significant long-lasting implications for the stroke survivor. Recovery of independent ambulation is a critical component of stroke rehabilitation, and those who recover ability to ambulate live longer [10]. Recovery of ambulation after stroke appears to be associated with initial time to lower extremity weight bearing activity [11], and training in ambulation seems to translate to increased independence in other functional skills such as toilet transfers [12]. More minutes per day spent in PT gait activities were associated with higher discharge FIM scores and increased rates of discharge to home [12]. Predictors of stepping activity after stroke seem to be associated with amount and intensity of the walking training [13]. There are two concerns in rehabilitation associated with determining dosage associated with activity based interventions: (1) the amount of practice/repetition needed to build skills necessary for independence, and (2) the intensity of the practice/repetition needed to improve the cardiovascular conditioning necessary to meet the physical demands of daily life tasks as well as improving fitness and reducing risks associated with disuse/deconditioning. It is unclear whether the inpatient rehabilitation experience accomplishes either of these goals.

If inpatient physical activity dosage with an emphasis on walking is critical to recovery of ambulation then an observation of the stroke rehabilitation environment may assist the rehabilitation team in optimizing an environment that will maximize outcomes. The purpose of this case report is to describe the physical demands of a person recovering from stroke in the early days of stroke recovery, admitted to an inpatient rehabilitation unit in the United States within 2 weeks of experiencing onset of first stroke. As a second objective the social interaction of the stroke rehabilitation is also reported.

## 2. Case Description

This case report was developed to test methods for a larger study designed to explore the relationship between physical activity intensity in inpatient stroke rehabilitation and mobility outcomes. To improve sensitivity of the testing materials, the person selected for the case had to be completing the first week of inpatient rehabilitation and meet the criteria of: (1) medical stability meaning not confined to bed rest or restricted mobility for medical reasons, (2) able to participate in some mobility training both seated (e.g., wheelchair propulsion) and upright (gait or pregait activities), (3) require speech therapy services, and (4) have family involved in discharge planning. A physical therapist collaborator identified the first individual meeting this criteria after methods had been developed to participate in this case report.

Data collection occurred in an inpatient stroke rehabilitation facility in a local teaching hospital representing the only stroke rehabilitation center accredited by the American Stroke Association in the geographic area.

*2.1. Patient.* At the time of the data collection, EA was a 67-year-old married man admitted to a local inpatient rehabilitation center/Stroke Unit four days prior to participating in the data collection. After the study was described, he gave his assent to participate. EA was diagnosed with a first ischemic right middle cerebral artery infarct 12 days prior to admission and 16 days prior to data collection. At the time of data collection, according to the initial examinations of the occupational therapist and physical therapist assigned to EA, he required minimal assistance and set up with self-cares if completed in a seated position. He required moderate assistance with all upright mobility including pregait activities and supervision with seated wheelchair mobility over short distances. He had active use of the affected lower extremity (LE) and some voluntary activity of the affected upper extremity (UE), but did not spontaneously use the affected extremity for self-care including brushing teeth and shaving. He was right hand dominant. He was described as having normal receptive language skills, but

Table 1: Percent time in physical activity during rehabilitation day[a].

| Description of activity | Percent time in activity | Activity code |
|---|---|---|
| Sitting supported engaged in cognitive activity | 35.92 | 1 |
| Sitting supported resting | 19.42 | 1 |
| Sitting supported using unaffected UE in therapeutic activity | 18.45 | 2 |
| Sleeping | 10.68 | 0 |
| Sitting unsupported, no activity | 3.88 | 3 |
| Sitting supported engaged in UE activity with affected extremity | 2.91 | 2 |
| Not observed | 2.91 | n/a |
| Walking or walking activity | 1.94 | 4 |
| Resting, laying in bed, but not sleeping | 1.94 | 0 |
| Independent seated mobility | .97 | 4 |
| Sitting in bed in ADL activity | 0.97 | 2 |

[a]Observations occurred between 7:30 AM and 5:00 PM. Activities from the appendix that were not witnessed are not included in this table.

slurred speech and mild short-term memory limitations by the speech pathologist.

Discharge goals for EA were to return home with support, able to complete seated self-care skills with set up and requiring minimal assistance for upright tasks including transfers. He was expected to require minimal assistance for household level ambulation using an assistive device and to be independent with wheelchair mobility over even and uneven surfaces for short distances. Therapists anticipated his discharge to be 2 weeks from the date of data collection.

*2.2. Methods.* A modification of methods used by Bernhardt et al. [6] was used to design the survey tool used for data collection. The original Bernhardt tool was presented to a small focus group consisting of 13 therapists: 9 physical therapists, 2 occupational therapists, and 2 speech therapists from the Stroke Unit. The tool was assessed by the focus group to determine whether any activities were missing, whether there was agreement on the intensity indicators, and for understanding of data collection methods. Revisions to the Bernhardt tool were based on the focus group feedback, and presented a second time to the focus group for consensus. The final version of the data collection tool used in this study is provided as an appendix.

Four evaluators recorded EA's activity intensity and social contacts from 7:30 AM until 5:00 PM on a weekday in the first week of inpatient rehabilitation. Observations were collected every ten minutes between 7:30–9:00 and every 5 minutes from 9:00 AM until 5:00 PM to increase sensitivity of the observations. Observations between 9:00 and 10:00 were completed by all four raters to assess interrater reliability (percent agreement) of the tool; otherwise all observations were by a single rater. At each observation the activity category, intensity of the activity, and presence of others was noted on the scoring form according to the template presented in the appendix. The raters did not interact directly with EA. For observations of EA in the room, the observer witnessed the activity from outside the room. For observations in the unit, observations were made from a distance that did not allow for physical or verbal interaction with EA.

The observation was recorded as unavailable if EA was off the unit, or if any person providing care or socializing with EA requested privacy. The highest level of activity witnessed at the observation moment (as opposed to the highest level of activity in the 5 minute observation window) was recorded. In total 103 observations were recorded; EA was off the unit for 3 observations resulting in 100 observations with data.

*2.3. Results.* Interrater reliability was evaluated using percent agreement; raters agreed 89% of the time on behavioral ratings indicating good reliability of the recording tool. Activity data are reported in Table 1.

Most (73.79%) of EA's day is spent in low-intensity activity typically involving sitting and engaging in self-care activities, cognitive rehabilitation, or upper extremity activities. Only 2.91% of EA's day is spent in activity that may present a significant aerobic challenge with a focus on mobility training. EA spent relatively little time resting in bed but not sleeping, but spent a large portion of the day sitting and resting. This may suggest that there is down time during the day where a transfer back to bed to rest may not be productive due to the rehabilitation schedule (i.e., in between therapy sessions). This time window may present opportunity for increasing physical activity participation independent of traditional therapy times.

While relatively inactive, the participant was rarely alone. EA was interacting with at least one other individual for 67% of the observations. Of this time, 55.5% of the observations recorded interactions with the therapy staff, 34.4% with family members and 10.1% with nontherapist/nonprofessional hospital staff. Two or more persons were present with the subject during 25% of the person-present observations.

## 3. Discussion

There are two issues facing optimizing of dosage of rehabilitation therapies and nontherapeutic activity: the dosage necessary to improve the cardiovascular conditioning of the patient to increase independent engagement in daily living skills and the dosage necessary to improve the functional mobility of the patient. The activity pattern for EA suggests that there is considerable "down time" during the rehabilitation day. Some of that down time provides needed rest between therapy sessions. However some time, especially that associated with the "seated but resting" category, may reflect a window that could be capitalized on to increase activity, especially that activity which could increase cardiovascular endurance. Independent seated physical activity (such as getting one's-self to therapies using independent wheelchair mobility, or seated low resistance, high repetition strength training) may be able to be increased in a way that does not require additional staff supervision or increase risk of injury due to falls.

Although EA receives rehabilitation services consistent with reported norms, it appears that the bulk of the rehabilitation delivered is provided at a relatively low intensity with an emphasis on seated activities. This is a bit surprising given EA's discharge goal of "some household ambulation." Other studies have reported more inactivity in the stroke recovery process, however, the intensity of services provided seem to be consistent with other reports [6, 7].

The examination of EA's activity intensity profile provides a window into the types of interventions delivered, and secondarily into the dosage of interventions targeted specifically to practice of ambulation. The relatively low-activity intensity suggests few upright-, gait-, or pregait-related activities were delivered. Although one explanation for the low physical activity intensity in this case may be attributed to EA's risk of injury with unsupervised upright activity, the activity profile suggests that therapeutic activities may not be challenging the ambulation goal. It is possible that the activity pattern reflects the prioritization of safety over upright mobility. As the therapists did not identify independent upright ambulation as the primary mobility goal after discharge from the stroke unit, a focus on seated mobility may have dominated the rehabilitation sessions. While independent seated mobility may be a very meaningful outcome for assuring safety at discharge, if this goal limits practice of upright ambulation (and thus discharge outcome) perhaps these strategies should be reconsidered.

Identifying ideal intensity for rehabilitation is a difficult challenge for therapists designing a comprehensive rehabilitation program for a person in the early stages of stroke recovery. Dosage and intensity are informed by many factors; some specific to the individual, some based on the experience of the therapist and team, and some based on resources and externally imposed regulations. In the absence of clear guidelines informing ideal intensity, however, the rehabilitation team should explore whether activity intensity in and outside of formalized rehabilitation sessions is adequate to advance behavioral change desired.

This case study begins to ask the question as to whether intensity of physical activity is adequate to sustain the long-term behavioral change and cardiovascular conditioning needed in stroke recovery. This particular case begs some interesting questions. EA spent approximately 13 percent of the rehabilitation day either sleeping or resting. While this number is not as high as reported in other studies, perhaps this down time needs further description to optimize outcomes. Additionally, absent more time to utilize, perhaps an increase physical activity of individual therapy sessions could be examined. A comprehensive assessment of rehabilitation from admission to the rehabilitation unit through discharge from rehabilitation should be considered to adequately assess the intensity of dosage of rehabilitation throughout the entire course of formalized stroke recovery.

This case also demonstrates some limitations to the understanding of stroke recovery. Although the impact of low intensity functional training in the post-acute window of stroke recovery appears to support improvement in functional performance without clear change in underlying cardiorespiratory fitness [14, 15], whether this effect holds in the acute phases of stroke recovery is unknown. By contrast, other authors seem to support an exercise dosage of moderate intensity and short duration (30 minutes) optimize coronary risk reduction for people in the post-acute phase of stroke recovery [16]. A "best" dosage may be dependent upon phase of stroke recovery and individual goals (enhanced function or enhanced fitness and reduced stroke risk).

Stroke rehabilitation is complex. Interventions promoting functional recovery need to be balanced with interventions designed to assure safety of the stroke survivor and primary caregiver, and interventions that optimize reduction of stroke. What may be best in the acute phases of stroke recovery may not be best in subacute phases of stroke recovery. These changing and sometimes competing needs are delivered in an environment defined by shorter lengths of stay and increased responsibility on the family to provide care. The acute recovery window needs further study to support the rehabilitation team in providing optimized care in a changing resource environment.

## 4. Conclusions

In the United States, inpatient rehabilitation after stroke is characterized by a short, intense bout of therapy provided with the goal of optimizing probability of discharge to home. In the case observed, the physical intensity of the rehabilitation seems relatively low compared to the mobility and self-care expectations of the patient upon return home. The relative inactivity raises questions about adequacy of activity dosage necessary to meet rehabilitation goals.

## Appendix

Physical activity, intensity, categorization, and social interaction are shown in Table 2.

Table 2

| Observed activity | Activity class (Intensity) | Category | People present (y/n)—classification[a] |
|---|---|---|---|
| No physical activity/resting | No activity | 0 | |
| No physical activity/resting but not sleeping (in bed) | No activity | 0 | |
| Supported in bed, engaged in therapeutic cognitive activity | Therapeutic activity | 1 | |
| Talking/reading/watching television while in bed supported | Nontherapeutic activity | 1 | |
| Eating with unaffected hand while in bed supported | Nontherapeutic activity | 1 | |
| Sitting in bed supported, ADL activity | Therapeutic activity, low intensity | 2 | |
| Sitting out of bed, supported, eating or exercising with the unaffected UE | Therapeutic activity, low intensity | 2 | |
| Sitting supported out of bed, resting | Therapeutic activity, low intensity | 1 | |
| Sitting supported out of bed, talking/reading/watching or engaged in other cognitive activity | Therapeutic activity, low intensity | 2 | |
| Sitting supported out of bed engaged in UE activity with the affected extremity | Therapeutic activity, moderate intensity | 3 | |
| Sitting unsupported | Therapeutic activity, moderate intensity | 3 | |
| Mobility training exercise (bed mobility, transfer training) | Therapeutic activity, moderate intensity | 3 | |
| Mat activities (4 point, kneeling, floor transfers or other core training exercises) | Therapeutic activity, high intensity | 4 | |
| Standing activities | Therapeutic activity, high intensity | 4 | |
| Walking or walking activities | Therapeutic activity, high intensity | 4 | |
| Independent seated mobility (e.g., wheelchair propulsion) | Therapeutic activity, high intensity | 4 | |
| Aquatic therapy | Therapeutic activity, high intensity | 4 | |

[a]Classification of persons present; 1: Family member, 2: Nurse, physician, or nontherapist member of the health care team, 3: hospital staff (transporter, aid, interpreter), 4: therapist (physical therapist, occupational therapist, speech pathologist), 5: Physical Therapist Aid or Student Physical Therapist, 6: Psychologist, 7: Certified Nursing Assistant.

## References


[1] M.-H. Hu, S.-S. Hsu, P.-K. Yip, J.-S. Jeng, and Y.-H. Wang, "Early and intensive rehabilitation predicts good functional outcomes in patients admitted to the stroke intensive care unit," *Disability and Rehabilitation*, vol. 32, no. 15, pp. 1251–1259, 2010.

[2] J. Karges and S. Smallfied, "A description of the outcomes, frequency, duration, and intensity of occupational, physical, and speech therapy in inpatient stroke rehabilitation," *Journal of Allied Health*, vol. 38, no. 1, pp. E1–E10, 2009.

[3] P. Langhorne, F. Coupar, and A. Pollock, "Motor recovery after stroke: a systematic review," *The Lancet Neurology*, vol. 8, no. 8, pp. 741–754, 2009.

[4] D. U. Jette, N. K. Latham, R. J. Smout, J. Gassaway, M. D. Slavin, and S. D. Horn, "Physical therapy interventions for patients with stroke in inpatient rehabilitation facilities," *Physical Therapy*, vol. 85, no. 3, pp. 238–248, 2005.

[5] W. D. Weerdt, B. Selz, G. Nuyens et al., "Time use of stroke patients in an intensive rehabilitation unit: a comparison between a Belgian and a Swiss setting," *Disability and Rehabilitation*, vol. 22, no. 4, pp. 181–186, 2000.

[6] J. Bernhardt, H. Dewey, A. Thrift, and G. Donnan, "Inactive and alone: physical activity within the first 14 days of acute stroke unit caree," *Stroke*, vol. 35, no. 4, pp. 1005–1009, 2004.

[7] W. H. Gage, K. F. Zabjek, K. M. Sibley, A. Tang, D. Brooks, and W. E. McIlroy, "Ambulatory monitoring of activity levels of individuals in the sub-acute stage following stroke: a case series," *Journal of NeuroEngineering and Rehabilitation*, vol. 4, article 41, 2007.

[8] Services CfMaM, *Inpatient Review Transition Fact Sheet*, 2007.

[9] S. R. O'Brien, "Trends in inpatient rehabilitation stroke outcomes before and after advent of the prospective payment system: a systematic review," *Journal of Neurologic Physical Therapy*, vol. 34, no. 1, pp. 17–23, 2010.

[10] K. B. Slot, E. Berge, P. Dorman, S. Lewis, M. Dennis, and P. Sandercock, "Impact of functional status at six months on long term survival in patients with ischaemic stroke: prospective cohort studies," *British Medical Journal*, vol. 336, no. 7640, pp. 376–379, 2008.

[11] E. Viosca, R. Lafuente, J. L. Martínez, P. L. Almagro, A. Gracia, and C. González, "Walking recovery after an acute stroke: assessment with a new functional classification and the Barthel Index," *Archives of Physical Medicine and Rehabilitation*, vol. 86, no. 6, pp. 1239–1244, 2005.

[12] S. D. Horn, G. DeJong, R. J. Smout, J. Gassaway, R. James, and B. Conroy, "Stroke rehabilitation patients, practice, and outcomes: is earlier and more aggressive therapy better?" *Archives of Physical Medicine and Rehabilitation*, vol. 86, no. 12, pp. S101–S114, 2005.

[13] J. L. Moore, E. J. Roth, C. Killian, and T. G. Hornby, "Locomotor training improves daily stepping activity and gait efficiency in individuals poststroke who have reached a "plateau" in recovery," *Stroke*, vol. 41, no. 1, pp. 129–135, 2010.

[14] M. C. Cramp, R. J. Greenwood, M. Gill, A. Lehmann, J. C. Rothwell, and O. M. Scott, "Effectiveness of a community-based low intensity exercise programme for ambulatory stroke survivors," *Disability and Rehabilitation*, vol. 32, no. 3, pp. 239–247, 2010.

[15] K. Michael, A. P. Goldberg, M. S. Treuth, J. Beans, P. Normandt, and R. F. Macko, "Progressive adaptive physical activity in stroke improves balance, gait, and fitness: preliminary results," *Topics in Stroke Rehabilitation*, vol. 16, no. 2, pp. 133–139, 2009.

[16] J. H. Rimmer, A. E. Rauworth, E. C. Wang, T. L. Nicola, and B. Hill, "A Preliminary Study to Examine the Effects of Aerobic and Therapeutic (Nonaerobic) Exercise on Cardiorespiratory Fitness and Coronary Risk Reduction in Stroke Survivors," *Archives of Physical Medicine and Rehabilitation*, vol. 90, no. 3, pp. 407–412, 2009.

# 12

# Paediatric Stroke: Review of the Literature and Possible Treatment Options, including Endovascular Approach

**Elisa F. Ciceri,[1] Valeria Cuccarini,[1] Luisa Chiapparini,[1] Veronica Saletti,[2] and Luca Valvassori[3]**

[1] *Neuroradiology Department, Fondazione Istituto "C. Besta", Via Celoria 11, 20133 Milan, Italy*
[2] *Paediatric Department, Fondazione Istituto "C. Besta", Via Celoria 11, 20133 Milan, Italy*
[3] *Neuroradiology Department, Ospedale Niguarda, Piazza Ospedale Maggiore 3, 20162 Milan, Italy*

Correspondence should be addressed to Elisa F. Ciceri, elisaciceri@yahoo.com

Academic Editor: Halvor Naess

Stroke is among the top 10 causes of death in childhood. More than half of the surviving children have long-term neurological sequelae. Ischemic stroke (IS) includes arterial ischemic stroke and cerebral venous thrombosis with venous infarction. Haemorrhagic stroke (HS) includes intracerebral haematoma or subarachnoid haemorrhage. Risk factors for stroke are different in children and in adults. 10–30% of IS have no identified risk factors. However, multiple risk factors are recognizable in the majority of stroke in children; thus, a comprehensive diagnostic evaluation is crucial. Vascular abnormalities, such as arteriovenous malformations, aneurysms, vessel dissection, stenosis, and moyamoya disease, are frequently associated with both IS and HS and lead to high recurrence rates. Endovascular and surgical treatment options are sometimes indicated, performed on the basis of expert opinion, and extrapolated from the adult procedures. In the present paper, we review the recent literature and we discuss the treatment in five cases managed at our institutions.

## 1. Introduction

In young population stroke is often an underestimated cause of neurological disturbances with different possible aetiologies and multiple treatment options. A thorough knowledge of the pathophysiology of the disease, of the natural history and of the possible different therapies including medical or surgical approaches, represents a necessary instrument in order to obtain a prompt and correct diagnosis and a successful recovery. Additionally, diagnosis of paediatric stroke is even more difficult, due to the limited expressive and interpretive skills of symptoms compared to the adult population.

Stroke is among the top 10 causes of death in childhood with an incidence of 2–13 per 100,000 children. More than half of the surviving children who had a stroke have long-term neurological sequelae [1].

Ischemic stroke (IS) refers to both arterial ischemic stroke (AIS) and cerebral venous thrombosis (CVT) resulting in venous infarction. Hemorrhagic stroke (HS) includes intracerebral haemorrhage and nontraumatic subarachnoid haemorrhage. Nearly half of paediatric strokes are hemorrhagic [2].

There are differences in the incidence of stroke during childhood, with incidence rate of 3/100,000 under the age of 1 year (even when neonatal or perinatal stroke, which is known to have a particularly high incidence rate, is excluded) and of 0.7/100,000 at 5–9 years. Another incidence peak is observed in male adolescents probably due to hormonal factors [3].

The risk factors for childhood stroke are markedly different from those in adults, including young adults. Childhood stroke in which no risk factors are identified represent 10–30% of cases [3].

In the next paragraphs we try to give a schematic presentation of the main risk factors for arterial, venous, and haemorrhagic stroke, an overview about the stroke outcome, and of the recurrence rate. In evaluating this complex pathology, it is always important to consider that the same risk factor can determine all the three situations and that multiple factors can differently combine each others in the same situation.

## 2. Risk Factors

### *2.1. Arterial Ischemic Stroke (AIS)*

*2.1.1. Arteriopathies.* In childhood AIS, abnormalities of the cerebral circulation (both intracranial and cervical) have been reported in up to 80% of the cases [3]. The most frequently identified form of arteriopathy is termed transient cerebral arteriopathy (TCA) or focal cerebral arteriopathy of childhood (FCA), defined as vascular stenosis not otherwise classified as dissection, moyamoya, sickle cell arteriopathy (SCA), postvaricella arteriopathy, vasculitis, or other specific diagnoses. TCA or FCA represents a monophasic transient arteriopathy affecting large- or medium-sized vessels that, on follow-up imaging few months after the infarct, generally shows regression or nonprogression. It seems that many cases of FCA have a postinfectious mechanism underlying the arteriopathy, particularly recent upper respiratory tract infections [3].

Craniocervical arterial dissection may be responsible for 7 to 20% of childhood AIS. In children, the anterior circulation is involved more frequently than the posterior circulation. There is a history of trauma in half of the cases although the trauma may be minor; in these cases the cervical arteries are most commonly affected, while intracranial dissection accounts for at least a quarter of the cases. In nontraumatic cases 60% of dissections are intracranial. In dissecting diseases, symptoms can be related either to mass effect, ischemia, or SAH. If all vascular layers of the intradural artery are dissected, a subarachnoid hemorrhagic will occur. Intramural clot formation can cause distal thromboembolic ischemia or occlusion of perforator branches and local ischemia. Chronic dissecting process may eventually lead to formation of a "giant partially thrombosed aneurysm" [4]. Unlike in the adult, an underlying condition predisposing to dissection is seldom found in children. Recurrence rate is about 10% [1, 3, 5].

Moyamoya is a noninflammatory nonatherosclerotic vasculopathy. It is characterized by progressive occlusion or stenosis of the cerebral vasculature particularly involving the vessels feeding the circle of Willis, most commonly of the distal internal carotid arteries, with compensation resulting in the development of an extensive network of hypertrophic arterial collaterals distal to the occlusion. Moyamoya can be idiopathic (disease) or secondary (syndrome) when associated with other causes of vasculopathy, such as sickle cell disease (SCD), Down's syndrome, neurofibromatosis, and previous cranial irradiation. Genetic polymorphisms of HLA class II genes have been associated with idiopathic moyamoya disease [6, 7].

Primary CNS vasculitis or systemic vasculitis (lupus erythematosus, Henoch-Schonlein purpura, Wegener granulomatosis, polyarteritis nodosa, Takayasu arteritis, and Kawasaki disease) have been linked to stroke.

Rare causes of cerebral arteriopathy in children include neurofibromatosis 1 (NF1) arterial dysplasia, postirradiation arteriopathy, fibromuscular dysplasia, and collagen disorders.

*2.1.2. Cardiac Diseases.* Cardiac disease is one of the most commonly identified risk factors in childhood IS, as it is identified in 15–30% of cases of AIS.

In children with preexisting major congenital cardiac malformations, embolic phenomena are the major cause of stroke. Other factors involved include hypoxia, hypotension, and polycytemia.

An association between IS and cardiac surgery or catheterization is found in about 40% of children with cardiac disease.

Patent foramen ovale (PFO) has been referred to as "the back door to the brain" through which small venous thrombi not filtered by the pulmonary vasculature enter the systemic circulation. In children and young adults with otherwise cryptogenic stroke, an increased prevalence of PFO has been found, even if there are not conclusive data demonstrating causality [8].

Children with AIS may have both cardiac disease and intracranial arteriopathy.

*2.1.3. Haematological Disorders.* In children with SCD the risk of stroke is about 200 times greater than in other children, and up to one-third of children with SCD have silent strokes (neuroimaging evidence without history of stroke) that frequently lead to cognitive deficits. $\beta$-thalassemia can also lead to IS.

Both of these conditions can cause stroke because of anemia and hypercoagulable state. Moreover, development of stenosis of the intracranial internal carotid artery (ICA) and of the proximal middle cerebral artery (MCA) in SCD determines a secondary moyamoya like vasculopathy due to repeated insults on the vessels' walls.

Iron-deficiency anaemia has been found to be present in 20% of previously healthy children with AIS.

A number of genetic thrombophilic traits have been associated with paediatric stroke: prothrombin G20210A, factor V Leiden G1691A, MTHFR C677T, lipoprotein(a), antiphospholipid antibodies/LLAC, protein S deficiency, antithrombin deficiency, protein C deficiency, different haplotypes of genes involved in the nitric oxide pathways and thus in possible endothelial impairment.

*2.1.4. Infections.* CNS infections, that is, meningitis and encephalitis, are present in 10% of cases of AIS, presumably due to vascular inflammation and thrombosis or due to reduced cerebral perfusion secondary to systemic hypotension, raised intracranial pressure, and low cerebrospinal fluid glucose.

Hypotension and hypercoagulable state as a consequence of bacteraemia or sepsis can lead to IS.

Focal cerebral artery stenosis with a history of varicella infection in the preceding year has been termed postvaricella angiopathy, thought to be due to viral invasion of the artery wall as already mentioned in the previous section on arteriopathies.

The most common risk factor identified in childhood stroke due to CVT is represented by middle-ear and paranasal sinus infections.

*2.1.5. Genetics.* An increased risk of stroke has been associated with numerous genetic diseases, such as the above-mentioned SCD and genetically inherited thrombophilic traits, Down's syndrome, NF1, Williams syndrome, homocystinuria, cerebral autosomal-dominant arteriopathy with subcortical infarcts and leukoencephalopathy (CADASIL) and Fabry disease, mitochondrial encephalomyopathy with lactic acidosis and stroke (MELAS) [9].

AIS and CVT share many of the above-mentioned risk factors.

*2.2. Cerebral Sinovenous Thrombosis (CVT).* CVT in childhood is a rare (incidence 0.4–0.7 per 100000 children per year, most occurring within the neonatal period) but underrecognized disorder, often of multifactorial aetiology, with neurologic sequelae in up to 40% of survivors and mortality approaching 10%. The spectrum of brain injury varies from venous congestion to parenchymal ischemia which may be cortical or subcortical and involve deep grey matter. The majority of the parenchymal infarcts are haemorrhagic. Subarachnoid and subdural haemorrhage are less frequent. In neonates there is a strong association between CVT and intraventricular haemorrhage. Infections appear to be the most common condition associated to CVT. Predisposing systemic comorbidity factors include fever, infection, dehydration, anaemia, and chronic medical conditions such as congenital heart disease, nephritic syndrome, autoimmune diseases, malignancy, and genetic and acquired prothrombotic disorders. Moreover, locoregional factors such as first of all otitis media and mastoiditis, then meningitis, head trauma, and recent intracranial surgery are strongly related to CVT [10].

*2.3. Haemorrhagic Stroke (HS)*

*2.3.1. Structural Lesions.* Structural lesions account for at least half of HS in children. Arteriovenous malformations (AVMs) are the most commonly identified structural lesions found in HS (30%), and 80% of the children with an AVM will declare their malformation by HS. Probability of a first haemorrhage is 2–4% per year [11].

The vast majority of arterial cerebral aneurysms in the paediatric age are symptomatic, and they account for 13% of HS, mostly presenting with subarachnoid haemorrhage (SAH). Aneurysms may be idiopathic (30%) or related to arterial dissection (50%), to bacterial or mycotic infections (15%), or to trauma (5–10%) [12]. In traumatic cases, HS often presents 2–4 weeks after the head injury.

HS is also related to SCD (25% of first strokes in children with SCD are haemorrhagic) and moyamoya, due to fragility of the dysplastic collateral vessels.

Cavernous malformations are found to be the cause of bleeding in 15% of HS paediatric cases.

Finally, intratumoral haemorrhage can be a rare feature of intracranial malignancy.

There is a threefold increased incidence of haemorrhage in the posterior circulation in children compared to adults and a fivefold increased incidence in involvement of the internal carotid artery termination [13, 14].

*2.3.2. Haematological Disorders.* Between 10 and 30% of childhood HS are caused by haematological disorders such as haemophilia, thrombocytopenia, von Willebrand's disease, coagulopathy secondary to hepatic dysfunction, or vitamin K deficiency [3].

About 25% of children have HS of undetermined cause.

## 3. Outcome

Fatality rates vary from 2 to 20% for IS and from 5 to 54% for HS. Male gender, black ethnicity, and stroke recurrence increase the risk of death. Neurological deficits are reported to be present in at least two-thirds of survivors.

Lesion location and extension is an important predictor of outcome.

Even if it is widely believed that brain plasticity can lead to improved outcome following acquired brain injury at an early age, there is increasing evidence to support the hypothesis that younger age at time of stroke is a predictor of a worse outcome, particularly for cognitive and neuropsychological domains [2, 3, 15, 16]. Mortality rate in paediatric group is reported to be 6 to 30% [17]. Therefore, children should be closely monitored over the time for possible recurrences.

These are aspects that should be taken into consideration also in children with silent infarctions.

## 4. Recurrence

Recurrence risk of AIS is about 1.2% in the perinatal age and 19% in later infancy and childhood, but probably a greater number of children have TIAs or silent reinfarctions. Five-year followup shows no recurrence in children with normal vascular imaging and up to 60% recurrence rate in children with vascular abnormalities [14].

HS recurrence rate is about 10% at 5-year followup. No recurrences are expected in idiopathic HS whereas 13% recurrence rate in children with vascular structural anomalies and in those with medical causes of HS; in the latter cases, recurrence tends to occur within the first week, while in the former it may occur years later [18].

Between 10% and 20% of children who have a CVT will experience a recurrent symptomatic venous event, half of which systemic rather than cerebral [10].

## 5. Diagnostic Imaging

Cerebral imaging includes computed tomography (CT) particularly when HS is suspected in order to rapidly discriminate between HS and IS and to distinguish between intracerebral haematoma or SAH. Magnetic resonance imaging (MRI) with angio-MR (MRA) helps to precisely identify the site of IS/HS, the involved structures, the presence of oedema, and/or mass effects. Diffusion MR (DWI) and

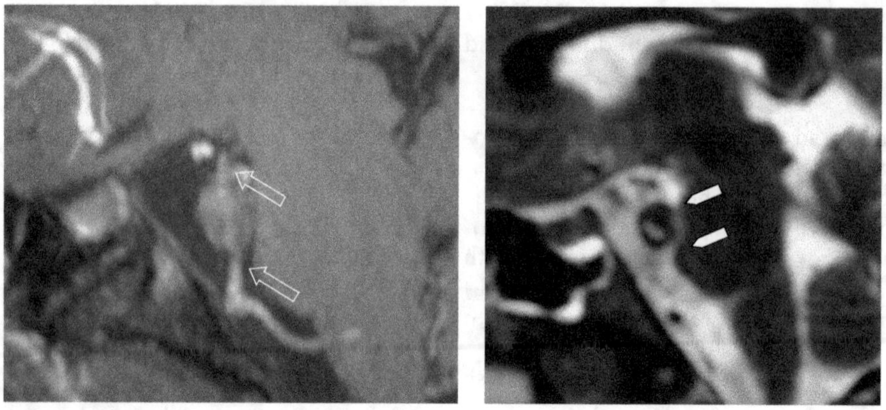

(a) (b)

FIGURE 1: MRA (a) and MRI sagittal sections (b), obtained 11 days after the initial symptoms, demonstrate the presence of a BA aneurysm with mass effect on the pons (arrowheads in (b)) and ischemic changes (not shown). At both edges of the aneurysm, stenosis of the BA is recognizable (arrows in (a)).

perfusion MR (PWI) are useful to evaluate the timing of the stroke and the cerebral blood flow in the surrounding areas. Gradient-echo and susceptibility-weighted images MR (GRE/SWI) are able to detect deoxyhaemoglobin in very recent bleeding when other sequences are unable to demonstrate the extent of the haematoma or to detect small amount of haemosiderin in old HS or in cryptic malformations, such as cavernous angiomas. Finally, in selected cases, digital subtraction cerebral angiography (DSA) is recommended to better evaluate the vascular tree. Specifically, dedicated cerebrovascular imaging with DSA is crucial when no cause for stroke is found via noninvasive vascular imaging. Sometimes vascular malformations are not immediately evident after the acute haemorrhage; therefore, when vascular imaging is normal or inconclusive, the studies should be repeated once the clot has been reabsorbed [1, 3, 14, 18].

## 6. Treatment

Three consensus papers suggest the guidelines for the evaluation and treatment of AIS in childhood [15, 19, 20], and one encompasses guidelines for the treatment or evaluation of paediatric HS [20].

*6.1. Medical Treatment.* Acute and chronic management of IS includes several options, depending on the aetiology of stroke, timing, extent, and so forth. Antioedema and antiplatelet treatments are often indicated. Anticoagulant therapies are usually employed in cardiac cause, CVT, dissection, and recurrent stroke while on antiplatelet therapy. Exchange transfusion (SCD), cerebral and systemic supportive care, and correction of specific conditions are always required. Paediatrics encompasses a wide range of ages with maturational differences. Optimal dosing is likely to differ as there are age-dependent differences in haemostasis, younger individuals demonstrating diminished specific indices of fibrinolysis and global, increased fibrinolytic capability [17].

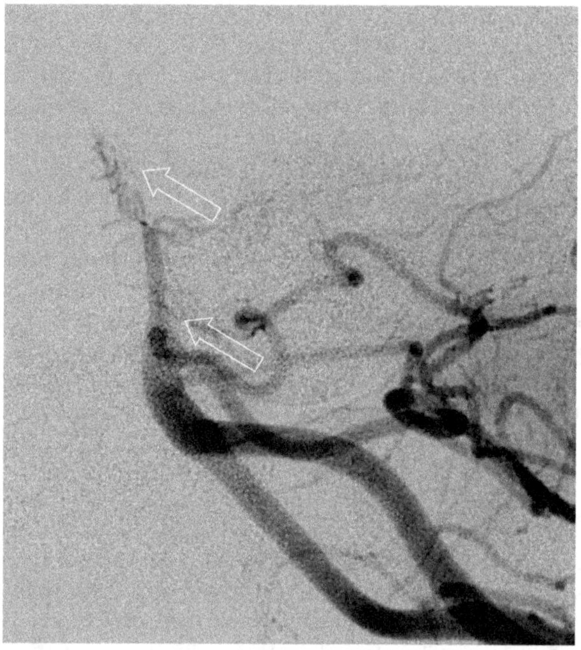

FIGURE 2: Follow-up angiogram, obtained 11 months after the onset of symptoms, shows complete obliteration of the BA at the level of the dissection, without any evidence of residual filling of the aneurysm.

CVT treatment includes general supportive measures and antithrombotic and nonantithrombotic therapies. Anticoagulant and antiplatelet treatment regimens vary between centers, and some of them prefer unfractioned heparin in the acute state, as the effects of heparin can be reversed if intracranial haemorrhage occurs. In the following 3 to 6 months, chronic anticoagulation is maintained with Low Molecular Weight Heparin (LMWH) or Coumadin [10]. Treatment of neonates with LMWH appears to be safe and should at least be considered. There are very few reports

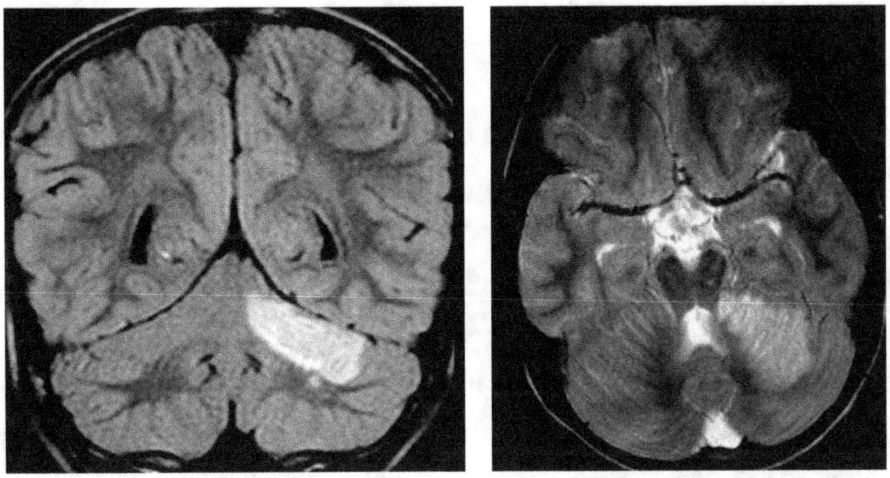

(a) (b)

FIGURE 3: MRI coronal FLAIR (a) and axial T2-weighted (b) images show an infarction in the left superior cerebellar hemisphere, in the territory of one hemispheric branch of the left SCA.

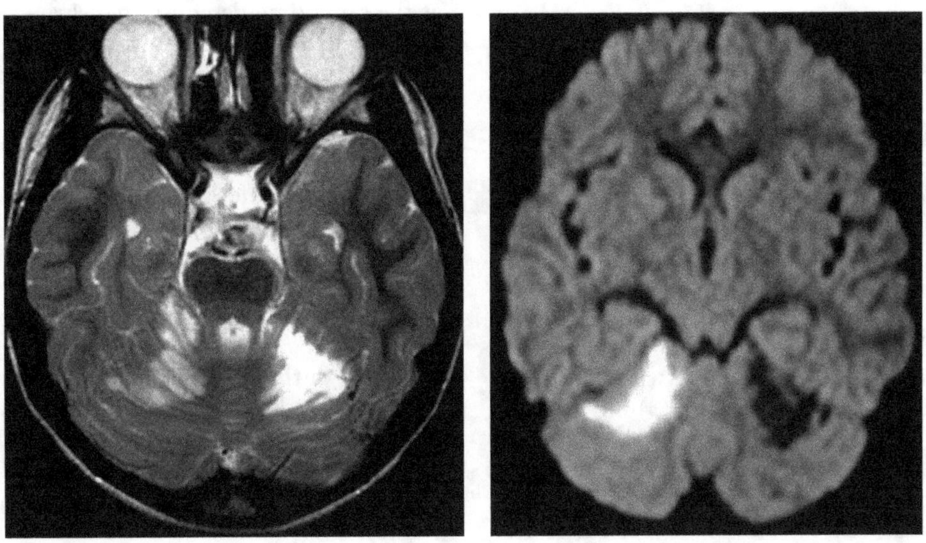

(a) (b)

FIGURE 4: MRI axial T2-weighted (a) and diffusion-weighted (DWI) (b) images demonstrate the old infarction in the left superior cerebellar hemisphere and the new lesion in the right superior cerebellar hemisphere with identical distribution. The restricted diffusivity (high signal intensity in (b)) indicates a recent infarction.

on the use of antiplatelet agents such as acetylsalicylic acid (ASA) or dipyridamole in the acute or chronic settings in paediatric age [10]. If significant ICH is associated with CVT, the use of anticoagulants is controversial. Septic situation requires antibiotics and may need surgical removal and drainage of the infection. Medical treatment of HS is mainly supportive, with correction of treatable haemorrhage risk factors or correction of specific conditions such as, for instance, antimicrobial treatment in infectious aneurysms.

While a neuroprotective role has been ascribed to hypertonic solutions of albumin, memantine HCl, and magnesium sulphate that are recommended for the treatment of adult ischemic stroke patients, no data are available in order to make recommendations regarding use in paediatric AIS [17].

*6.2. Surgical Options.* Within the management of paediatric stroke, invasive treatments are rarely performed in selected cases, based on expert opinion [11, 12, 16, 21–27].

Surgical revascularization procedures include direct surgical bypass or indirect procedures to encourage development of collateral blood vessels such as the encephaloduroarteriomyosinangiosis in moyamoya. In case of massive cerebellar oedema or haematoma, decompressive craniectomy and haematoma evacuation can be performed to prevent tonsillar herniation. Decompressive surgery is

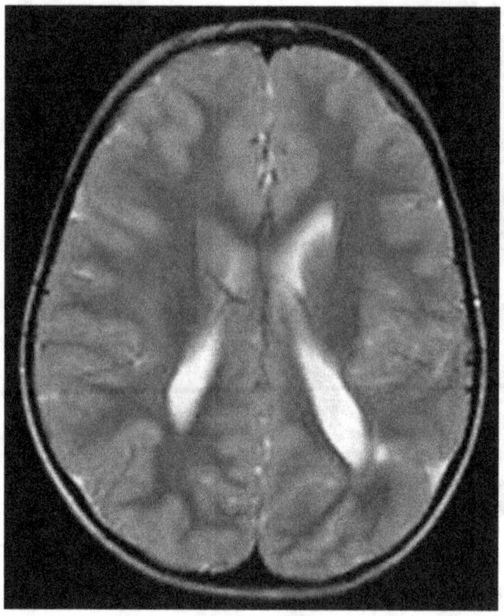

Figure 5: MRI axial T2 weighted shows the cortical-subcortical abnormalities in the left temporo-parietal-occipital region.

required in supratentorial large cerebral lesions with mass effect and transtentorial herniation. In hydrocephalus, after intraventricular haemorrhage or SAH, external ventricular drainage may be required. In vascular malformations such as aneurysms or AVMs, open surgery represents a possible treatment.

*6.3. Endovascular Options.* The endovascular options in case of IS comprise (1) intra-arterial thrombolysis and/or mechanical revascularization in thromboembolic lesions, (2) revascularization procedures with stenting with or without angioplasty in stenoses or dissections, and (3) intra-arterial administration of vasodilator drugs in vessels spasm. In cases of HS due to bleeding from vascular malformations, endovascular repair with platinum detachable coils or flow diverter for aneurysms, and histoacrylic or polymeric glue injections in AVM are possible alternatives. In selected cases, surgical and endovascular approaches can be combined. An additional option for the treatment of small AVM is represented by radiosurgery [28]. In case of cardiac disease (i.e., PFO), correction of the cardiac defect should be considered.

## 7. Illustrative Cases

*7.1. Case 1 (Figures 1 and 2).* A 15-year-old female patient was admitted to our hospital for angiographic followup and possible treatment of a partially thrombosed basilar artery (BA) dissecting aneurysm extending from the mid-basilar portion to the origin of the superior cerebellar arteries (SCAs). One week before her first hospitalization the patient had complained of sudden nuchal headaches sometimes associated with nausea, vomiting, and visual changes, which disappeared without any treatment. No history of previous trauma was reported. Physical and neurological examinations were within normal limits. Four-vessel cerebral digital subtraction angiography (DSA) and MRA (Figure 1) demonstrated the presence of the BA aneurysmal dilatation measuring 5 mm in its patent portion with an extension of 2 cm in length. Stenosis of the BA was recognizable proximal and distal to the aneurysm (Figure 1). Both SCAs were injected from the BA. MR imaging also visualized small ischemic areas in the left lower part of the pons and in the left cerebral peduncle (Figure 1). The patient was discharged on antiplatelet therapy (ticlopidine 250 mg/dL) to prevent further thrombotic events. The 2- and 4-month follow-up MR imaging with MRA showed further progression of the BA stenosis. Due to the good clinical condition of the patient, endovascular revascularization was not performed because of the high procedural risks. Finally, the follow-up angiogram (Figure 2) obtained 11 months after the initial symptoms demonstrated complete obliteration of the BA at the level of the dissection (arrows) without any evidence of filling of the aneurysmal pouch and adequate collateral flow to the upper BA, posterior cerebral arteries (PCAs), and SCAs provided by the internal carotid arteries via the posterior communicating arteries. MR imaging performed at the same time demonstrated shrinkage of the aneurysm without new ischemic lesions. The 19-month follow-up MR imaging ruled out the presence of new ischemic areas. At the present time, 6 years later, the patient remains clinically stable and neurologically intact. The extensive workup for suspected collagenopathy, including genetic research for the type 4 Ehlers-Danlos and collagen biopsy, was negative.

*7.2. Case 2 (Figures 3 and 4).* A 7-year-old roller-skater male was first admitted at a primary medical center with a 4-hour history of acute onset of unstable gait and left-limb weakness during a play fight with his sister, followed by diffuse headache. A brain CT scan was normal. Over the next 12 hours the patient's balance disorder improved, while left-limb weakness remained stable and a mild left cerebellar syndrome. Brain MRI and magnetic resonance angiography (MRA) showed a left cerebellar ischemic stroke and absence of the left superior cerebellar artery (SCA). Cardiac disorders were initially excluded by transthoracic echocardiogram.

The patient was admitted to our institute 5 days after symptoms onset. Anti-platelet treatment was started. Head and neck angio-CT and brain MRI revealed an infarction in the left superior cerebellar hemisphere (Figure 3) and the presence of a possible dissection of the left vertebral artery close to the foramen magnum. The cerebral DSA showed a lumen margin irregularity consistent with a fresh thrombus in the proximal tract of the left SCA. Laboratory findings excluded haematological disorders such as thrombophilias and SCD.

Over the next 7 days the patient's neurological symptoms gradually improved. Then, one week later, he abruptly developed headache, repeated vomiting, disturbance of consciousness with drowsiness, and right limb weakness. Brain MRI demonstrated a new cerebellar ischemic lesion in the superior right cerebellar hemisphere (Figure 4). Anticoagulant medication (low molecular weight heparin) was initiated. Over the following days the patient had

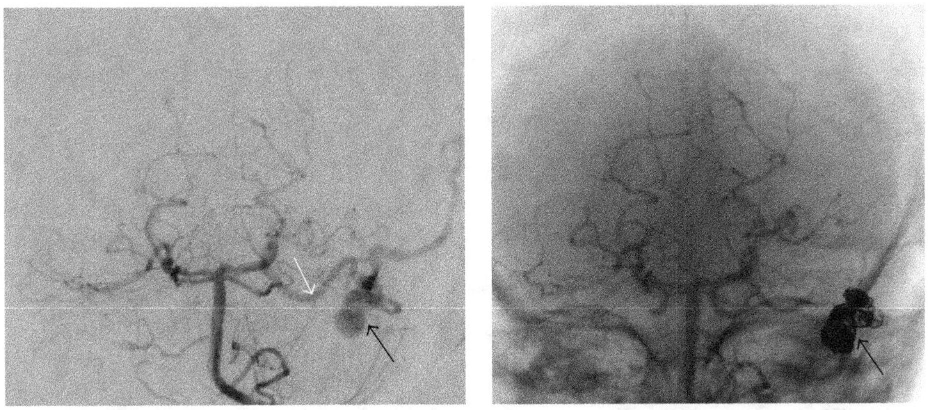

(a) (b)

FIGURE 6: Anteroposterior view of the left vertebral angiography showing a direct arteriovenous shunt between the anterior temporal branch of the left PCA (white arrow) and a superficial temporal vein with an interposed irregular aneurysmal dilatation (black arrow in (a)). The posttreatment angiography (b) demonstrates the complete resolution of the shunt obtained utilizing detachable platinum coils and histoacrylic glue (arrow in (b)).

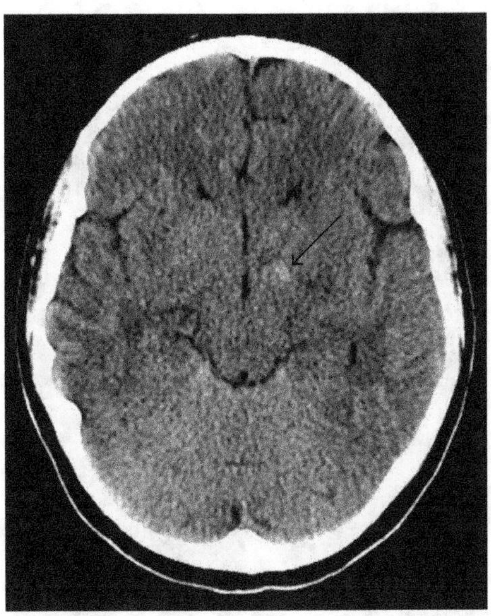

FIGURE 7: A small, well-defined hyperdense lesion in the left frontal basal area, just below the basal nuclei, is recognizable at the emergency CT (arrow). There is no evidence of subarachnoid haemorrhage.

a dramatic clinical improvement, and neurological examination demonstrated only a mild right cerebellar syndrome. Repeated transoesophageal echocardiography during Valsalva maneuver revealed an atrial septal defect that was repaired via percutaneous endovascular approach due to significant resting shunts. Clinical and neuroradiological followups since then were unremarkable.

*7.3. Case 3 (Figures 5 and 6).* A 4-year-old female, with a strong family history (father and grandfather) of hereditary hemorrhagic telangiectasia (HHT) or Rendu-Osler-Weber disease, was first evaluated at our institute at the age of 3 months for left temporal lobe hemorrhagic lesions detected elsewhere in the neonatal period. Neonatal history was complicated by tremors and generalized seizures that started on the second day of life after normal pregnancy and delivery.

On first admission at our institute, she was severely hypotonic; epilepsy was well controlled by antiepileptic monotherapy. Serial brain MRI and MRA studies (Figure 5) revealed left cortical-subcortical temporo-parietal-occipital gliotic-malacic areas associated with a cortical malformation.

A possible vascular malformation was also suspected in the left temporal hemisphere. Due to the age and the clinical condition of the patient, DSA was not performed at that time.

The patient presented psychomotor and language delay, and at the age of 4 years she started having recurrent episodes of epistaxis. Genetic analysis confirmed the HHT diagnosis with a mutation in the endoglin gene (ENG) on chromosome 9. Abdominal and pulmonary artero-venous malformations were excluded after adequate screening.

Four vessels DSA was then performed under general anesthesia, showing a left temporal arteriovenous shunt with an abnormal vascular dilatation, probably consistent with a venous varix (Figure 6(a)). It was successfully treated via endovascular approach with a superselective catheterization of the left anterior temporal artery, obliterating the venous varix and the shunt, utilizing detachable platinum coils and histoacrylic glue (Figure 6(b)).

*7.4. Case 4 (Figures 7 and 8).* A 12-year-old girl, who complained of a sudden headache with no other neurological deficit, was brought to the Emergency Room of another hospital. CT scan showed a small, round area of hyperdensity in the left basal frontal lobe, just below the basal ganglia (arrow in Figure 7). No subarachnoid blood was depicted. The patient was referred to our hospital for further examinations. At admittance, the patient was awake, well oriented, with no neurological deficit, but suffering

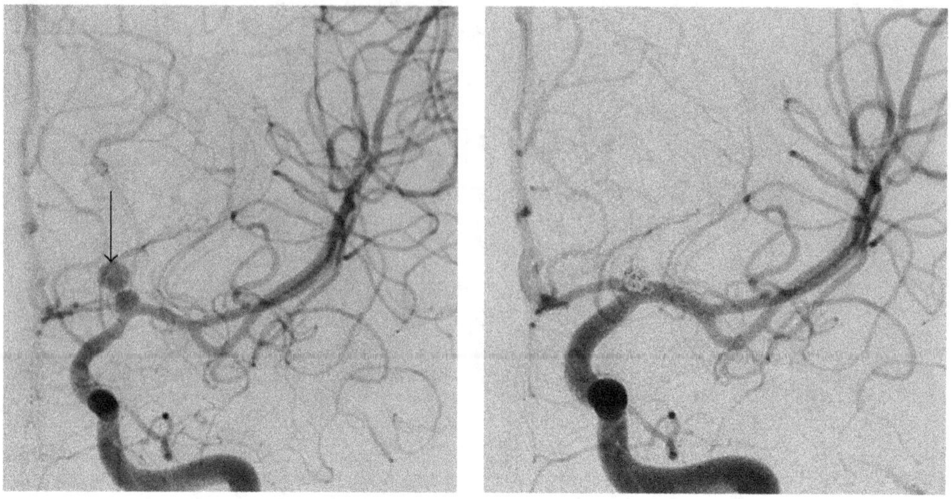

FIGURE 8: Anteroposterior view of the left internal carotid artery angiography shows a blister-like aneurysm at the intracranial bifurcation (a). Note the small pseudoaneurysm (arrow in (a)) at the dome of the aneurysmal sac, corresponding to the image seen on the CT (Figure 7), and the spasm in the supraclinoid portion of the carotid artery. The posttreatment angiography shows successful obliteration of the aneurysm with stent and a single platinum coil (b).

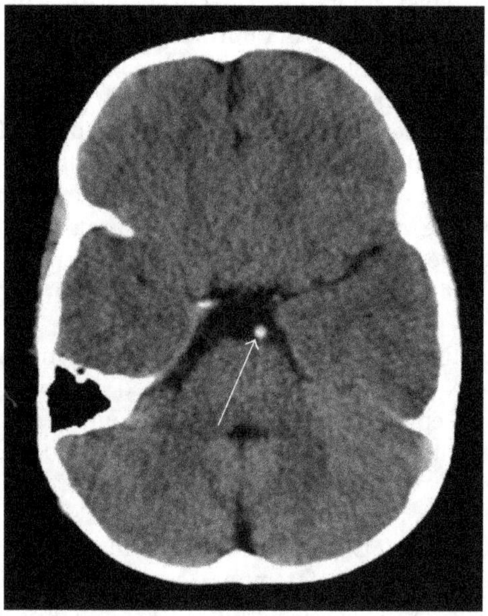

FIGURE 9: CT at admittance to Emergency Room shows a hyperdensity of the basilar artery, consistent with a thrombus (arrow).

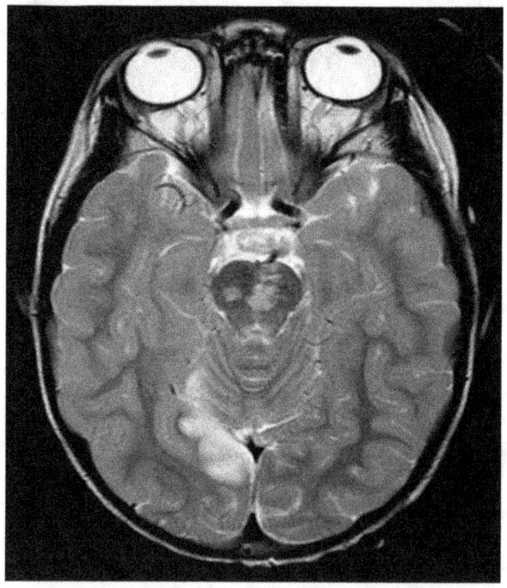

FIGURE 10: The axial T2 MR study performed 3 days after symptoms onset demonstrates the ischemic lesions in the pons and right occipital cortex.

from intense headache. DSA showed a small "blister-like" aneurysm at the left internal carotid artery bifurcation with a pseudoaneurysm just above it (arrow in Figure 8(a)). The patient was treated by endovascular approach, considering the neurosurgical approach more risky due to the presence of many perforating vessels in the area. Since the neck of the aneurysm was wide, a neuroform stent was deployed and a single platinum coil detached after passing through the struts of the stent. The final control showed the occlusion of the sac and the normal flow in the carotid artery (Figure 8(b)), with contrast stagnation inside the pseudoaneurysm. After the stent deployment, antiplatelet therapy was started and kept for 6 weeks. The patient had no deficit. Headache progressively decreased in the following days.

No recurrence of the aneurysm was observed at the 6-month follow-up angiography.

*7.5. Case 5 (Figures 9–11).* A 3-year-old African boy presented with sudden onset of nausea and vomiting. He was admitted to the Emergency Room hypotonic, hyporeactive, with abnormal ocular movements and recurrent seizures. In the recent past medical history, only sporadic headache was reported, after a varicella infection. At brain CT a hyperdense basilar artery was visible (arrow in Figure 9). At MRI with MRA, ischemic lesions in the vertebrobasilar territory with severe obstruction of the basilar and right posterior cerebral arteries were observed. As some hours had already passed from symptoms onset and the experience as well as the literature data on thrombolysis in children were poor, it was decided not to proceed to thrombolysis neither by venous nor arterial route. In addition, clinical conditions, though severe, did not seem to be life-threatening at that moment. Over the next few days, patient clinical conditions slowly but progressively improved. An MRI control at day 3 showed a new lesion in the pons (Figure 10). A DSA performed at day 12 confirmed the MRI findings: occlusion of the basilar artery from the vertebrobasilar (VB) junction to the tip, with good collaterals supplying the brainstem perforators and partial revascularization of the superior cerebellar arteries (arrows in Figure 11).

In the diagnostic workup, a patency of the foramen ovale was found, as the cardiologists did not consider the thromboembolic source causing the occlusion. At day 22, at discharge, no neurological deficits were present except for a very slight difficulty in walking with a preferred use of the left limbs.

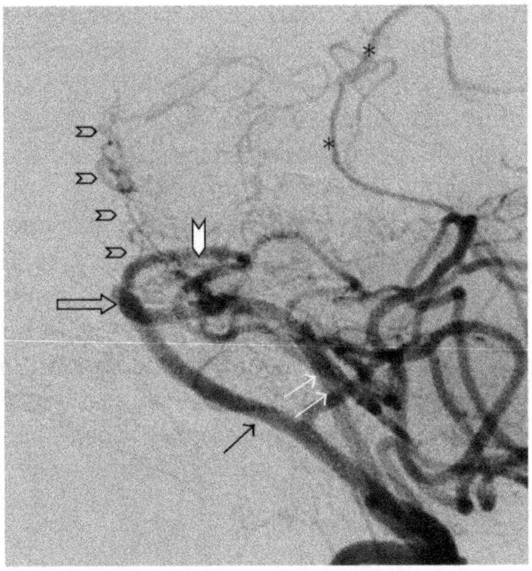

Figure 11: Cerebral angiography (lateral view) with injection of the left vertebral artery (arrow) shows occlusion of the basilar artery (open arrow) at the vertebrobasilar junction, just above the origin of the right superior cerebellar artery (white arrowhead). There are many tiny collaterals that supply the territory of the brainstem perforators (small arrowheads) and wider collaterals that reconstitute the superior cerebellar artery (asterisks). There is also retrograde filling of the right vertebral artery (white arrows) and of the right PICA.

## 8. Discussion and Conclusion

Stroke in paediatric population is associated with relative high morbidity, mortality, and recurrence rates. Silent stroke can be responsible for neuropsychological disability not otherwise recognizable.

If a stroke is suspected in a child, the diagnostic workup should include systemic blood tests (haematological disorders, infections), genetic and cardiac examinations (see our case 2). The neuroradiological diagnosis comprehends CT scan, MR imaging, and DSA. CT scan may demonstrate the presence and site of the intracranial bleeding (SAH or intracerebral haematoma) in case of HS. MR imaging with MRA better delineates the brain tissue status, the presence, the nature, and sometime the timing of possible structural lesions, for both HS and IS. They represent crucial tools both for treatment planning and followup. DSA is an invasive exam that should be performed by expert operators and only in selected cases. MRI and DSA in childhood are commonly performed in general anaesthesia to ensure a good quality imaging without any discomfort for the young patient.

In the appropriate setting, besides medical treatment, invasive procedures including endovascular approach should be considered. In cases of structural lesions a thorough risk/benefit analysis in order to decide the best treatment option is mandatory. Timing of invasive treatment can also represent a troublesome factor in a very young patient in whom fluid balance is a critical aspect in the anesthesiological and surgical management. In very small children, for this reason, it may be necessary to delay treatment waiting for a more favourable clinical status such as in our case 3.

In case of aneurysm the endovascular approach includes the obliteration of the fundus utilizing detachable coils associated with an intracranial stent in case of large neck, such as in our case 4. Experience in stent placement in children is limited; double antiplatelet therapy in case of stent deployment is recommended; since there are not specific trials for antiplatelet treatment for intracranial stenting in children, medical treatment is reasonably based on the adult's literature data. Another concern with paediatric intracranial stenting is the ongoing growth of the vessels over the time [11, 12, 23].

Dissecting aneurysm represents a typical vascular malformation in which the treatment must be tailored case by case. In case of a large dissecting aneurysm in a distal vascular territory, the obliteration of the arterial feeder with coils or glue should be taken into consideration. A balloon occlusion test to verify the possible collateral network can be previously performed. In case of a large thrombotic dissecting aneurysm in a vital territory, a precise preoperatory planning should be carried out, balancing benefits and risks. In our case 1, where a nonruptured large partially thrombosed aneurysm of the basilar artery causes a critical stenosis of the vessel, we preferred to delay the management of the aneurysm and of the BA stenosis because of the good clinical condition of the patient. Therefore, we followed the patient with MRI and MRA every 2–4 months. The spontaneous occlusion of the BA with repair of the aneurysm occurred asymptomatically.

Detachable coils and glue can be successfully utilized to occlude arteriovenous fistulas or AVM, such as in our case 3 in whom the direct AV fistula was related to HHT; in fact the presence of a cerebral AVM is one of the four diagnostic criteria for HHT [27].

In childhood, revascularization procedures in thrombotic vessels utilizing an endovascular approach are anecdotic (our case 5), likewise for the new flow-diverters devices that are indicated for aneurysmal repair in adult, and no literature data or specific recommendations are available as already discussed in the Treatment section.

In conclusion, stroke in childhood represents a challenging disease in which a correct diagnostic conduct may lead to the most appropriate treatment. A decision-making process should be carried out case by case by a multispecialist group, including the neuropaediatrician, neurosurgeon, and neuroradiologist. Future trials focused on treatment of vascular diseases in the youngest population are necessary to better understand the disease and, therefore, to improve the treatment.

## Conflict of Interests

The authors declare that they have no conflict of interests.

## References

[1] L. A. Beslow and L. C. Jordan, "Pediatric stroke: the importance of cerebral arteriopathy and vascular malformations," *Child's Nervous System*, vol. 26, no. 10, pp. 1263–1273, 2010.

[2] L. C. Jordan, "Assessment and treatment of stroke in children," *Current Treatment Options in Neurology*, vol. 10, no. 6, pp. 399–409, 2008.

[3] A. A. Mallick and F. J. K O'Callaghan, "Risk factors and treatment outcomes of childhood stroke," *Expert Review of Neurotherapeutics* , vol. 10, no. 8, pp. 1331–1346, 2010.

[4] T. Krings and I. S. Choi, "The many faces of intracranial arterial dissections," *Interventional Neuroradiology*, vol. 16, no. 2, pp. 151–160, 2010.

[5] C. Amlie-Lefond, T. J. Bernard, G. Sebire et al., "Predictors of cerebral arteriopathy in children with arterial ischemic stroke: results of the international pediatric stroke study," *Circulation*, vol. 119, no. 10, pp. 1417–1423, 2009.

[6] H. J. Cho, Y. H. Jung, Y. D. Kim, H. S. Nam, D. S. Kim, and J. D. Heo, "The different infarct patterns between adulthood-onset and childhood-onset moyamoya disease," *Journal of Neurology, Neurosurgery & Psychiatry*, vol. 82, no. 1, pp. 38–40, 2011.

[7] D. M. Ibrahimi, R. J. Tamargo, and E. Ahn, "Moyamoya disease in children," *Child's Nervous System*, vol. 26, no. 10, pp. 1297–1308, 2010.

[8] D. Kenny, M. Turner, and R. Martin, "When to close a patent foramen ovale," *Archives of Disease in Childhood*, vol. 93, no. 3, pp. 255–259, 2008.

[9] C. Tzoulis and L. A. Bindoff, "Serial diffusion imaging in a case of mitochondrial encephalomyopathy, lactic acidosis, and stroke-like episodes," *Stroke*, vol. 40, no. 2, pp. e15–e17, 2008.

[10] N. Diamini, L. Billinghurst, and F. J. Kirkham, "Cerebral venous sinus (sinovenous) thrombosis in children," *Neurosurgery Clinics of North America*, vol. 21, no. 3–5, pp. 511–527, 2010.

[11] T. Krings, S. Geibprasert, and K. TerBrugge, "Classification and endovascular management of pediatric cerebral vascular malformations," *Neurosurgery Clinics of North America*, vol. 21, no. 3, pp. 463–482, 2010.

[12] T. Krings, S. Geibprasert, and K. G. TerBrugge, "Pathomechanisms and treatment of pediatric aneurysms," *Child's Nervous System*, vol. 26, no. 10, pp. 1309–1318, 2010.

[13] L. C. Jordan, S. C. Johnston, Y. W. Wu, S. Sidney, and H. J. Fullerton, "The importance of cerebral aneurysms in childhood hemorrhagic stroke a population-based study," *Stroke*, vol. 40, no. 2, pp. 400–405, 2009.

[14] H. J. Fullerton, Y. W. Wu, S. Sidney, and S. C. Johnston, "Risk of recurrent childhood arterial ischemic stroke in a population-based cohort: the importance of cerebrovascular imaging," *Pediatrics*, vol. 119, no. 3, pp. 495–501, 2007.

[15] Paediatric Stroke Working Group, "Stroke in childhood: clinical guidelines for diagnosis, management and rehabilitation," 2004.

[16] A. Kirton, J. H. Wong, J. Mah et al., "Successful endovascular therapy for acute basilar thrombosis in an adolescent," *Pediatrics*, vol. 112, no. 3, pp. e248–e251, 2003.

[17] J. Irazuzta and K. J. Sullivan, "Hyperacute therapies for childhood stroke: a case report and review of the literature," *Neurology Research International*, vol. 2010, Article ID 497326, 2010.

[18] H. J. Fullerton, Y. W. Wu, S. Sidney, and S. C. Johnston, "Recurrent hemorrhagic stroke in children: a population-based cohort study," *Stroke*, vol. 38, no. 10, pp. 2658–2662, 2007.

[19] P. Monagle, E. Chalmers, A. Chan et al., "Antithrombotic therapy in neonates and children: american college of chest physicians evidence-based clinical practice guidelines (8th edition)," *Chest*, vol. 133, no. 6, pp. 887S–968S, 2008.

[20] E. S. Roach, M. R. Golomb, and R. Adams, "Management of stroke in infants and children: a scientific statement from a special writing group of the american heart association stroke council and the council of cardiovascular disease in the young," *Stroke*, vol. 39, no. 9, pp. 2644–2691, 2008.

[21] S. Grigoriadis, J. M. Gomori, N. Grigoriadis, and J. E. Cohen, "Clinically successful late recanalization of basilar artery occlusion in childhood: what are the odds? Case report and review of the literature," *Journal of the Neurological Sciences*, vol. 260, no. 1-2, pp. 256–260, 2007.

[22] Y. Y. Lee, K. L. Lin, H. S. Wang et al., "Craniocervical arterial dissection: a cause of childhood arterial ischemic stroke in Taiwan," *Journal of the Formosan Medical Association*, vol. 109, no. 2, pp. 156–162, 2010.

[23] Y. J. Lai, F. C. Chang, C. J. Lin, T. C. Hsieh, and K. L. Wang, "Endovascular therapy in pediatric intracranial carotid artery dissection," *Pediatric Neurology*, vol. 42, no. 4, pp. 291–294, 2010.

[24] R. Gupta, H. J. Yi, T. G. Jovin, and M. B. Horowitz, "Three unusual arteriovenous fistulas presenting in young children successfully treated with transarterial endovascular embolization," *Pediatric Neurosurgery*, vol. 41, no. 6, pp. 328–333, 2005.

[25] E. F. Ciceri, C. Regna-Gladin, A. Erbetta et al., "Iatrogenic intracranial pseudoaneurysms: neuroradiological and therapeutical considerations, including endovascular options," *Neurological Sciences*, vol. 27, no. 5, pp. 317–322, 2006.

[26] V. K. Sharma, H. L. Teoh, L. Y. Wong, J. Su, B. K. Ong, and B. P. Chan, "Recanalization therapies in acute ischemic stroke: pharmacological agents, devices, and combinations," *Stroke Research and Treatment*. In press.

[27] T. Krings, S. M. Chng, A. Ozanne, H. Alvarez, G. Rodesch, and P. L. Lasjaunias, "Hereditary hemorrhagic telangiectasia in children: endovascular treatment of neurovascular malformations," *Neuroradiology*, vol. 47, no. 12, pp. 946–954, 2005.

[28] D. Kondziolka, H. Kano, H. C. Yang, J. C. Flickinger, and L. Lunsford, "Radiosurgical management of pediatric arteriovenous malformations," *Child's Nervous System*, vol. 26, no. 10, pp. 1359–1366, 2010.

13

# Incidental Thrombus in Transit Causing Embolic Stroke

**Brian Malm,[1,2] Paul Hermany,[1] and Alan Morrison[3]**

[1] *Section of Cardiovascular Medicine, Department of Internal Medicine, Yale University School of Medicine, Yale University, New Haven, CT, USA*
[2] *Department of Cardiology, VA Connecticut Healthcare System, West Haven, CT, USA*
[3] *Warren Alpert School of Medicine, Brown University, Providence, RI, USA*

Correspondence should be addressed to Brian Malm; brian.malm@yale.edu

Academic Editor: Hisao Ogawa

Thrombus in transit leading to paradoxical systemic arterial embolism is a rare echocardiographic finding in patients presenting with embolic stroke. We present a case of a patient who had an atrial thrombus in transit discovered incidentally and later suffered a fatal stroke. Etiologies of cardioembolic stroke and the use of echocardiography in diagnosis and management are briefly discussed.

## 1. Case Presentation

A 68-year-old male with Parkinson's disease was referred for an echocardiogram by his primary care physician as part of an outpatient work-up for intermittent hypotension and bradycardia. He denied any other cardiovascular or transient neurological symptoms. He uses a walker for ambulation. His past medical history is also notable for hypertension, hyperlipidemia, and osteoarthritis. He has had no prior cardiac testing. His current medications include alprostadil, amantadine, carbidopa/levodopa, entacapone, loratadine, midodrine, oxybutynin, ropinirole, and simvastatin. He also receives botulin toxin injections for muscular rigidity. He is an ex-smoker and drinks alcohol in moderation. His family history is notable only for hypertension. He previously worked as an accountant. His physical exam was notable for slow gait and resting tremor and was otherwise unremarkable including normal blood pressure. His transthoracic echocardiogram demonstrated a large highly mobile elongated mass consistent with thrombus (asterisk Figure 1(a)) in the right atrium which crosses the interatrial septum, presumably through a patent foramen ovale (arrow Figure 1(a)) into the left atrium. The thrombus also prolapses across both the tricuspid and mitral valves during diastole (Figure 1(b)) and measures greater than 10 cm in length. The patient was sent to the nearest emergency department, started on heparin and admitted to the hospital for further management. Shortly after admission the patient suffered a massive and ultimately fatal, left middle cerebral artery stroke.

## 2. Case Discussion

Cerebrovascular events are a leading cause of morbidity and mortality in the United States and the majority of these are ischemic in etiology [1]. Cardioembolic etiology of ischemic stroke accounts for approximately 20% of all cases and occurs most often in the setting of high risk conditions including, but not limited to, atrial fibrillation, intracardiac mass/thrombus, rheumatic mitral valve disease, prosthetic heart valves, complex aortic atheroma, and dilated cardiomyopathies [2, 3]. In patients with cryptogenic stroke where a causal cardioembolic source has not been identified on routine evaluation, there is an increased incidence of patent foramen ovale (PFO) implicating paradoxical embolization as a potential causative mechanism for stroke in these patients, though this is often challenging to demonstrate, especially considering the prevalence of PFO is >25% of the population [4, 5]. Treatment options for patients with cardioembolic stroke in the setting of a PFO include antithrombotic therapy and percutaneous or surgical closure. Selection of appropriate candidates for, and the utility of, percutaneous PFO closure remains uncertain given conflicting evidence for benefit from randomized clinical trials [6, 7], though recently presented 10-year results from the RESPECT trial demonstrate

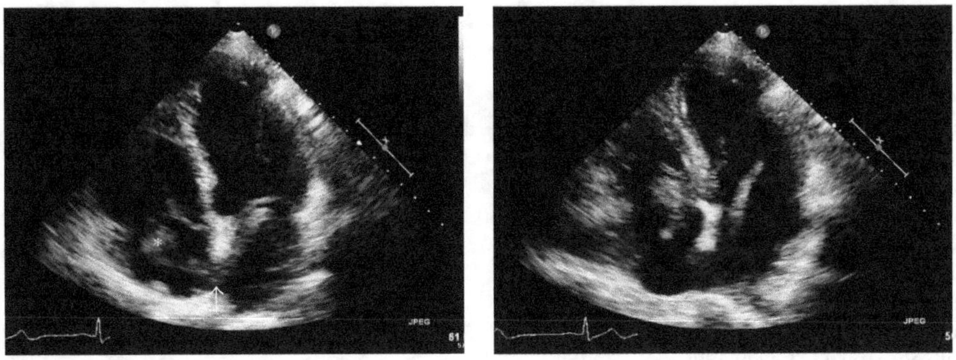

(a) (b)

FIGURE 1: (a) Transthoracic echocardiogram apical four-chamber view in diastole showing a large thrombus (asterisk) extending from the right atrium to the left atrium via a patent foramen ovale (arrow). (b) Apical four-chamber view in diastole demonstrating prolapse of the thrombus across the mitral and tricuspid valves.

significant stroke reduction with PFO closure compared to medical therapy alone [8]. This finding led to subsequent FDA approval of the Amplatzer PFO occluder device.

Diagnostic imaging remains the cornerstone for accurate diagnosis and risk stratification in patients with cerebrovascular disease and stroke. Echocardiography is widely available and remains the current standard imaging modality for the evaluation of stroke patients with a suspected cardioembolic source. Use of transthoracic echocardiography with harmonic imaging and agitated saline contrast allows for the accurate diagnosis of suspected right-to-left shunt through a PFO/ASD in patients diagnosed with cardioembolic stroke [9]. In selected cases, transesophageal echocardiography is necessary for diagnosis of interatrial shunt and accurate characterization of the atrial septal anatomy, particularly when device closure is being considered [10]. In addition, atrial septal aneurysms have been associated with cryptogenic stroke and right-to-left shunting and may be missed on TTE [11, 12].

Thrombus in transit leading to systemic arterial embolism is a rare echocardiographic finding in patients presenting with embolic stroke. These thrombi typically originate from the deep veins of the pelvis and proximal lower extremities but may also be seen in patients with certain malignancies such as renal cell carcinoma. Arterial embolization in this setting requires communication between the right and left heart, most commonly through a PFO. Paradoxical embolization is most often reported in the setting of pulmonary embolism which may lead to acutely increased right heart pressures favoring right-to-left shunting through a PFO [13]. Reports of thrombus in transit in the literature are most often described in patients undergoing diagnostic testing in the setting of a stroke [14]. This case is unique as the interatrial thrombus in transit was discovered incidentally on transthoracic echocardiography ordered for an unrelated indication. Management options include anticoagulation, inferior vena cava filter placement, and prompt consideration for surgical removal. Despite these interventions, the reported 30-day mortality of this finding approaches 20% [13].

## Conflicts of Interest

The authors declare that they have no conflicts of interest.

## References

[1] Writing Group Members, V. L. Roger, A. S. Go et al., "Heart disease and stroke statistics—2012 Update: A Report From the American Heart Association," *Circulation*, vol. 125, pp. e2–e220, 2012.

[2] E. Doufekias, A. Z. Segal, and J. R. Kizer, "Cardiogenic and aortogenic brain embolism," *Journal of the American College of Cardiology*, vol. 51, no. 11, pp. 1049–1059, 2008.

[3] H. Ay, K. L. Furie, A. Singhal, W. S. Smith, A. G. Sorensen, and W. J. Koroshetz, "An evidence-based causative classification system for acute ischemic stroke," *Annals of Neurology*, vol. 58, no. 5, pp. 688–697, 2005.

[4] H. Hara, R. Virmani, E. Ladich et al., "Patent foramen ovale: current pathology, pathophysiology, and clinical status," *Journal of the American College of Cardiology*, vol. 46, no. 9, pp. 1768–1776, 2005.

[5] I. Meissner, J. P. Whisnant, B. K. Khandheria et al., "Prevalence of potential risk factors for stroke assessed by transesophageal echocardiography and carotid ultrasonography: the SPARC study," *Mayo Clinic Proceedings*, vol. 74, no. 9, pp. 862–869, 1999.

[6] A. J. Furlan, M. Reisman, J. Massaro et al., "Closure or medical therapy for cryptogenic stroke with patent foramen ovale," *The New England Journal of Medicine*, vol. 366, no. 11, pp. 991–999, 2012.

[7] J. D. Carroll, J. L. Saver, D. E. Thaler et al., "Closure of patent foramen ovale versus medical therapy after cryptogenic stroke," *The New England Journal of Medicine*, vol. 368, no. 12, pp. 1092–1100, 2013.

[8] D. E. Thaler on behalf of the RESPECT Investigators, "Randomized Evaluation of Recurrent Stroke Comparing PFO Closure to Established Current Standard of Care Treatment—RESPECT trial long-term follow-up" Presented at Transcatheter Cardiovascular Therapeutics (TCT) Meeting 2016, Washington, DC, USA.

[9] J.-W. Ha, M.-S. Shin, S. Kang et al., "Enhanced detection of right-to-left shunt through patent foramen ovale by transthoracic contrast echocardiography using harmonic imaging," *American Journal of Cardiology*, vol. 87, no. 5, pp. 669–671, 2001.

[10] R. N. Belkin, B. D. Pollack, M. L. Ruggiero, L. L. Alas, and U. Tatini, "Comparison of transesophageal and transthoracic echocardiography with contrast and color flow Doppler in the detection of patent foramen ovale," *American Heart Journal*, vol. 128, no. 3, pp. 520–525, 1994.

[11] A. C. Pearson, D. Nagelhout, R. Castello, C. R. Gomez, and A. J. Labovitz, "Atrial septal aneurysm and stroke: a transesophageal echocardiographic study," *Journal of the American College of Cardiology*, vol. 18, no. 5, pp. 1223–1229, 1991.

[12] L. Cabanes, J. L. Mas, A. Cohen et al., "Atrial septal aneurysm and patent foramen ovale as risk factors for cryptogenic stroke in patients less than 55 years of age: a study using transesophageal echocardiography," *Stroke*, vol. 24, no. 12, pp. 1865–1873, 1993.

[13] P. O. Myers, H. Bounameaux, A. Panos, R. Lerch, and A. Kalangos, "Impending paradoxical embolism: systematic review of prognostic factors and treatment," *Chest*, vol. 137, no. 1, pp. 164–170, 2010.

[14] K. Aggarwal, V. K. Jayam, M. A. Meyer, A. K. Nayak, and S. Nathan, "Thrombus-in-transit and paradoxical embolism," *Journal of the American Society of Echocardiography*, vol. 15, no. 9, pp. 1021-1022, 2002.

# 14

# Pacemaker Placement in Patients with Stroke-Mediated Autonomic Dysregulation

**Ali A. Alsaad,[1] Christopher O. Austin,[2] Maisha T. Robinson,[3] and Michael B. Phillips[1]**

[1]*Department of Internal Medicine, Mayo Clinic, Jacksonville, FL 32224, USA*
[2]*Division of Cardiovascular Diseases, Mayo Clinic, Jacksonville, FL 32224, USA*
[3]*Department of Neurology, Mayo Clinic, Jacksonville, FL 32224, USA*

Correspondence should be addressed to Michael B. Phillips; phillips.michael2@mayo.edu

Academic Editor: Omer Faruk Dogan

Lateral medullary syndrome (LMS) is an ischemic disease of the medulla oblongata, which involves the territory of the posterior inferior cerebellar artery. Lateral medullary syndrome is often missed as the cause of autonomic dysregulation in patients with recent brain stem stroke. Due to the location of the baroreceptor regulatory center in the lateral medulla oblongata, patients with LMS occasionally have autonomic dysregulation-associated clinical manifestations. We report a case of LMS-associated autonomic dysregulation. The case presented as sinus arrest and syncope, requiring permanent pacemaker placement. A dual-chamber pacemaker was placed, after failure of conservative measures to alleviate the patient's symptoms. Our case shows the importance of recognizing LMS as a potential cause for life-threatening arrhythmias, heart block, and symptomatic bradycardia. Placement of permanent pacemaker may be necessary in some patients with LMS presenting with syncope, secondary to sinus arrest.

## 1. Introduction

Lateral medullary syndrome, also known as Wallenberg's syndrome, is an ischemic disease of the medulla which involves the territory of the posterior inferior cerebellar artery [1]. The clinical triad typically consists of contralateral sensory deficit, ipsilateral ataxia, and ipsilateral Horner's syndrome. Due to the location of the baroreceptor regulatory center in the lateral medulla oblongata, patients with Wallenberg's syndrome occasionally have autonomic dysregulation [2]. Infarction of this intricate territory can lead to lability of vascular tone and heart rate, resulting in recurrent syncope [1, 3]. We report a case of LMS with autonomic dysregulation in a patient with sinus arrest and syncope, treated successfully by permanent pacemaker placement.

## 2. Case Report

An 85-year-old man, with a history of normal pressure hydrocephalus, treated with ventriculoperitoneal shunt, coronary artery disease, hypertension, and mild dementia, presented with severe, intractable nausea, vomiting, and hoarseness associated with ataxia and recurrent syncopal episodes. Magnetic resonance imaging (Figure 1) revealed an acute infarction in the left cerebellar tonsil, left cerebellar hemisphere, and left medullary restiform body, in the territory of the left posterior inferior cerebellar artery (PICA). Radiologic findings were consistent with lateral medullary infarction. The clinical picture was suggestive of lateral medullary syndrome (LMS).

The exact reason for the brainstem and cerebellar stroke remained unclear, as diagnostic testing including transesophageal echocardiography and carotid ultrasound failed to reveal any significant abnormalities. Also, cardiac telemetry monitoring did not reveal any evidence of supraventricular arrhythmias, including atrial fibrillation.

During hospitalization, the patient experienced multiple syncopal episodes. The syncopal episodes were brief and predominately associated with postural changes, as well as significant nausea and vomiting. No seizure-like activity was noted and both the patient and his caregiver denied any history of similar episodes of nausea, vomiting, or syncope prior to this admission.

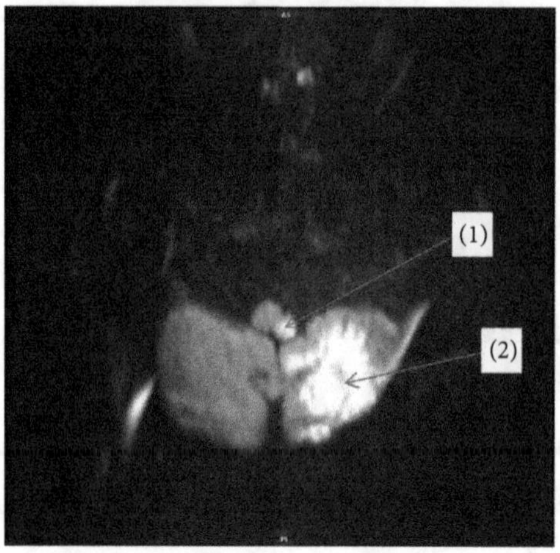


FIGURE 1: Axial diffusion weighted imaging sequence of a magnetic resonance imaging scan of the brain demonstrates hyperintensity in various brain areas. Those findings are consistent with an acute stroke in the left medullary restiform body (1) and left cerebellar hemisphere (2).

During the events, the patient was witnessed to have sinus arrest, lasting up to 6 seconds, with an intermittent junctional escape rhythm (Figure 2). Otherwise, the baseline electrocardiography and cardiac telemetry was sinus rhythm, with heart rate 50–60 beats per minute and right bundle branch block. The patient had documented blood pressure lability during the syncopal episodes, with a peak of 218/92 mm Hg. This represented a substantial difference from prior baseline blood pressure of 130/70 mm Hg. Physical examination was remarkable for cerebellar ataxia and nystagmus. No sensory loss or signs of Horner syndrome were found to suggest a full constellation of lateral medullary syndrome. No significant abnormalities were found in laboratory tests results. The patient's medication regimen at the time of the initial events included metoprolol, bethanechol, and clonidine, all of which possess potential atrioventricular nodal blocking properties. Therefore, all of those medications were discontinued. Lisinopril was administered daily to control hypertension.

Functional assessment of the Codman® Hakim® shunt (Codman/Johnson & Johnson, Raynham, Massachusetts) by fluoroscopic shunt evaluation revealed a pressure of 140 cm $H_2O$ from the last recorded setting, which was 130 cm $H_2O$. However, adjustment of the shunt settings to 130 cm $H_2O$ failed to control his autonomic symptoms or prevent recurrent syncope and associated sinus arrest. This finding excluded Cushing reflex as an etiology for symptomatic bradycardia, secondary to elevated intracranial pressure.

The patient's symptoms continued to occur over the course of the next few days, despite the discontinuation of all potential medications with chronotropic and/or dromotropic effects. Five days after the initial symptoms and due to these persistent events, the patient underwent placement of a dual-chamber pacemaker. An L101 Essentio® pacemaker (Boston Scientific, Marlborough, Massachusetts) was placed with two leads, to right atrium and right ventricle with DDD mode, with resolution of syncopal events. However, his nausea and

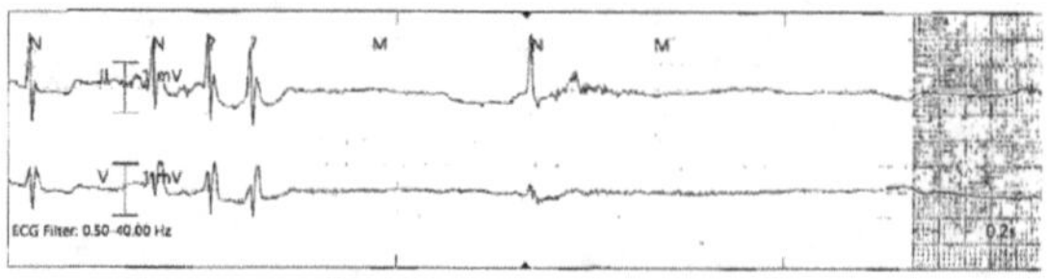


FIGURE 2: Telemetry strip during one of the syncope episodes showing a junctional escape beat overlaying a sinus arrest (6-second pause) proceeded by premature atrial contractures.

vomiting persisted. The patient was subsequently discharged to poststroke rehabilitation center, with prescribed antiemetic medications to control nausea and vomiting.

Follow-up at 1, 3, and 6 months revealed that the patient had no syncopal or presyncope episodes after the placement of the pacemaker. Interrogation of the pacemaker revealed normal device and lead function with no recorded arrhythmia.

## 3. Discussion

Lateral medullary, or Wallenberg's, syndrome was originally described by Adolf Wallenberg more than 100 years ago. It was described as a constellation of signs and symptoms, including nausea, vomiting, hoarseness, ataxia, vertigo, and sensory loss secondary to lateral medullary infarction [1, 2]. Horner syndrome of unilateral miosis, ptosis, and anhidrosis may also be seen. Dysphonia and hoarseness are well described in LMS and they were present in our patient. The mechanism of the stroke in LMS is usually atherosclerotic, secondary to plaque rupture in the vertebral artery or the posterior inferior cerebellar artery. Cardiac and carotid emboli are also potential mechanisms for this disease. Rarely, LMS can be caused by vertebral artery dissection, involving the distribution of posterior inferior cerebellar artery [3]. Anatomically, the medulla encompasses the baroreceptor regulatory center and its impairment may result in labile blood pressures and bradycardia [1, 4]. Autonomic dysregulation may be secondary to the involvement of several medullary nuclei, including nucleus tractus solitarius and nucleus ambiguus, which aid in regulation of autonomic function [4–6].

Previous case reports have described autonomic dysfunction in patients with medullary infarctions. Hong et al. [4] reported cases of autonomic dysfunction, specifically parasympathetic, in patients with infarctions of the ventrolateral right medulla [6]. Sinus arrest, requiring placement of permanent cardiac pacemaker, has also been described in the literature in association with LMS [7, 8].

Cushing reflex, the classic triad of systemic hypertension, bradycardia, and increased intracranial pressure, would be a plausible explanation for our patient's presentation. However, no symptomatic benefit was achieved after adjustment of intracranial pressure using the Codman Hakim system, making this an unlikely explanation for the patient's presentation.

Although our patient did not have prototypical LMS, with associated Horner syndrome and sensory loss, he did have clear evidence of lateral medullary infarction localized to the cerebellum and inferior cerebellar peduncle (restiform body) on MRI. More importantly, our patient had persistent syncope, ataxia, and nystagmus, despite appropriate medical therapy, secondary to parasympathetic tone dysregulation from lateral medullary infarction. Fortunately, the syncopal episodes responded to permanent cardiac pacing, supporting the hypothesis that syncope was predominately the result of sinus arrest (cardioinhibitory response), as opposed to dysautonomia-associated hypotension (vasodepressor response), for which the role of cardiac pacing is poorly defined.

It is important to note that the patient had no prior history of stroke and his MRI indicated no areas of old infarctions. In particular, insular and hypothalamic regions appeared to be free of acute and previous strokes on MRI. Those areas are especially known to be associated with autonomic dysregulation [9, 10]. This point suggests a different localization of the stroke-mediated autonomic dysregulation in our index case, specifically the medullary restiform body and left cerebellar hemisphere.

A transient episode of atrial fibrillation and sinus arrhythmia could have been the etiology for his symptoms, as well as stroke. However, there were neither reported symptoms of nausea, vomiting, or syncope, nor any episodes of supraventricular arrhythmia on continuous cardiac telemetry. Whether the stroke was cardioembolic or atherosclerotic, resolution of recurrent syncope after pacemaker placement suggests symptomatic benefit, which may be applicable in selected cases.

In conclusion, lateral medullary syndrome is a potential cause for life-threatening arrhythmias, heart block, and symptomatic bradycardia. In-hospital telemetric monitoring is recommended following stroke, with associated LMS. Placement of a permanent pacemaker may be necessary for some patients with medullary infarcts, in order to control sinus arrest secondary to dysautonomia. Based on this case experience, we recommend placing a pacemaker if no symptomatic benefit is obtained by conservative measures alone.

## Conflicts of Interest

All authors declare that there are no conflicts of interest regarding the publication of this paper.

## References

[1] J. S. Kim, "Pure lateral medullary infarction: clinical-radiological correlation of 130 acute, consecutive patients," *Brain*, vol. 126, no. 8, pp. 1864–1872, 2003.

[2] S. Vaidyanathan, R. Capper, and D. Chadha, "Stridor: an unusual presentation of lateral medullary syndrome," *The Journal of Laryngology and Otology*, vol. 121, no. 7, article e9, 2007.

[3] J. S. Kim, J. H. Lee, and C. G. Choi, "Patterns of lateral medullary infarction: vascular lesion-magnetic resonance imaging correlation of 34 cases," *Stroke*, vol. 29, no. 3, pp. 645–652, 1998.

[4] J. M. Hong, T. J. Kim, D. H. Shin, J. S. Lee, and I. S. Joo, "Cardiovascular autonomic function in lateral medullary infarction," *Neurological Sciences*, vol. 34, no. 11, pp. 1963–1969, 2013.

[5] P. von Heinemann, O. Grauer, G. Schuierer et al., "Recurrent cardiac arrest caused by lateral medulla oblongata infarction," *BMJ Case Reports*, 2009.

[6] J. T. Korpelainen, K. A. Sotaniemi, and V. V. Myllylä, "Autonomic nervous system disorders in stroke," *Clinical Autonomic Research*, vol. 9, no. 6, pp. 325–333, 1999.

[7] M. Kushner and R. W. Peters, "Prolonged sinus arrest complicating a thrombotic stroke," *Pacing and Clinical Electrophysiology*, vol. 9, no. 2, pp. 248–249, 1986.

[8] S. Koay and B. Dewan, "An unexpected Holter monitor result: multiple sinus arrests in a patient with lateral medullary syndrome," *BMJ Case Reports*, vol. 2013, 2013.

[9] Z. A. Al-Qudah, H. A. Yacoub, and N. Souayah, "Disorders of the autonomic nervous system after hemispheric cerebrovascular disorders: an update," *Journal of Vascular and Interventional Neurology*, vol. 8, no. 4, pp. 43–52, 2015.

[10] S. Oppenheimer, "Cerebrogenic cardiac arrhythmias: cortical lateralization and clinical significance," *Clinical Autonomic Research*, vol. 16, no. 1, pp. 6–11, 2006.

# 15

# Rehabilitation of the Upper Extremity after Stroke: A Case Series Evaluating REO Therapy and an Auditory Sensor Feedback for Trunk Control

**G. Thielman[1] and P. Bonsall[2]**

[1] *Department of Physical Therapy, University of the Sciences, Philadelphia, PA 19104-4495, USA*
[2] *Department of Occupational Therapy, Magee Rehabilitation Hospital, Philadelphia, PA 19106, USA*

Correspondence should be addressed to G. Thielman, g.thielm@usp.edu

Academic Editor: Marco Iosa

*Background and Purpose.* Training in the virtual environment in post stroke rehab is being established as a new approach for neurorehabilitation, specifically, ReoTherapy (REO) a robot-assisted virtual training device. Trunk stabilization strapping has been part of the concept with this device, and literature is lacking to support this for long-term functional changes with individuals after stroke. The purpose of this case series was to measure the feasibility of auditory trunk sensor feedback during REO therapy, in moderate to severely impaired individuals after stroke. *Case Description.* Using an open label crossover comparison design, 3 chronic stroke subjects were trained for 12 sessions over six weeks on either the REO or the control condition of task related training (TRT); after a washout period of 4 weeks; the alternative therapy was given. *Outcomes.* With both interventions, clinically relevant improvements were found for measures of body function and structure, as well as for activity, for two participants. Providing auditory feedback during REO training for trunk control was found to be feasible. *Discussion.* The degree of changes evident varied per protocol and may be due to the appropriateness of the technique chosen, as well as based on patients impaired arm motor control.

## 1. Background and Purpose

Stroke is the leading cause of long-term disability in the United States, as there are estimated 6.4 million Americans that have survived a stroke and are now living with minor-to-severe activity limitations [1]. Activity limitations are often associated with persistent impairment of the upper limb. Specific impairments in this group can range from loss of range of motion, to impaired force generation, to decreased reaction times. These impairments can all lead to loss of arm function and further deficits in motor control, severely affecting a person's ability to live independently [2].

Training utilizing repetitive task practice strategies in poststroke rehab is an evolving method of treatment with a variety of treatment regimens possible. Recently, the application of various robotic systems to incorporate repetitive task practice and facilitate real-world tasks in stroke rehabilitation has been investigated [3–6]. However, since this groundbreaking form of treatment is so new, protocols are not well established and the differences between the robotic devices being used have led to difficulty in establishing specificity within protocols.

In 2 recent reviews evaluating the effect of robotic therapy on the upper limb of individuals after stroke, the high variability of all the work completed to date limited the determination of the effectiveness of this type of therapy [3, 4]. One report indicated that even with robotic training, compensatory movement strategies were still a confluence and needed to be controlled [3]. According to prior robotic therapy investigations in this realm, the ideal candidates are those individuals who are quite impaired in their movement and are unable to perform the forward reaching movement without having the arm supported from the elbow to the hand [3–6]. However, individuals after stroke in the acute phase [5] as well as in the chronic phase [5] with mild-to-moderately severe impairments, have been shown to benefit from robotic therapy through various measures.

One delving question in poststroke rehabilitation is what is beneficial with individuals who are quite impaired and how great is the level of impairment where one can still benefit from the therapy [6]? One investigation that attempted to answer this question trained individuals at least 6 months after stroke onset, who were considered moderate to severe (average upper extremity Fugl Meyer {FMA} 9/66) and utilized passive supported therapy in a gravity-eliminated position [7]. The results for that investigation revealed impairment and disability level changes (functional changes were not assessed). One multicenter, randomized controlled trial evaluating the effectives of robotics in long-term upper-limb impairment led to no improvement in motor function immediately after training, but did show improved outcomes 9 months after therapy was complete (as compared to usual care with nondescript therapy) [8]. There was a third comparative group in that investigation that led to similar changes as the robotic group. Thus, more intense analysis of robotic therapy is necessary to help us understand how these results can translate into regularly used training protocols.

The robot-aided device REO has had only one pilot investigation and one feasibility study completed to date [9, 10]. This REO system involves the patient being securely constrained to a device that can facilitate passive, active assisted, and active movement while avoiding compensatory trunk movement. Similar to the robotic devices discussed previously, the REO provides visual and auditory feedback as a means to enhance motor learning. In addition, this device forces the restriction of the trunk movement by use of a strap across the shoulder connected to the chair. The one pilot investigation mentioned did result in changes for a variety of patient levels on various outcome measures (FMA, strength, spasticity, and pain); however, no control condition was utilized [9]. The feasibility investigation noted that moderately impaired individuals after stroke (FMA 35/66) that were in inpatient rehab were accepting of the device and demonstrated significant changes on the FMA, but again there was no control condition [10].

Several investigations that have controlled the compensatory strategies of individuals after stroke onset have been undertaken recently [11–13]. A review paper [11] and a proof of concept paper [12] evaluated how controlling compensatory movements through feedback was incorporated into upper-limb recovery. The limited randomized controlled investigations that were found in that review, suggested that individuals who have had a stroke benefit from performance feedback in the physical environment (such as motor control deficits involving the controlling of trunk movement) to preserve motor learning abilities [11]. In other words, if the individuals can learn to control their trunk movements, motor recovery of the upper limb as evidenced by kinematic changes, can be made. The proof of concept paper noted clinical improvements on the FMA in more severely impaired poststroke individuals, when given proprioceptive feedback about the involved arm [12]. Thus, incorporating controlling trunk and/or arm movements has been shown to be an effective training method for individuals at various levels of impairment after stroke.

Systematic reviews of task-specific training have indicated that intensity and task specificity are primary indicators of effective treatment for individuals after stroke [3, 14]. Upper-limb training investigations for individuals who have suffered a stroke have shown improved arm movement ability after completing the task-related training (TRT) with the impaired upper limb [15–17]. One particular method investigated showed that restricting trunk use, as is also used with the REO, has some short-term functional benefits as well as benefits to recovery of the impaired arm (interjoint coordination via reorganization of the arm versus trunk degrees of freedom), but no functional benefits [15, 18]. The concern reported is that the trunk stabilizer becomes a dependent force on which the patient relies to achieve greater arm movement. Additionally, the present protocols using the REO, as mentioned previously, have not been adapted to the recent findings addressing the minimal functional effects of training with the trunk strapped down. Lastly, the appropriate level of patient to most benefit from unrestrained TRT has previously been defined in the literature as moderately impaired on the FMA (scoring between 20 and 40), and TRT has been well tested out in terms of trunk stabilization feedback, thus making for a solid control condition [15, 17].

The present case series utilized TRT as a control condition in a crossover comparison design, to obtain preliminary data for establishing a REO protocol for the upper limb. The purpose of this case series was to measure changes that can be made by incorporating a novel form of feedback to control trunk movements and auditory trunk sensor feedback during robot assisted arm therapy in moderate to severely impaired individuals after stroke. It was expected that all subjects would exhibit having learned to reach with greater use of their arm/less use of their trunk, exhibiting less dependency than with the stabilizer feedback.

## 2. Case Descriptions

Individuals with the following were excluded: receptive aphasia, apraxia, or other significant cognitive deficits (determined by the primary investigator during interview question and answer, as well as during command following during the screening sessions). Additional exclusions were (a) sensory/perceptual or orthopedic problems that limit one's ability to reach at the table without sliding the arm on the tabletop (discerned during initial physical exam screening using the Motor Assessment Scale {MAS} [19], a simple classification of arm and hand movements using the involved upper extremity) and (b) any cardiac or pulmonary conditions that limited exercise (physician clearance). The MAS cutoff was at level 4 for upper arm and 1 for hand, allowing for scapular stability/mobility and some grasping activity.

*Inclusion criteria*: demonstrating severe and moderately severe arm movement impairments, defined between 20 and 44 on the upper-arm subsection of the FMA (a series of functional multitask arm/hand movements, out of a possible score of 66) [20]. Individuals scoring below this range have previously been determined to be unable to participate in unrestrained TRT, receiving no benefit from the training [17] and individuals scoring greater than 50 have been considered only mildly impaired [21]. Written approval was obtained from the subject's physician after individual's consent; prior to actual participation and after subjects signed the informed consent the patient's primary physician was sent a letter describing the investigation, their patient's involvement, and asking for medical clearance via a waiver.

Three individuals after stroke voluntarily chose to be evaluated for the investigation, were ultimately included, and were randomized as to which protocol was given initially. All 3 individuals had a goal to be able to use their impaired arm for activities of daily living (ADLs). Subject (1): 63-year-old male, 3 years after onset of left-sided cerebrovascular accident (parietal lobe/basal ganglia), right side (dominant) sensorimotor deficits; subject (2): 68-year-old male 18 months after left-sided parietal lobe CVA that led to right side (dominant) sensorimotor deficits, subject (3): 56-year-old male 16 months after onset of right-sided parietal lobe CVA led to left-sided (nondominant) sensorimotor weakness.

*2.1. Design.* The institutional review boards at both the University of the Sciences and Magee Rehabilitation Hospital approved the study. Using a crossover design, four weeks of real-world TRT was first completed for 2 subjects, and then 4 weeks of REO therapy was completed after a 3-4-week washout period where no training was performed. The reverse sequence was utilized for the third subject; REO followed by a 3-4-week washout and 4-week real-world TRT. This clinical trial is registered with the NIH clinical trials registry as NCT000844870.

*2.2. Testing.* Several standardized outcome measures were collected no longer than five days before the start of each training and within five days after completion of each training period. Due to the proximity of the testing in between the crossover period/washout period the initial postesting data was utilized as the subsequent pretesting data. Subjects were advised to continue to use their "new found" movement as much as possible, just as they had been advised during the training timeframe. The rehabilitative effects were measured according to the International Classification of Functioning, Disability and Health model (ICF) [22]. Body structure and function typically include motor impairment, while activity is measured by daily task performance, and participation measured by life situations.

The FMA [20] as well as the Reaching Performance Scale (RPS—measure of trunk movement used in reaching) [21], were used to determine body function and structure changes of the arm and trunk, respectively. Clinical measures of elbow and shoulder active range of motion (AROM) were assessed using a goniometer [23] (shoulder flexion was measured in sitting against gravity, while elbow extension was measured with gravity eliminated; the patients participating were not all able to complete elbow motion against gravity), and grip strength was measured using a dynamometer [24]. The average or 3 trials were used for all clinical measures. The MAS [19], used in pretest screening, was again collected at posttest as an additional body function and structure measure. Wolf Motor Function Test (WMFT—total time score to complete a number of tasks with impaired upper extremity) [25] was used as an activity measure, as well as the Motor Activity Log (MAL—patient's perception of function related to certain arm activities) [26]. Lastly, cognitive changes via the minimental status exam (MMSE—23 or lower is indicative of cognitive impairment, with a max score of 30) were collected [27].

*2.3. Intervention.* The rehabilitative sessions lasted 40–45 minutes, 2-3 days a week for up to 6 weeks (12 sessions). Subjects were seated with trunk-motion free. Both protocols were arranged to train with a wireless sensor pad draped across the back of the chair, cueing the subjects to keep their back against the pad whenever the back came off of the chair (see Figure 1). Figure 1 displays the individual with their back off of the sensor pad, initiating the auditory signal. Intermittent feedback for both groups was arranged by use of a faded feedback protocol in which the first third of the training trials were without the feedback 20% of the time, the second third of trials were without feedback for 40% of the time, and the final third was without feedback for 60% of the time [28]. This feedback protocol has previously been utilized in a TRT investigation [17].

REO allowed patients to perform robot-assisted activities, which involved continuous reaching with the arm placed in the device (see Figure 2). Visual feedback from the video monitor yielded the perceived best path to complete each motion. This marked path was overlaid by the subject's actual path taken. Verbal and some tactile feedback by the therapist was given during initial REO training, as the auditory sensor device proved to add a higher dimension of concentration for controlling trunk movement. Although the REO device has a shoulder restraint to control trunk movement, the goal was to not utilize this restraint. The goal was to complete motions while avoiding compensatory trunk movement, during passive, active-assisted, and active movement.

Variable practice TRT involved reaching to contact or grasp objects variably placed on the workspace, requiring arm movements of different amplitudes across all quadrants of the tabletop [15–17]. Common objects were used that varied in size, shape, and weight (e.g., cups, mugs, writing and eating utensils). Training activities included, sliding the arm across the tabletop with objects in hand and reaching to grasp/transport objects. As training progressed, subjects were encouraged to increase speed. Subjects received an auditory signal for feedback when the back came off of the pad. Instructions given were to move at preferred speed, and as training progressed subjects were encouraged to increase speed. If a session lasted less than 45 min, subsequent sessions employed more complex tasks. As REO incorporated some active-assisted and some passive movements the time spent in therapy was the best way to equate the sessions and therefore, REO required 10–20% more training trials per session. During each session, 180–220 movements

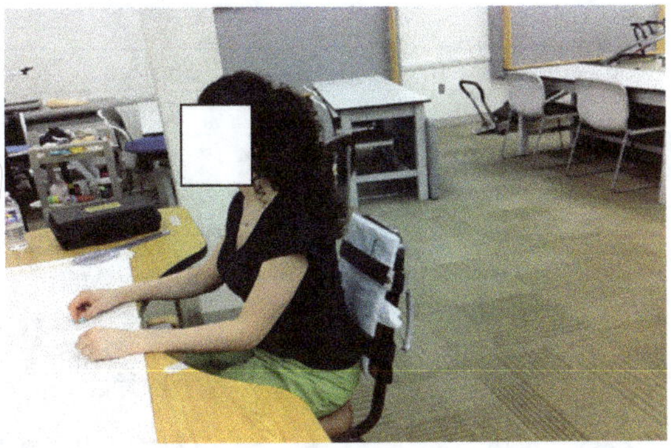

FIGURE 1: TRT workstation with sensor pad placed on anterior surface of chair back.

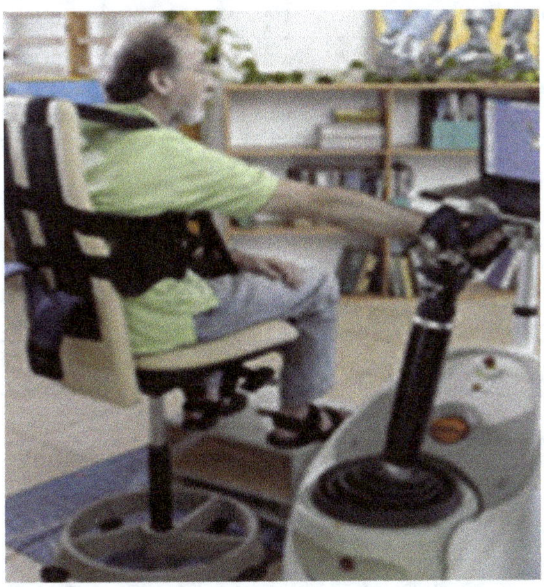

FIGURE 2: REO therapy training device (with trunk strap attached).

were performed for the TRT group, and 240–260 robotic movements (recording only movements reaching out away from the body in each protocol) were performed for the REO group, using the hemiparetic arm. Equivalent training time and feedback were controlled for with both protocols.

*2.4. Analysis.* Postests taken after each training bout, on each method, were completed and compared to pretraining scores. Significant changes were evident by relative change scores of 30% or greater. Based off of findings from other stroke investigations where minimal clinically important differences (MCID) after stroke revealed a 16% to 30% change as being meaningful for a number of the ICF measures we tested [29, 30], we conservatively used 30% for our results. A recent systematic review of outcome measures used for the evaluation of robot-assisted upper-limb exercise in stroke [31] has further details regarding the MCID for the FMA, grip strength, and WMFT, indicating a MCID of 7 for the FMA, 2.9 Kg for grip strength, and 12 for the WMFT. We were only able to use the FMA and the grip strength since the WMFT score in their calculations was a calculated mean rate of performance score (functional ability scale), not the performance times as we used. We used the MAL as an equivalent measure to their mean rate of performance score.

## 3. Results

*3.1. REO Performance.* Subject 1 performed approximately the same amount of time on guided (passive) and initiated (active assisted) movement (40% each), with only 20% on the most difficult step-initiated (active) movement. Subject 2 performed about 30% of the time on the guided movement and 45% of the time on the initiated movement, and then 25% of the time on the most difficult step initiated activities. Subject 3 followed the same pattern as subject 1 for guided and initiated movement, but the percentages were 45% each therefore, leaving only 10% of the training on the most difficult step-initiated movement. The rationale for determining each of the programs and progress is a clinical decision based on biomechanics of the joint, capsular tightness, movement smoothness, and the ability to appropriately recruit the needed muscle pattern throughout the normal reaching pattern with no excessive compensatory mechanisms observed. The program progression is always to push the individual to the edges of their movement in which he or she is still able to maintain good reaching mechanics.

*3.2. Outcome Measures.* REO and TRT led to changes for all 3 participants (see Table 1). Table 1 notes the training order on the $x$-axis and the particular outcome measure on the $y$-axis, which are arranged according to ICF classification. Particular significant MCID training changes are highlighted for each subject.

Subject 1 displayed body function and structure level changes only after TRT for the MAS hand (65% improvement), with no improvement apparent after the REO. Further body function and structure changes were indicated by the RPS (far and near), yielding 30% improvement after REO, and this was maintained after TRT. Following this body function and structure level trend were elbow extension and grip strength (30% improvement for each), both maintained after REO and TRT. Lastly, activity measure changes after REO were noted by the WMFT at 45% improvement, again maintained after TRT.

Subject 2 displayed activity level changes that were only apparent after TRT, indicated by the WMFT (45% improvement). Subject 3 yielded body function and structure level changes after TRT that were maintained after REO (30% improvement on RPS near and far). Additionally, subject 3 presented with activity level changes indicated by the WMFT, evident after TRT (35% improvement) and maintained after REO. All other changes were below 30% and were not considered to be as relevant as the findings reported here.

Observationally, the one initial body function and structure impairment that was limiting to a subject was the poor scapular stability, and capsular tightness/impingement of subject 3, exhibited by limited amount of shoulder flex and elbow extension; this permitted much less active

TABLE 1: Outcome tests.

| | Subject 1 (REO first) | Subject 2 (TRT first) | Subject 3 (TRT first) |
|---|---|---|---|
| ***Impairments** pre-MAS-* | Upper Arm = 5/6<br>Hand = 1/6 | Upper Arm = 5/6<br>Hand = 1/6 | Upper Arm = 5/6<br>Hand = 6/6 |
| *Posttraining 1/pretraining 2* | 5/6, 2/6 | 5/6, 1/6 | 5/6, 6/6 |
| *Posttraining 2* | 5/6, 5/6 (after TRT only)* | 5/6, 1/6 | 5/6, 6/6 |
| ***Impairment** pre-RPS(close)* | 8/18 | 8/18 | 11/18 |
| *Posttraining 1/pretraining 2* | 13/18 (after each)* | 9/18 | 17/18 (after each)* |
| *Posttraining 2* | 13/18 (after each)* | 9/18 | 16/18 (after each)* |
| ***Impairments** pre-RPS (far)* | 8/18 | 9/18 | 11/18 |
| *Posttraining 1/pretraining 2* | 13/18 (after each)* | 8/18 | 17/18 (after each)* |
| *Posttraining 2* | 13/18 (after each)* | 10/18 | 15/18 (after each)* |
| ***Impairments** pre-FMA* | 30/66 | 26/66 | 37/66 |
| *Posttraining 1/pretraining 2* | 27/66 | 26/66 | 36/66 |
| *Posttraining 2* | 27/66 | 25/66 | 40/66 |
| ***Impairment** pre-shld. Flex* | 98 deg | 106 deg | 83 deg |
| *Posttraining 1/pretraining 2* | 104 deg | 133 deg | 89 deg |
| *Posttraining 2* | 97 deg | 114 deg | 90 deg |
| ***Impairment** pre-elbow ext* | 40 deg | 66 deg | 57 deg |
| *Posttraining 1/pretraining 2* | 69 deg (after each)* | 63 deg | 66 deg |
| *Posttraining 2* | 71 deg (after each)* | 70 deg | 64 deg |
| ***Impairment** pre-grip str.* | 12 lbs. | 5 lbs. | 10 lbs. |
| *Posttraining 1/pretraining 2* | 20 lbs. (after each)* | 5 lbs. | 12 lbs. |
| *Posttraining 2* | 21 lbs. (after each)* | 2 lbs. | 10 lbs. |
| ***Activity** pre-WMFT-* | 216.94 sec | 300.33 sec | 179.24 sec |
| *Posttraining 1/pretraining 2* | 112.97 sec (after each)* | 164.38 sec (after TRT only) | 53.18 sec (after each)* |
| *Posttraining 2* | 128.61 sec (after each)* | 403.10 sec | 49.76 (after each)* |
| ***Activity** pre-MAL* | 5/70 | 7/70 | 18/70 |
| *Posttraining 1/pretraining 2* | 7/70 | 16/70 | 30/70 |
| *Posttraining 2* | 11/70 | 14/70 | 39/70 |
| ***Cognition** pre-MMSE* | 28/30 | 29/30 | 27/30 |
| *Posttraining 1/pretraining 2* | 29/30 | 29/30 | 27/30 |
| *Posttraining 2* | 29/30 | 29/30 | 28/30 |

MAS: Motor Assessment Scale, RPS: Reaching Performance Scale, FMA: Fugl Meyer Assessment, WMFT: Wolf Motor Function Test, MMSE: Minimental Status Exam, MAL: Motor Activity Log.
Asterisk after parentheses indicate at least 30% change, after the particular therapy.

movement training (step initiated), as compared to the other 2 subjects. Conversely, subject 1 was especially able to utilize the REO for active movement, as his general scapular stability permitted extensive step-initiated movement.

## 4. Discussion

Both protocols used environmental feedback as a means to enhance motor learning. However, it became apparent during initial training that using the sensor to limit trunk movement during REO therapy was sensory overload for the subjects, and thus verbal and some tactile feedback from the therapist was necessary (at first) to control shoulder movement/compensatory movements of the trunk while completing the movement path outlined on the computer screen. The traditional method of forcibly restricting the trunk during REO has limited long-term functional use due to the poor carryover of trunk control once the restraint is removed, detracting from the ultimate goal of these protocols [16, 18, 32, 33]. Conversely, using the REO with the trunk restraint can be very advantageous, allowing independent interaction with the REO, when clinicians are working on repetitive task practice and treating more than one patient at a time [34]. However, as the training therapist discovered during initial controlled training sessions, the modification in the training movement set by the REO device can also be used to limit the motion to a safe distance that does not cause any substitution.

Two out of three participants with moderate levels of body function and structure motor impairment were able to utilize a robotic therapy device, with these training modifications, to benefit the impaired upper limb. Particular REO performance guidelines can be gathered from this case series as all 3 subjects were trained with general training progression patterns, demonstrating that a moderately impaired patient would be able to perform at least 200 training movements reaching out away from one's body during the course of a typical training session. It was apparent that 10–20% more arm movements per session with robotic therapy allowed for equivalent training session time, compared to more established TRT.

All 3 subjects made activity level changes as indicated by the WMFT, with subjects 1 and 3 maintaining these changes after each of the protocols. Subjects 1 and 3 also displayed body function and structure changes (RPS near and far), that were maintained after each of the protocols. Subject 2 made the least amount of changes, while no subject made changes on the other activity level measure (MAL), perhaps not being as sensitive as the WMFT.

As all 3 subjects did yield WMFT activity level changes, this is perhaps the best indicator of the benefits of these additional structured activities engaging their impaired arm in training. The RPS level changes for subjects 1 and 3 that were maintained for either therapy are a credit to the generalized focus of both types of therapy assisting in controlling arm versus trunk disassociation of movement. The focus of improving the problem of arm control in this population is clearly indicated with these impairments and addressable with the REO. Conversely, subject 2 made no changes as a result of the REO activities; in fact, the gains made on the WMFT and shoulder flexion were back to baseline after the completion of the training on the REO. The treating therapist felt that this was due to scapular immobility and capsular tightness. Thus, despite meeting the minimal criteria to be included in the investigation, the compensatory abilities may have initially masked the poor function of the scapula. Furthermore, subject 2 made no changes on the MAS hand score or with elbow extension. Thus, in comparison to the changes made by subjects 1 and 3 on these measures and in conjunction with the trunk control changes (RPS), we were able to confirm that compensatory trunk movement is used to assist arm reach, as well as hand orientation for grasping.

Clinically, the activity level change (MAL) represents a strong indicator of the patient's belief that they are benefiting from therapy, and with no subject perceiving this benefit, it may be a limitation of the measure. However, there were no changes on the FMA, which is often cited as a measure of motoric change and notably, both other published reports that utilized the REO demonstrated positive findings on the FMA as well as a high level of patient satisfaction [8, 9]. Evaluating the changes that subject 1 made on the MAS hand section that were not seen on the FMA score is perhaps due to the fact that the body function and structure changes made were at the elbow, arm control (RPS), and grip strength, not on some of the finer hand and wrist activities tested out by the FMA.

The result that this auditory feedback training modification is not just possible with TRT but also with REO for this level of patient is promising and warrants further investigative evaluation. The benefits that are carried over from the initial training protocol to the next can be seen as a limitation, as it is unknown with such a short washout period if the overall benefit is the cumulative effect of additional therapy or the true effect of the actual therapy just received. Conversely, the progression of REO to TRT as a training protocol may be the ideal protocol for a patient with the level of impairments as subject 1, as this was the most number of changes evidenced.

The use of Kinematic analysis in future investigations should lead to a differentiation of upper arm, lower arm movement, and trunk control as well as assist in determining control strategies that are developed as a result of training. A randomized controlled investigation with a population of subjects with similar deficits and perhaps similar time after stroke (as well as subsequent similar baseline measurements) would better clarify what impairments are better trained with REO, what impairments are better trained with more established protocols such as TRT, and the appropriate length of training of each.

## Conflict of Interests

The authors declare there are no competing interests in this paper.

## Acknowledgments

This paper was presented in part at the 2010 Combined Sections Meeting of the American Physical Therapy Association, San Diego, CA. Project funding is provided by USciences Office of Academic Affairs. Nicole Walsh, OTR/L assisted with the REO training at Magee Rehabilitation Hospital and the following USP Graduate Students assisted in writing the methodology, and performing the training on the subjects: Greg Oomen and Dave Sen.

## References

[1] A. Tennant, J. M. L. Geddes, J. Fear, M. Hillman, and M. A. Chamberlain, "Outcome following stroke," *Disability and Rehabilitation*, vol. 19, no. 7, pp. 278–284, 1997.

[2] S. J. Page, G. D. Fulk, and P. Boyne, "Clinically important differences for the Upper-extremity fugl-meyer scale in people with minimal to moderate impairment due to chronic stroke," *Physical Therapy*, vol. 92, no. 6, pp. 791–798, 2012.

[3] G. Kwakkel, B. J. Kollen, and H. I. Krebs, "Effects of robot-assisted therapy on Upper limb recovery after stroke: a systematic review," *Neurorehabilitation and Neural Repair*, vol. 22, no. 2, pp. 111–121, 2008.

[4] J. Mehrholz, T. Platz, J. Kugler, and M. Pohl, "Electromechanical and robot-assisted arm training for improving arm function and activities of daily living after stroke," *Stroke*, vol. 40, no. 5, pp. e392–e393, 2009.

[5] S. Masiero, A. Celia, G. Rosati, and M. Armani, "Robotic-assisted rehabilitation of the Upper limb after acute stroke," *Archives of Physical Medicine and Rehabilitation*, vol. 88, no. 2, pp. 142–149, 2007.

[6] G. Morone, M. Iosa, M. Bragoni et al., "Who may have durable benefit from robotic gait training? A 2 year follow up randomized controlled trial in patients with subacute stroke," *Stroke*, vol. 43, no. 4, pp. 1140–1142, 2012.

[7] L. R. MacClellan, D. D. Bradham, J. Whitall et al., "Robotic Upper-limb neurorehabilitation in chronic stroke patients,"

*Journal of Rehabilitation Research & Development*, vol. 42, no. 6, pp. 717–722, 2005.

[8] A. C. Lo, P. D. Guarino, L. G. Richards et al., "Robot-assisted therapy for long-term Upper-limb impairment after stroke," *The New England Journal of Medicine*, vol. 362, no. 19, pp. 1772–1783, 2010.

[9] F. Bovolenta, M. Goldoni, P. Clerici, M. Agosti, and M. Franceschini, "Robot therapy for functional recovery of the Upper limbs: a pilot study on patients after stroke," *Journal of Rehabilitation Medicine*, vol. 41, no. 12, pp. 971–975, 2009.

[10] I. Treger, S. Faran, and H. Ring, "Robot-assisted therapy for neuromuscular training of sub-acute stroke patients. A feasibility study," *European Journal of Physical and Rehabilitation Medicine*, vol. 44, no. 4, pp. 431–435, 2008.

[11] S. K. Subramanian, C. L. Massie, M. P. Malcolm, and M. F. Levin, "Does provision of extrinsic feedback result in improved motor learning in the Upper limb poststroke? A systematic review of the evidence," *Neurorehabilitation and Neural Repair*, vol. 24, no. 2, pp. 113–124, 2010.

[12] M. Casadio, P. Giannoni, P. Morasso, and V. Sanguineti, "A proof of concept study for the integration of robot therapy with physiotherapy in the treatment of stroke patients," *Clinical Rehabilitation*, vol. 23, no. 3, pp. 217–228, 2009.

[13] P. Lam, D. Hebert, J. Boger et al., "A haptic-robotic platform for Upper-limb reaching stroke therapy: preliminary design and evaluation results," *Journal of NeuroEngineering and Rehabilitation*, vol. 5, article 15, 2008.

[14] G. Kwakkel, B. Kollen, and E. Lindeman, "Understanding the pattern of functional recovery after stroke: facts and theories," *Restorative Neurology and Neuroscience*, vol. 22, no. 3-4, pp. 281–299, 2004.

[15] G. Thielman, T. Kaminski, and A. M. Gentile, "Rehabilitation of reaching after stroke: comparing 2 training protocols utilizing trunk restraint," *Neurorehabilitation and Neural Repair*, vol. 22, no. 6, pp. 697–705, 2008.

[16] G. Thielman, "Rehabilitation of reaching poststroke: a randomized pilot investigation of two types of trunk control," *Journal of Neurologic Physical Therapy*, vol. 34, no. 3, pp. 138–144, 2010.

[17] G. T. Thielman, C. M. Dean, and A. M. Gentile, "Rehabilitation of reaching after stroke: task-related training versus progressive resistive exercise," *Archives of Physical Medicine and Rehabilitation*, vol. 85, no. 10, pp. 1613–1618, 2004.

[18] S. M. Michaelsen, R. Dannenbaum, and M. F. Levin, "Task-specific training with trunk restraint on arm recovery in stroke: randomized control trial," *Stroke*, vol. 37, no. 1, pp. 186–192, 2006.

[19] J. H. Carr, R. B. Shepherd, L. Nordholm, and D. Lynne, "Investigation of a new motor assessment scale for stroke patients," *Physical Therapy*, vol. 65, no. 2, pp. 175–180, 1985.

[20] D. J. Gladstone, C. J. Danells, and S. E. Black, "The fugl-meyer assessment of motor recovery after stroke: a critical review of its measurement properties," *Neurorehabilitation and Neural Repair*, vol. 16, no. 3, pp. 232–240, 2002.

[21] S. M. Michaelsen, S. Jacobs, A. Roby-Brami, and M. F. Levin, "Compensation for distal impairments of grasping in adults with hemiparesis," *Experimental Brain Research*, vol. 157, no. 2, pp. 162–173, 2004.

[22] *International Classification of Function in Disability and Health: ICF*, World Health Organization, Geneva, Switzerland, 2001.

[23] C. Norkin and D. White, *Measurement of Joint Motion: A Guide To Goniometry*, F. A. Davis Company, Philadelphia, Pa, USA, 1995.

[24] J. E. Harris and J. J. Eng, "Paretic Upper-limb strength best explains arm activity in people with stroke," *Physical Therapy*, vol. 87, no. 1, pp. 88–97, 2007.

[25] S. L. Wolf, P. A. Catlin, M. Ellis, A. L. Archer, B. Morgan, and A. Piacentino, "Assessing Wolf motor function test as outcome measure for research in patients after stroke," *Stroke*, vol. 32, no. 7, pp. 1635–1639, 2001.

[26] S. W. Park, S. L. Wolf, S. Blanton, C. Winstein, and D. S. Nichols-Larsen, "The EXCITE trial: predicting a clinically meaningful motor activity log outcome," *Neurorehabilitation and Neural Repair*, vol. 22, no. 5, pp. 486–493, 2008.

[27] F. Özdemir, M. Birtane, R. Tabatabaei, G. Ekuklu, and S. Kokino, "Cognitive evaluation and functional outcome after stroke," *American Journal of Physical Medicine & Rehabilitation*, vol. 80, no. 6, pp. 410–415, 2001.

[28] R. Schmidt and D. L. Lee, *Motor Control and Learning: A Behavioral Emphasis*, Human Kinetics Books, Champaign, Ill, USA, 2005.

[29] A. J. Vickers and D. G. Altman, "Analysing controlled trials with baseline and follow up measurements," *BMJ*, vol. 323, no. 7321, pp. 1123–1124, 2001.

[30] C. E. Lang, D. F. Edwards, R. L. Birkenmeier, and A. W. Dromerick, "Estimating minimal clinically important differences of Upper-extremity measures early after stroke," *Archives of Physical Medicine and Rehabilitation*, vol. 89, no. 9, pp. 1693–1700, 2008.

[31] M. Sivan, R. J. O'Connor, S. Makower, M. Levesley, and B. Bhakta, "Systematic review of outcome measures used in the evaluation of robot-assisted Upper limb exercise in stroke," *Journal of Rehabilitation Medicine*, vol. 43, no. 3, pp. 181–189, 2011.

[32] S. M. Michaelsen and M. F. Levin, "Short-term effects of practice with trunk restraint on reaching movements in patients with chronic stroke," *Stroke*, vol. 35, no. 8, pp. 1914–1919, 2004.

[33] S. M. Michaelsen, R. Dannenbaum, and M. F. Levin, "Task-specific training with trunk restraint on arm recovery in stroke: randomized control trial," *Stroke*, vol. 37, no. 1, pp. 186–192, 2006.

[34] N. G. Kutner, R. Zhang, A. J. Butler, S. L. Wolf, and J. L. Alberts, "Quality-of-life change associated with robotic-assisted therapy to improve hand motor function in patients with subacute stroke: a randomized clinical trial," *Physical Therapy*, vol. 90, no. 4, pp. 493–504, 2010.

16

# Effectiveness of Thrombolytic Therapy in Acute Embolic Stroke due to Infective Endocarditis

**Siva P. Sontineni, Aryan N. Mooss, Venkata G. Andukuri, Susan Marie Schima, and Dennis Esterbrooks**

*Division of Cardiology, Creighton University, Omaha, NE 68131, USA*

Correspondence should be addressed to Siva P. Sontineni, ssontineni@gmail.com

Academic Editor: Raymond T. F. Cheung

*Objective.* To identify the role of thrombolytic therapy in acute embolic stroke due to infective endocarditis. *Design.* Case report. *Setting.* University hospital. *Patient.* A 70-year-old male presented with acute onset aphasia and hemiparesis due to infective endocarditis. His head computerized tomographic scan revealed left parietal sulcal effacement. He was given intravenous tissue plasminogen activator with significant resolution of the neurologic deficits without complications. *Main Outcome Measures.* Physical examination, National Institute of Health Stroke Scale, radiologic examination results. *Conclusions.* Thrombolytic therapy in selected cases of stroke due to infective endocarditis manifesting as major neurologic deficits can be considered as an option after careful consideration of risks and benefits. The basis for such favorable response rests in the presence of fibrin as a major constituent of the vegetation. The risk of precipitating hemorrhage with thrombolytic therapy especially with large infarcts and mycotic aneurysms should be weighed against the benefits of averting a major neurologic deficit.

## 1. Introduction

The safety and efficacy of thrombolytic treatment of acute ischemic stroke due to septic brain embolism is not well established [1]. Large trials of thrombolytic therapy of acute ischemic stroke have excluded patients with septic embolization. Published systematic reviews do not address the role of the thrombolytic therapy in the setting of septic embolization to the brain, such as in infective endocarditis [2].

Stroke is the most common of neurologic complications associated with infective endocarditis [3]. The treatment and prevention strategies of this complication are still in evolution. The prevention rests on initiating early antibiotic therapy and consideration of surgery for recurrent events. The role of thrombolytic therapy for acute ischemic strokes in addition to antiplatelet therapy for the prevention of recurrent strokes has increasingly been recognized. We present here our experience of thrombolytic treatment of acute ischemic stroke in a patient with unsuspected infective endocarditis and the available evidence in the literature.

## 2. Clinical Summary

A 70-year-old Caucasian male with history of hypertension and hyperlipidemia presented to a remote emergency room with altered mental status, right hemiparesis, and aphasia. On initial evaluation his National Institutes of Health Stroke Scale (NIHSS) score was 13. A computed tomography scan of the head revealed left parietal hypodense area without haemorrhage. Two and half-hour after the onset of symptoms, intravenous tissue plasminogen activator (t-PA) was started at the outlying emergency room and then transported to our University hospital for further management. On presentation, patient had already finished his t-PA infusion. On physical exam he had fever (39.7°C) and cardiac auscultation revealed a blowing 3/6-holosystolic murmur at the apex. A transthoracic echocardiogram revealed left ventricular ejection fraction of 60–65% with moderate mitral regurgitation. Transesophageal echocardiogram revealed 1.6 × 1.2 cm vegetation on the anterior mitral valve leaflet (Figure 1). Blood cultures returned positive for *Streptococcus pneumoniae* and he was started on penicillin

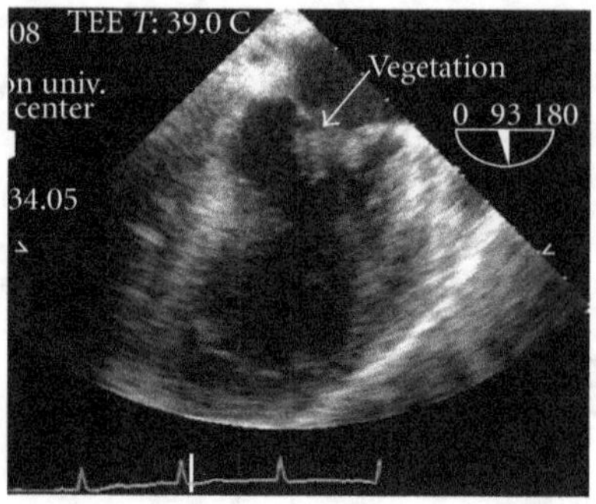


Figure 1: Transesophageal echocardiogram revealing vegetation on the mitral valve leaflets.

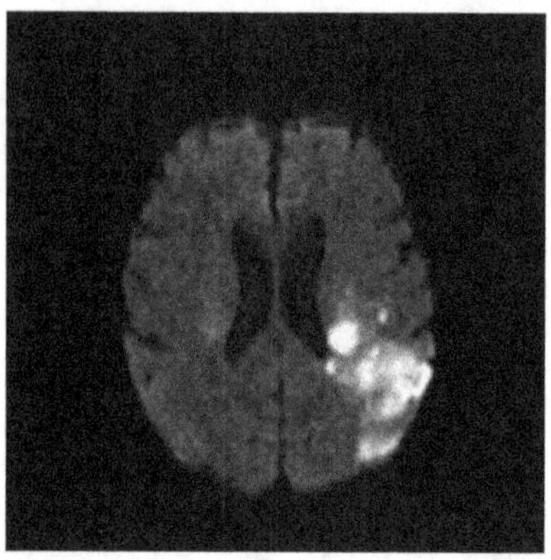

Figure 2: Diffusion weighted MRI after thrombolysis showing left parietal hyperintensities. Areas of focal intensities were also identified in other location including the right cerebral hemisphere, consistent with embolic source as a likely cause of these bilateral and sporadic hyperintense lesions.

G intravenous $5 \times 10^6$ units every four hours. A diffusion weighted MRI of the brain (Figure 2) revealed bilateral acute ischemic areas (left parietal and frontal regions in the left middle cerebral artery distribution and in the right corona radiata and right occipital lobe) and magnetic resonance angiography was normal. Aspirin (81 mg) was started one day after thombolysis and penicillin G was continued for 6 weeks, followed by steady clinical improvement with the continued care of physical, occupational, and speech therapists. The NIHSS score was 5 at discharge with minimal residual aphasia. Two months later, he was evaluated for weight loss, anemia, and melena and was diagnosed with carcinoma of the colon for which he successfully underwent right hemicolectomy without any complication.

## 3. Discussion

The use thrombolytic therapy in patients with infective endocarditis suffering from embolic events is not well studied. Treatment with intravenous thrombolysis within 3 hours of symptom onset has become the standard of care in acute ischemic stroke [4]. Other treatment modalities such as intra-arterial thrombo lysis and catheter-based mechanical thrombus disruption therapies have been studied in the treatment of acute ischemic stroke with variable success [5–7]. The value and safety of these therapies in acute stroke caused by embolism related to infective endocarditis is evolving. Whether the increased risk of intracranial hemorrhage in patients with infective endocarditis is to be considered a contraindication for thrombolysis is unclear. Most of these strokes are ischemic and therefore may respond to thrombolysis. Our case example along with other reported cases of successful intravenous thrombolysis in patients meeting the standard criteria for intravenous t-PA could spur further studies to address this clinical scenario. Similar reports of successful intra-arterial thrombolysis of basilar artery and left internal carotid artery thrombosis in two subjects with infective endocarditis need further evaluation by well designed studies [1, 8]. We summarize the outcomes of these four cases in Table 1. Publication bias is a concern with such reports in the literature with only favourable outcomes being reported.

Infective endocarditis is an endovascular microbial infection of cardiovascular structures, including large intrathoracic vessels and intracardiac foreign bodies. The commonly accepted pathogenetic theory is from endothelial injury with deposition of noninfective sterile thrombotic vegetations to transient bacteremia with microorganism adhesion (injury-thrombus-infection theory). The characteristic lesions consist of vegetations composed of platelets, fibrin, microorganisms, and inflammatory cells [9]. Thus fibrinolytic therapy may be helpful in thrombus resolution by their action on the fibrin present in the vegetation itself or new fibrin that may develop after embolization. Local destructive effects, distant haematogenous seeding, immunologic and embolic phenomena can complicate the clinical course of infective endocarditis.

Embolism occurs in 20–40% of infective endocarditis cases, but its incidence decreases to 9–21% after initiation of antibiotic treatment. The risk of embolism is especially high with large vegetations (>10 mm), mobile vegetations and during the early course of endocarditis therapy. The brain and spleen are the most frequent sites of embolism in infective endocarditis [10].

The overall incidence of stroke in patients with infective endocarditis is about 10% and can result either from embolic infarction or haemorrhage. Patients with mitral valve endocarditis are at a greater risk of stroke than patients with aortic valve endocarditis [3]. Cerebral embolism may manifest as a stroke of varying severity associated with fever, or may be asymptomatic [10]. In a retrospective analysis by Hart et al. [11], 74% of ischemic strokes were noted in native-valve endocarditis at presentation, 13% occurred within 48 hours after diagnosis, and 9% of infarcts are large. Hemorrhagic stroke in patients with infective endocarditis occurs during the early stages (60% within 48 hours) of clinical course and the mechanisms responsible can be septic arteritis, secondary hemorrhagic transformation of infarction, accompanying anticoagulation and mycotic aneurysms [12]. Hemorrhagic conversion of the ischemic infarct due to septic emboli is the most frequent mechanism followed by the rupture of pyogenic arteritis and mycotic aneurysms [13]. The presence of pathologic lesions such as

Table 1: Clinical characteristics and outcomes of reported cases of thrombolysis in infective endocarditis.

| Ref. no | Year | Age | Gender | IE suspected | Organism | Fever | Symptoms | Admission NIHSS Score | Imaging prior to thrombolysis | Thrombolytic used | Time interval | Microaneurysms | Discharge NIHSS score Bleeding complication |
|---|---|---|---|---|---|---|---|---|---|---|---|---|---|
| 1 | 2003 | 31 | F | Prethrombolysis | *Streptococcus mitis* | Absent | Limb weakness Vertigo Tinnitus Gaze palsies | 13 | CT scan: hypodensity of thalamus | Intra-arterial urokinase | 5h | None on CT | NIHSS score 5, no hemorrhage |
| 8 | 2009 | 12 | F | Post thrombolysis | *Streptococcus pneumoniae* | Present | Acute hemiparesis Aphasia | 18 | MRI: multiple diffusion-restricted lesions; MRA absent flow in the left internal carotid artery | Intra-arterial t-PA | 6h | None on MRI | NIHSS score 5, no hemorrhage |
| 19 | 2007 | 56 | M | Post thrombolysis | *Beta-hemolytic streptococcus* | Present | Acute hemiparesis Aphasia | 15 | CT scan: loss of insular ribbon with indistinctness of lentiform nuclei, no hypodensity | Intravenous t-PA | 2h, 36 min | Unknown | NIHSS score 4, no hemorrhage |
| Our case | 2009 | 70 | M | Post thrombolysis | *Streptococcus pneumonia* | Present | Acute hemiparesis Aphasia | 13 | CT scan: hypodensity | Intravenous t-PA | 2h, 30 min | None on MRA | NIHSS score 5, no hemorrhage |

IE: infective endocarditis; M: male; F: female; NIHSS: National Institute of Health Stroke Scale; CT: computed tomography; MRI: magnetic resonance imaging; MRA: magnetic resonance angiography.

pyogenic arteritis, mycotic aneurysms, and large infarcts due to cerebral embolism increases the risk of hemorrhage with thrombolytics in patients with infective endocarditis. The relatively low incidence of 6% of intracranial hemorrhage [11] and the fact that the fibrin thrombus constitutes most of the vegetation according to pathological studies [9] raise the question whether infective endocarditis should be a relative rather than an absolute contraindication in carefully selected patients who may potentially benefit from thrombolytic therapy, in the absence of mycotic aneurysm and large infarcts [8].

The cornerstone of medical treatment of infective endocarditis is to institute effective antibiotic therapy as soon as possible to reduce the mortality and morbidity from embolic complications and heart failure [10, 14]. The role of antiplatelet agents in the therapy of infective endocarditis has been increasingly recognized. Anavekar et al. [15] evaluated the effects of preceding antiplatelet therapy (aspirin, dipyridamole, clopidogrel, ticlopidine, or any of combination) on the risk of embolism in a cohort of 600 cases of infective endocarditis. In this retrospective study, embolic events occurred in 12.0% of patients who had received prior antiplatelet therapy compared to 28% patients who had not received therapy. This analysis demonstrates that the risk of symptomatic emboli associated with infective endocarditis is reduced in patients who received continuous daily antiplatelet therapy before onset of infective endocarditis.

Anticoagulation is still a matter of debate in infective endocarditis, since it can increase the risk of complications, mostly neurological. In a study of patients with native and prosthetic valve endocarditis, stroke was significantly more frequent among anticoagulated patients (20% versus 7%) than nonanticoagulated patients [16]. In a similar analysis, patients who were already on anticoagulation for prosthetic valves had the same embolic risk as compared to those who are not on anticoagulation [14]. Oral anticoagulation is ineffective in stroke prophylaxis, and their use may even be associated with an increased case fatality rate, especially for patients with *Staphylococcus aureus* infective endocarditis [17]. Thus the indications for anticoagulation in infective endocarditis remain similar to those in valvular heart disease, and anticoagulation with heparin should be maintained whenever a brain infarct is present, unless it is large and/or haemorrhagic [16]. European society of cardiology guidelines recommend to discontinue coumadin therapy and replace by heparin soon after the diagnosis of infective endocarditis [18].

In spite of these positive outcomes in these selected case reports, the mainstay of therapy of infective endocarditis remains prompt antibiotic therapy. In all cases of acute ischemic strokes, especially those with a history of fever, infective endocarditis need to be considered and promptly investigated with blood cultures and echocardiographic evaluation. Whenever the clinical suspicion is high for infective endocarditis, careful clinical judgement is required before instituting thrombolytic therapy, weighing the benefits of averting a major neurologic deficit with high NIHSS score versus precipitating cerebral hemorrhage. Prior imaging to identify the presence of mycotic aneurysm can be considered whenever feasible to guide the decision to some extent, however prior pathologic studies of infective endocarditis attributed only a minority of cerebral hemorrhages to the mycotic aneurysms [13]. Although current evidence is lacking for the effects of thrombolytic therapy on the clinical course of mycotic aneurysms, it is intuitive to consider increase the risk of cerebral hemorrhage with thrombolytic therapy in the presence of mycotic aneurysm. Additionally we believe publication bias in the literature on this subject is a significant issue with only favourable cases being reported.

In conclusion, thrombolytic therapy in cases of stroke due to infective endocarditis manifesting with major neurologic deficits is a subject of controversy and needs careful evaluation in a randomized trial. The beneficial effects of therapy can be greatly jeopardised by the serious complications of intracranial hemorrhage.

## References


[1] M. Siccoli, D. Benninger, B. Schuknecht, R. Jenni, A. Valavanis, and C. Bassetti, "Successful intra-arterial thrombolysis in basilar thrombosis secondary to infectious endocarditis," *Cerebrovascular Diseases*, vol. 16, no. 3, pp. 295–297, 2003.

[2] A. Furlan, R. Higashida, L. Wechsler, et al., "Intra-arterial prourokinase for acute ischemic stroke. The PROACT II study: a randomized controlled trial. Prolyse in Acute Cerebral Thromboembolism," *The Journal of the American Medical Association*, vol. 282, no. 21, pp. 2003–2011, 1999.

[3] D. J. Anderson, L. B. Goldstein, W. E. Wilkinson, et al., "Stroke location, characterization, severity, and outcome in mitral vs aortic valve endocarditis," *Neurology*, vol. 61, no. 10, pp. 1341–1346, 2003.

[4] "Tissue plasminogen activator for acute ischemic stroke. The National Institute of Neurological Disorders and Stroke rt-PA Stroke Study Group," *The New England Journal of Medicine*, vol. 333, no. 24, pp. 1581–1587, 1995.

[5] P. Mandava and T. A. Kent, "Intra-arterial therapies for acute ischemic stroke," *Neurology*, vol. 68, no. 24, pp. 2132–2139, 2007.

[6] R. Jahan, G. R. Duckwiler, C. S. Kidwell, et al., "Intraarterial thrombolysis for treatment of acute stroke: experience in 26 patients with long-term follow-up," *American Journal of Neuroradiology*, vol. 20, no. 7, pp. 1291–1299, 1999.

[7] I. Ikushima, H. Ohta, T. Hirai, et al., "Balloon catheter disruption of middle cerebral artery thrombus in conjunction with thrombolysis for the treatment of acute middle cerebral artery embolism," *American Journal of Neuroradiology*, vol. 28, no. 3, pp. 513–517, 2007.

[8] M. Tan, D. Armstrong, C. Birken, et al., "Bacterial endocarditis in a child presenting with acute arterial ischemic stroke: should thrombolytic therapy be absolutely contraindicated?" *Developmental Medicine and Child Neurology*, vol. 51, no. 2, pp. 151–154, 2009.

[9] G. Thiene and C. Basso, "Pathology and pathogenesis of infective endocarditis in native heart valves," *Cardiovascular Pathology*, vol. 15, no. 5, pp. 256–263, 2006.

[10] G. Habib, "Management of infective endocarditis," *Heart*, vol. 92, no. 1, pp. 124–130, 2006.

[11] R. G. Hart, J. W. Foster, M. F. Luther, and M. C. Kanter, "Stroke in infective endocarditis," *Stroke*, vol. 21, no. 5, pp. 695–700, 1990.

[12] R. G. Hart, K. Kagan-Hallet, and S. E. Joerns, "Mechanisms of intracranial hemorrhage in infective endocarditis," *Stroke*, vol. 18, no. 6, pp. 1048–1056, 1987.

[13] J. Masuda, C. Yutani, R. Waki, J. Ogata, Y. Kuriyama, and T. Yamaguchi, "Histopathological analysis of the mechanisms of intracranial hemorrhage complicating infective endocarditis," *Stroke*, vol. 23, no. 6, pp. 843–850, 1992.

[14] C. Paschalis, W. Pugsley, R. John, and M. J. G. Harrison, "Rate of cerebral embolic events in relation to antibiotic and anticoagulant therapy in patients with bacterial endocarditis," *European Neurology*, vol. 30, no. 2, pp. 87–89, 1990.

[15] N. S. Anavekar, I. M. Tleyjeh, N. S. Anavekar, et al., "Impact of prior antiplatelet therapy on risk of embolism in infective endocarditis," *Clinical Infectious Diseases*, vol. 44, no. 9, pp. 1180–1186, 2007.

[16] J. P. Delahaye, P. Poncet, V. Malquarti, J. Beaune, J.-P. Gare, and J. M. Mann, "Cerebrovascular accidents in infective endocarditis: role of anticoagulation," *European Heart Journal*, vol. 11, no. 12, pp. 1074–1078, 1990.

[17] B. Piechowski-Jóźwiak and J. Bogousslavsky, "Infectious endocarditis and stroke: any lessons learned since William Osler's Gulstonian lectures?" *Neurology*, vol. 61, no. 10, pp. 1324–1325, 2003.

[18] D. Horstkotte, F. Follath, E. Gutschik, et al., "Guidelines on prevention, diagnosis and treatment of infective endocarditis executive summary: the task force on infective endocarditis of the european society of cardiology," *European Heart Journal*, vol. 25, no. 3, pp. 267–276, 2004.

# Long-Term Survival of Young Stroke Patients: A Population-Based Study of Two Stroke Registries from Tartu, Estonia

**R. Vibo,[1] S. Schneider,[2] and J. Kõrv[1]**

[1] *Department of Neurology and Neurosurgery, University of Tartu, 51014 Tartu, Estonia*
[2] *Department of Neurology, North Estonia Medical Center, 13419 Tallinn, Estonia*

Correspondence should be addressed to S. Schneider, siim.schneider@regionaalhaigla.ee

Academic Editor: Halvor Naess

The aim of this paper was to evaluate the long-term survival of young stroke patients in Estonia, analyse time trends of survival, and compare the results with other studies. We have used 2 population-based first-ever stroke registry data (1991–1993 and 2001–2003) to analyse the 1-, 5-, and 7-year outcome of young stroke patients by the Kaplan-Meier method of analysis. From the group of 1206 patients, 129 (11%) were aged under 55 years. The overall survival rate at 1, 5, and 7 years was 0.70 (95% CI 0.62–0.78), 0.63 (95% CI 0.55–0.72), and 0.61 (95% CI 0.53–0.70), respectively. The survival was significantly worse for patients with intracerebral haemorrhage ($P < 0.01$) and for those aged from 45 to 54 years compared to the younger age group from 0 to 44 years ($P = 0.03$). For patients with ischemic stroke, aged from 15 to 44 years, the 1-, 5-, and 7-year survival rate was 0.89 (95% CI 0.79–1.00), 0.75 (95% CI 0.61–0.93), and 0.75 (0.61–0.93), respectively. There was no difference in overall survival between the two studied periods. We report a low long-term survival rate among young stroke patients in Estonia. Increasing age and hemorrhagic stroke subtype were associated with lower survival. We have previously shown a worse outcome for 1-year survival compared to other studies and currently this trend continues for 5- and 7-year survival rates. In fact, these are the lowest survival rates for the combined and separate stroke subtypes reported so far.

## 1. Introduction

A young patient with a stroke is always a challenge, even for a stroke physician. Although the outcome of a stroke in the young is believed to be better, it still has a significant impact on the person's quality of life and moreover can be fatal. Data about long-term survival of young stroke patients are scarce and are usually collected retrospectively or are hospital-based [1–20]. Most of these studies have included ischemic strokes and have reported a rather good prognosis but some of the studies were performed years ago when the diagnostic criteria for stroke differed considerably.

Stroke incidence is known to be higher in developing countries, and also in Eastern Europe, compared to the Western countries. In Estonia, the total first-ever stroke incidence is comparable to that of other European countries, but is higher for the younger age groups [21]. The incidence declined by 2001–2003, but it was still 13 per 100 000 for the subjects aged 0 to 44 and 118 per 100 000 for subjects aged 45 to 54 years in Tartu, Estonia [22]. In addition, the 1-year outcome of stroke in terms of functional deficit and survival has also been worse compared to the data from several other study centres [23].

The aim of this paper was to evaluate long-term survival of young stroke patients in Estonia, analyse changes in survival between 1991 to 2003, and compare the results with other studies.

## 2. Methods

Data from the two population-based stroke registries [21, 25] from Tartu, Estonia, were used. The first registry included all first-ever in a lifetime strokes from 1991 to 1993 (3 years) and the other registry included patients from 2001 to 2003 (2 years). These registries included both hospitalised and nonhospitalised cases and prospective "hot pursuit" case-finding methods were used to assure the inclusion of all stroke patients in the area. The more detailed description

TABLE 1: Median survival rates by age group, stroke subtype, and gender.

| Time | Survival | 95% CI | Survival | 95% CI | Survival | 95% CI | $P$ value |
|---|---|---|---|---|---|---|---|
| | All | | Men | | Women | | |
| 1 year | 0.70 | 0.62–0.78 | 0.73 | 0.63–0.83 | 0.65 | 0.53–0.80 | |
| 5 years | 0.63 | 0.55–0.72 | 0.61 | 0.52–0.73 | 0.65 | 0.53–0.80 | 0.45 |
| 7 years | 0.61 | 0.53–0.70 | 0.59 | 0.49–0.71 | 0.65 | 0.53–0.80 | |
| | | | 0–44 years ($n$ = 41) | | 45–54 years ($n$ = 88) | | |
| 1 year | | | 0.85 | 0.75–0.97 | 0.63 | 0.53–0.74 | |
| 5 years | | | 0.73 | 0.61–0.89 | 0.58 | 0.49–0.69 | 0.03 |
| 7 years | | | 0.73 | 0.61–0.89 | 0.56 | 0.46–0.67 | |
| | BI ($n$ = 91) | | ICH ($n$ = 26) | | UND ($n$ = 12) | | |
| 1 year | 0.79 | 0.71–0.88 | 0.39 | 0.24–0.63 | 0.67 | 0.45–0.99 | |
| 5 years | 0.71 | 0.63–0.81 | 0.31 | 0.17–0.55 | 0.67 | 0.45–0.99 | <0.001 |
| 7 years | 0.69 | 0.60–0.79 | 0.31 | 0.17–0.55 | 0.67 | 0.45–0.99 | |
| | | | BI 0–44 years ($n$ = 30) | | BI 45–54 years ($n$ = 61) | | |
| 1 year | | | 0.90 | 0.80–1.00 | 0.74 | 0.64–0.86 | |
| 5 years | | | 0.77 | 0.63–0.93 | 0.69 | 0.58–0.82 | 0.15 |
| 7 years | | | 0.77 | 0.63–0.93 | 0.66 | 0.55–0.79 | |

of methods used for data collection, definitions, and other criteria for these registries have been published earlier [21, 22, 25].

In this current study, patients aged <55 years at stroke onset were included in the analysis. The Estonian Population Register was used for obtaining survival data. The cut-off point for survival data was February 2001 for the first and January 2011 for the second registry for the evaluation of the 7-year outcome.

The study was approved by the Ethics Review Committee on Human Research of the University of Tartu.

*2.1. Statistical Methods.* Survival rate was estimated by the Kaplan-Meier method (1-, 5-, and 7-year survival rate). Survival distributions were compared using the log-rank test. $P$ values less than 0.05 were considered significant. The analysis was carried out by the statistical software package R.

## 3. Results

A total of 1280 patients, (501 men and 779 women) with first-ever stroke, were registered during the 5-year study period, with 829 patients from 1991 to 1993 and 451 patients from 2001 to 2003. Patients with subarachnoid haemorrhage (64 patients) were excluded from this current analysis and additionally 10 patients were lost for the long-term followup. From the group of 1206 patients, 129 (11%) were <55 years of age (38% women and 62% men), and these were included in the survival analysis. The mean age of patients was 46.1 (±9.6) years (range 1 to 55 years). Of them, 91 (71%) had a brain infarction (BI), 26 (20%) an intracerebral haemorrhage (ICH), and 12 (9%) had an undefined type of stroke (UND). Only 3 patients were <15 years of age (2 of them with BI and one with ICH). Perinatal strokes were not included.

Sixty-four of 129 patients (50%) had hypertension, 4 (3%) atrial fibrillation, 17 (13%) diabetes mellitus, 20 (16%) ischemic heart disease, and 7 (5%) had had a previous transient ischemic attack. In 48 patients (38%), no cardiovascular risk factors were identified at stroke onset. The survival rates by age, gender, and stroke subtypes are shown in Table 1. For comparison with previous studies we also calculated the survival rates for patients with ischemic stroke aged 15 to 44 years. The 1-, 5-, and 7-year survival rates were 0.89 (95% CI 0.79–1.00), 0.75 (95% CI 0.61–0.93), and 0.75 (0.61–0.93), respectively.

As expected, the survival rate was worse for patients with ICH and for the older age group. There was no significant difference in overall survival rates between the two studied periods ($P$ = 0.8) nor in young ischemic stroke survival between the two study periods ($P$ = 0.6).

## 4. Discussion

The main finding of our study is the low long-term survival rate among young first-ever stroke patients. At the same time most previous reports agree that although the survival of young stroke patients is lower than in the general population, it is still comparatively high [17, 26]. Our previous study [23] has shown a worse outcome for 1-year survival compared to other studies and currently this trend continues for 5- and 7-year survival rates. In fact, these are the lowest survival rates for combined and separate stroke subtypes reported so far. In our study increasing age (0–44 years versus 45–54 years) and hemorrhagic stroke subtype were associated with lower long-term survival. Earlier studies have also found an association between the male gender and higher mortality in young stroke patients [2, 4]. Although this trend can also be seen in our study, it did not reach statistical significance. The more recent study by Putaala et al. [16] could also not

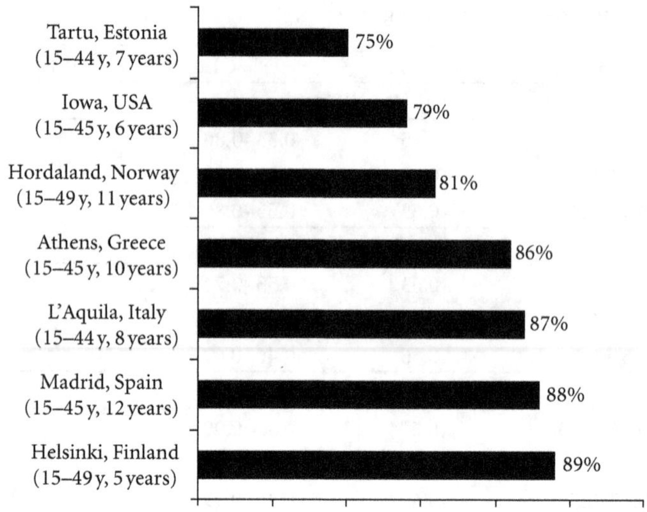


FIGURE 1: Survival of young patients with ischaemic stroke in different studies [1, 2, 4, 16, 18, 24].

identify this association. Quite surprisingly, the survival rate for women remained unchanged after 1 year.

The survival rates for young ischaemic stroke patients from several studies are summarized in Figure 1. The general annual survival rate follows the pattern of earlier studies being clearly lowest in the first year and significantly increases thereafter, but is constantly lower than other studies. The differences in survival rates across the studies could be associated with several aspects. The study type, inclusion criteria, follow-up period, and type of data analysis differ across studies. All, with the exception of three [2, 17, 18], have been hospital based and do not represent a defined population. Although the follow-up periods in these studies are variable, the trend of outcome is still obvious. The results of our study come from two prospective population-based registries. However, a limitation of our study is the small sample size.

The main factor for low survival may be severe stroke, and although there are no comparative data, we speculate that stroke cases are more severe in Estonia. This may be related to a higher prevalence of risk factors leading to a worse outcome. However, in 38% of cases no cardiovascular risk factors were identified despite extensive diagnostic tests. This points to the fact that there may be also other possible causes for higher stroke incidence and lower survival among young subjects in Estonia, for example, genetics, lifestyle, or environmental factors. However, these hypotheses are difficult to prove. And finally, the life expectancy in Estonia was 75.8 years in 2010, 70.6 years for men and 80.8 years for women. Although this rate has constantly grown during the past decade, it is still 3 to 4 years less for women and 5 to 7 years less for men, compared to that of most other European countries [27]. Still, there was no significant difference in stroke survival between the two study periods.

Unfortunately, we were not able to identify the causes of death of young stroke patients because of the strict Estonian data protection legislation. The causes of death are confidential and coded linking between registries is not allowed. As the cardiovascular mortality and deaths, due to accidents and excess alcohol intake, are high in the young Estonian population (especially in men), a number of our young stroke patients might die due to other causes rather than from stroke.

## 5. Conclusion

Long-term survival rates of young stroke patients differ significantly across the world. The causes of high stroke incidence and low survival rates in Eastern Europe can be explained in some terms, but the proportion of stroke patients with no identifiable risk factors is high. Future studies and everyday clinical practice should focus on thorough detection of the etiology of stroke, promoting a healthy lifestyle, optimizing primary and secondary prevention strategies thus decreasing the incidence of stroke and achieving a better outcome for young stroke patients.

## Acknowledgment

The study was supported by targeted financing from the Estonian Ministry of Education and Research (Grant no. SF0180064s07).

## References

[1] L. J. Kappelle, H. P. Adams, M. L. Heffner, J. C. Torner, F. Gomez, and J. Biller, "Prognosis of young adults with ischemic stroke: a long-term follow-up study assessing recurrent vascular events and functional outcome in the Iowa Registry of Stroke in Young Adults," *Stroke*, vol. 25, no. 7, pp. 1360–1365, 1994.

[2] C. Marini, R. Totaro, and A. Carolei, "Long-term prognosis of cerebral ischemia in young adults," *Stroke*, vol. 30, no. 11, pp. 2320–2325, 1999.

[3] D. Leys, L. Bandu, H. Hénon et al., "Clinical outcome in 287 consecutive young adults (15 to 45 years) with ischemic stroke," *Neurology*, vol. 59, no. 1, pp. 26–33, 2002.

[4] J. F. Varona, F. Bermejo, J. M. Guerra, and J. A. Molina, "Long-term prognosis of ischemic stroke in young adults: study of 272 cases," *Journal of Neurology*, vol. 251, no. 12, pp. 1507–1514, 2004.

[5] B. Hindfelt and O. Nilsson, "The prognosis of ischemic stroke in young adults," *Acta Neurologica Scandinavica*, vol. 55, no. 2, pp. 123–130, 1977.

[6] J. M. Ferro and M. Crespo, "Prognosis after transient ischemic attack and ischemic stroke in young adults," *Stroke*, vol. 25, no. 8, pp. 1611–1616, 1994.

[7] J. Bogousslavsky and F. Regli, "Ischemic stroke in adults younger than 30 years of age. Cause and prognosis," *Archives of Neurology*, vol. 44, no. 5, pp. 479–482, 1987.

[8] G. Lanzino, A. Andreoli, G. di Pasquale et al., "Etiopathogenesis and prognosis of cerebral ischemia in young adults. A survey of 155 treated patients," *Acta Neurologica Scandinavica*, vol. 84, no. 4, pp. 321–325, 1991.

[9] M. Camerlingo, L. Casto, B. Censori et al., "Recurrence after first cerebral infarction in young adults," *Acta Neurologica Scandinavica*, vol. 102, no. 2, pp. 87–93, 2000.

[10] J. Matias-Guiu, J. Alvarez-Sabin, and R. Falip, "Prognosis of ischaemic stroke in young adults," in *Proceedings of the ECST Collaborators Meeting*, Edinburgh, UK, September 1991.
[11] A. B. Grindal, R. J. Cohen, R. F. Saul, and J. R. Taylor, "Cerebral infarction in young adults," *Stroke*, vol. 9, no. 1, pp. 39–42, 1978.
[12] B. D. Snyder and M. Ramirez Lassepas, "Cerebral infarction in young adults. Long term prognosis," *Stroke*, vol. 11, no. 2, pp. 149–153, 1980.
[13] K. Srinivasan, "Ischemic cerebrovascular disease in the young. Two common causes in India," *Stroke*, vol. 15, no. 4, pp. 733–735, 1984.
[14] A. M. Chancellor, G. L. Glasgow, P. A. Ockelford, A. Johns, and J. Smith, "Etiology, prognosis, and hemostatic function after cerebral infarction in young adults," *Stroke*, vol. 20, no. 4, pp. 477–482, 1989.
[15] R. Musolino, P. La Spina, A. Granata et al., "Ischaemic stroke in young people: a prospective and long-term follow-up study," *Cerebrovascular Diseases*, vol. 15, no. 1-2, pp. 121–128, 2003.
[16] J. Putaala, S. Curtze, S. Hiltunen, H. Tolppanen, M. Kaste, and T. Tatlisumak, "Causes of death and predictors of 5-year mortality in young adults after first-ever ischemic stroke: the Helsinki young stroke registry," *Stroke*, vol. 40, no. 8, pp. 2698–2703, 2009.
[17] K. Nedeltchev, T. A. der Maur, D. Georgiadis et al., "Ischaemic stroke in young adults: predictors of outcome and recurrence," *Journal of Neurology, Neurosurgery and Psychiatry*, vol. 76, no. 2, pp. 191–195, 2005.
[18] H. Naess, H. I. Nyland, L. Thomassen, J. Aarseth, and K. M. Myhr, "Long-term outcome of cerebral infarction in young adults," *Acta Neurologica Scandinavica*, vol. 110, no. 2, pp. 107–112, 2004.
[19] U. Waje-Andreassen, H. Naess, L. Thomassen, G. E. Eide, and C. A. Vedeler, "Long-term mortality among young ischemic stroke patients in Western Norway," *Acta Neurologica Scandinavica*, vol. 116, no. 3, pp. 150–156, 2007.
[20] J. L. Ruiz-Sandoval, C. Cantu, and F. Barinagarrementeria, "Intracerebral hemorrhage in young people: analysis of risk factors, location, causes, and prognosis," *Stroke*, vol. 30, no. 3, pp. 537–541, 1999.
[21] R. Vibo, J. Kõrv, and M. Roose, "The third stroke registry in Tartu, Estonia, from 2001 to 2003," *Acta Neurologica Scandinavica*, vol. 116, no. 1, pp. 31–36, 2007.
[22] R. Vibo, J. Kõrv, and M. Roose, "The third stroke registry in Tartu, Estonia: decline of stroke incidence and 28-day case-fatality rate since 1991," *Stroke*, vol. 36, no. 12, pp. 2544–2548, 2005.
[23] R. Vibo, J. Kõrv, and M. Roose, "One-year outcome after first-ever stroke according to stroke subtype, severity, risk factors and pre-stroke treatment. A population-based study from Tartu, Estonia," *European Journal of Neurology*, vol. 14, no. 4, pp. 435–439, 2007.
[24] K. Spengos and K. Vemmos, "Risk factors, etiology, and outcome of first-ever ischemic stroke in young adults aged 15 to 45—the Athens young stroke registry," *European Journal of Neurology*, vol. 17, no. 11, pp. 1358–1364, 2010.
[25] J. Kõrv, M. Roose, and A. E. Kaasik, "Stroke registry of Tartu, Estonia, from 1991 through 1993," *Cerebrovascular Diseases*, vol. 7, no. 3, pp. 154–162, 1997.
[26] J. F. Varona, "Long-term prognosis of ischemic stroke in young adults," *Stroke Research and Treatment*, vol. 2011, Article ID 879817, 2011.
[27] Selection of EU statistics, "Life expectancy at birth," Statistics Estonia, 2011, http://www.stat.ee/29928.

# 18

# Intracranial Vertebrobasilar Artery Dissection Associated with Postpartum Angiopathy

**James S. McKinney,[1,2] Steven R. Messé,[1] Bryan A. Pukenas,[3] Sudhakar R. Satti,[3] John B. Weigele,[3] Robert W. Hurst,[3] Joshua M. Levine,[1,4,5] Scott E. Kasner,[1] and Lauren H. Sansing[1]**

[1] *Department of Neurology, The Hospital of the University of PA, 3400 Spruce Street, Philadelphia, PA, 19104, USA*
[2] *Department of Neurology, Robert Wood Johnson Medical School, University of Medicine & Dentistry of New Jersey, 97 Patterson Street, New Brunswick, NJ 08901, USA*
[3] *Department of Neuroradiology, The Hospital of the University of Pennsylvania, 3400 Spruce Street, Philadelphia, PA, 19104, USA*
[4] *Department of Neurosurgery, The Hospital of the University of Pennsylvania, 3400 Spruce Street, Philadelphia, Pennsylvania, 19104, USA*
[5] *Department of Anesthesiology and Critical Care, The Hospital of the University of Pennsylvania, 3400 Spruce Street, Philadelphia, Pennsylvania, 19104, USA*

Correspondence should be addressed to James S. McKinney, mckinnjs@umdnj.edu

Academic Editor: Turgut Tatlisumak

*Background.* Cervicocephalic arterial dissection (CCAD) is rare in the postpartum period. To our knowledge this is the first reported case of postpartum angiopathy (PPA) presenting with ischemic stroke due to intracranial arterial dissection. *Case.* A 41-year-old woman presented with blurred vision, headache, and generalized seizures 5 days after delivering twins. She was treated with magnesium for eclampsia. MRI identified multiple posterior circulation infarcts. Angiography identified a complex dissection extending from both intradural vertebral arteries, through the basilar artery, and into both posterior cerebral arteries. Multiple segments of arterial dilatation and narrowing consistent with PPA were present. Xenon enhanced CT (Xe-CT) showed reduced regional cerebral blood flow that is improved with elevation in blood pressure. *Conclusion.* Intracranial vertebrobasilar dissection causing stroke is a rare complication of pregnancy. Eclampsia and PPA may play a role in its pathogenesis. Blood pressure management may be tailored using quantitative blood flow studies, such as Xe-CT.

## 1. Case Report

A 41-year-old pregnant woman with no other past medical history presented to a community hospital with pre-eclampsia at 36-week gestation. She had a systolic blood pressure (SBP) of 160 mmHg with proteinuria but no neurologic signs or symptoms. Twins were delivered by emergent Cesarean section under spinal anesthesia without apparent complications. She was discharged home on hospital day 5.

The following day she developed a severe headache, blurred vision, and SBP >160 mmHg. She had a generalized tonic-clonic seizure in the emergency department. She was orotracheally intubated for airway protection, treated with magnesium sulfate, levetiracetam, and labetalol. She had no further clinical seizures. A noncontrast CT of the head was normal. After extubation the following day, she became lethargic, and her mental status rapidly declined. MRI of the brain showed several areas of acute infarction in the posterior circulation. She was transferred to our neurological intensive care unit (NeuroICU) for further evaluation on the third day of hospitalization.

On presentation to our facility, she was lethargic and opened her eyes only to repeated tactile stimulation. She was oriented to name, could follow simple commands, and was severely dysarthric with incomprehensible speech. She had a right homonymous hemianopia, disconjugate gaze, and was quadriparetic. She was treated with a magnesium infusion, intravenous levetiracetam, aspirin 325 mg daily, and a

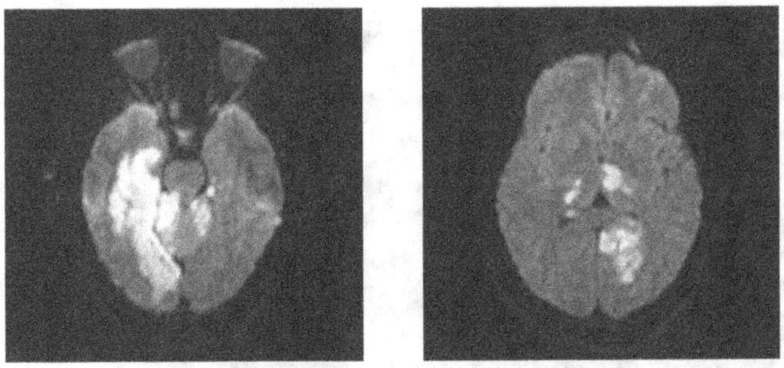

(a) (b)

Figure 1: Diffusion weighted MRI demonstrates several confluent areas of restricted diffusion, consistent with infarction, confined to the bilateral posterior circulation (a,b). This was confirmed on apparent diffusion coefficient maps (not shown). No restricted diffusion was present in the anterior circulation (not shown).

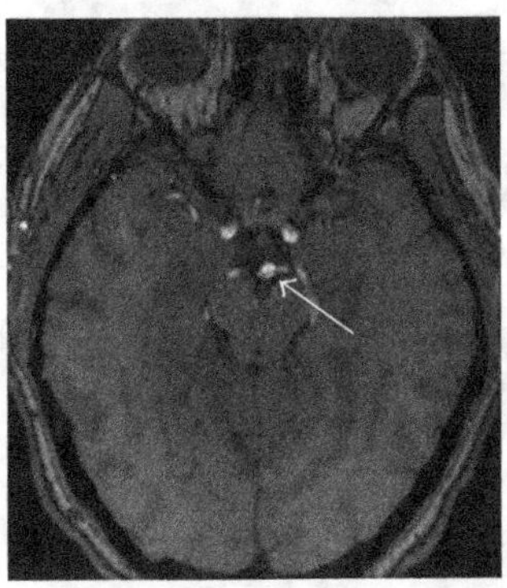

Figure 2: 3D Time of Flight MRA source images demonstrate a linear filling defect (white arrow) in the distal basilar artery with extension into the right posterior cerebral artery (PCA) P1 segment. Additional images (not shown) demonstrated this defect also extending into the left PCA P1 segment.

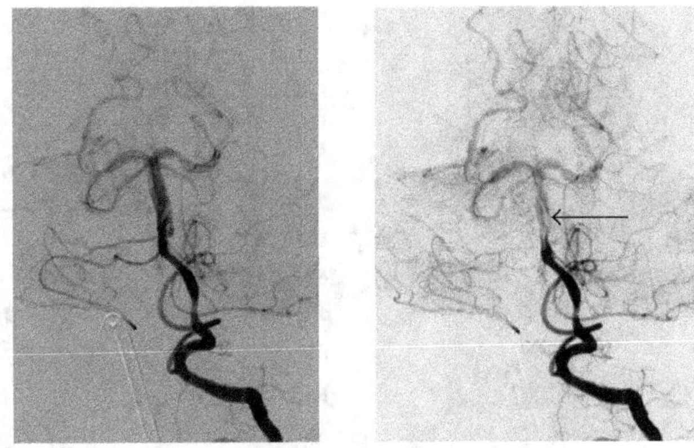

(a) (b)

Figure 3: Left vertebral artery injection demonstrates poor opacification of the basilar artery and posterior cerebral arteries (PCAs) despite an adequate contrast bolus. There is marked enlargement of the distal vertebral artery in the vicinity of the vertebrobasilar junction, extending into the basilar artery and the P1 segments of both PCAs. A linear filling defect is noted originating in, and spiraling around the basilar artery and extending into the proximal bilateral PCAs, consistent with a dissection (arrow B). There are also multiple segments of vascular dilatation and narrowing in the bilateral superior cerebellar arteries and distal PCAs consistent with postpartum angiopathy.

nicardipine infusion which was titrated to maintain a goal SBP less than 120 mmHg. On the third day of hospitalization at our institution she became comatose, and her SBP was persistently >130 mmHg despite aggressive medical therapy. Continuous EEG showed diffuse slowing but no epileptiform activity. MRI of the brain redemonstrated multiple acute infarcts isolated to the posterior circulation (Figure 1).

There was a small area of hemorrhagic transformation of the left occipital lobe infarct seen on gradient echo images (not shown). MRA of the head and neck revealed patent cervical arteries with an apparent dissection flap visualized throughout the basilar artery (Figure 2).

A conventional angiogram confirmed a "double lumen" within the basilar artery with possible involvement of both intradural vertebral arteries, a finding specific for a vertebrobasilar dissection [1, 2]. In addition, distinct from the vertebrobasilar dissection, there were multiple regions of segmental narrowing and dilatation of the intracranial arteries predominantly in the posterior circulation, consistent with concomitant PPA (Figure 3).

Given the radiographic findings there was uncertainty whether the patient's elevated blood pressure was contributing to her clinical deterioration or whether it was a compensatory mechanism to improve perfusion of ischemic tissue. To better direct management of her blood pressure, a Xenon enhanced CT (Xe-CT) was performed to quantify cerebral blood flow (CBF) at different blood pressures. This study showed areas of decreased relative cerebral blood volume in the bilateral posterior cerebral, right middle cerebral, and left anterior cerebral vascular territories at an SBP of 120 mmHg which improved by allowing the SBP to rise above 130 mmHg (Figure 4).

The Mg infusion was discontinued at that time, and her blood pressure target was changed to an SBP of 130 mmHg. Her neurological examination improved slowly over the next several weeks. She was discharged to an acute rehabilitation facility on hospital day 30. At the time of discharge, she was awake, alert, and oriented to person, place, and year. She had a dense right homonymous hemianopia and a moderate right hemiparesis. She required intermittent enteral feeding through a percutaneous gastrostomy tube.

Three months after hospital discharge, she remained in an acute rehabilitation facility. She continued to clinically improve. The gastrostomy tube had been removed, and she could walk with assistance. She continued to have significant memory difficulties and vision loss.

## 2. Discussion

Cervicocephalic arterial dissection (CCAD) is a rare postpartum complication only previously described in case reports and one recent small case series, involving a total of 6 patients [3–7]. The general annual incidence of symptomatic spontaneous CCAD is reported to be about 2.6 cases per

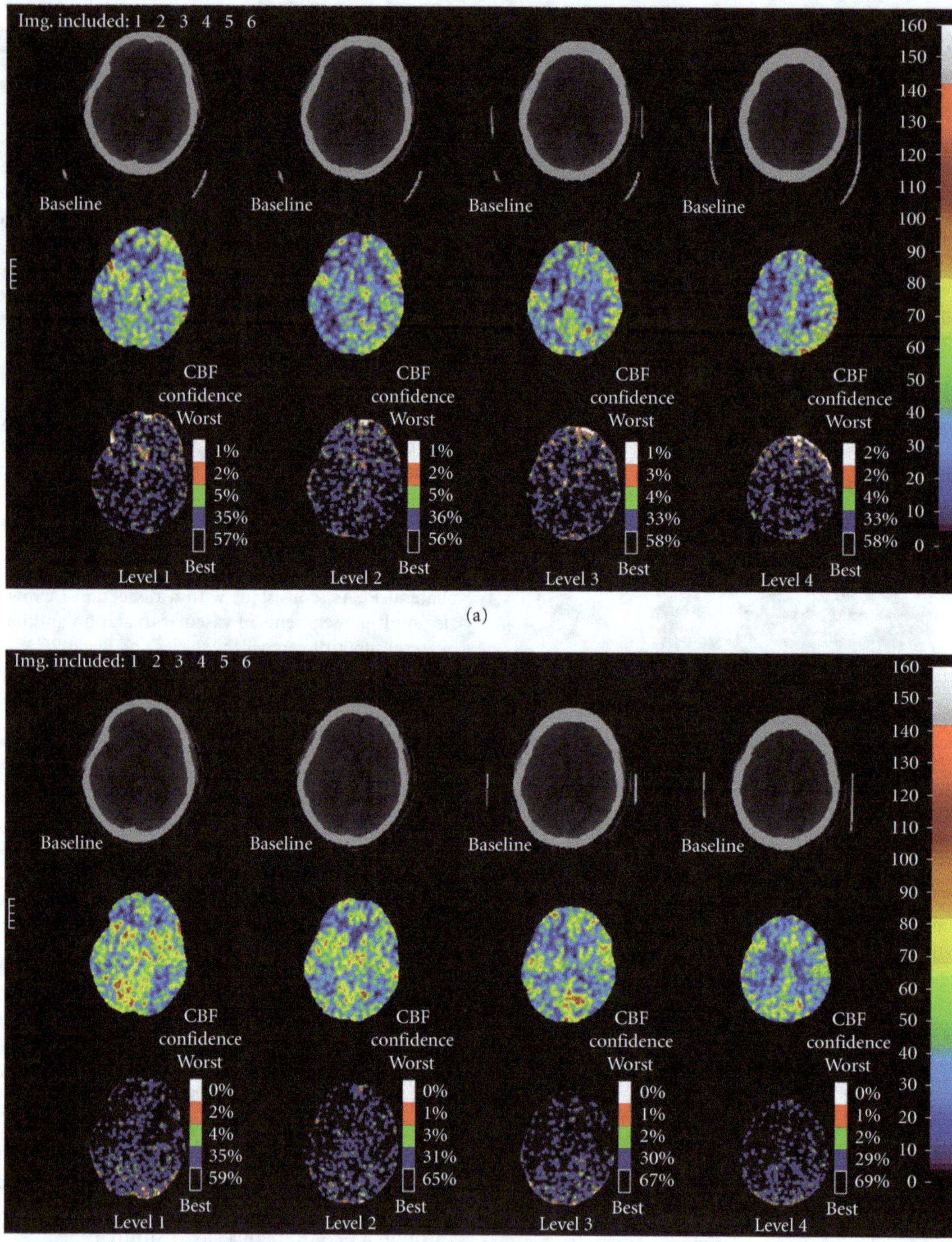


FIGURE 4: (a) Baseline Xenon perfusion study (SBP 120 mm Hg) demonstrates decreased cerebral blood flow (CBF) in both posterior cerebral artery (PCA) territories as well as in the right middle cerebral artery (MCA) and left anterior cerebral artery(ACA) territories. (b) With elevation of SBP (130 mm Hg), there is improvement in CBF in the right parietal region, but no significant improvement in the left PCA territory. There is increased perfusion in the right MCA and left ACA distributions. Increased perfusion is seen within the right occipital and left parietal lobe infarctions.

100000 [8]. A recent registry database identified 2.4% of cases of spontaneous CCAD occurred in the postpartum period [7]. Extrapolating this data would indicate that postpartum CCAD is as rare as 6.2 cases per 10000000 annually. In general, ischemic stroke complicating pregnancy and the postpartum period is also an uncommon condition with a reported incidence of 4.3 cases per 100000 deliveries [9]. In a series of 348295 consecutive deliveries, the most common cause of ischemic stroke was identified as eclampsia in 7 (47%) cases. The remaining etiologies were reported to be one case, each of extracranial vertebral artery dissection, PPA, amniotic fluid embolism with disseminated intravascular coagulation, and protein S deficiency. No etiology was determined in four cases.

The relationship between CCAD and the postpartum period remains unclear. A traumatic mechanism from strenuous labor is unlikely to be the mechanism in most cases. All 6 of the patients reported by Arnold et al. had uneventful deliveries with symptomatic dissection occurring at least 5 days postpartum, as did our patient who delivered via C-section and did not become symptomatic until day 6. A more likely association exists between CCAD and an acquired vasculopathy. In the prior series of spontaneous CCAD, 4/6 (67%) of patients who were postpartum had neuroimaging characteristics consistent with reversible cerebral vasoconstriction syndrome (RCVS), reversible posterior leukoencephalopathy (RPLS), or cortical subarachnoid hemorrhage (cSAH) without associated intradural dissection, while only 3/96 (3%) patients in the age and sex matched controls had similar findings [7]. Literature suggests that conditions such as pre-eclampsia/eclampsia, RCVS, PPA, and RPLS are all likely variable expressions of a common disease, but the underlying pathophysiology is poorly understood [10]. A common unifying theme is that surges in blood pressure and vasoactive or angiogenic substances damage the endothelial lining of vessels causing blood-brain-barrier dysfunction and accumulation of extracellular vasogenic edema. Placental growth factor (PlGF), soluble PlGF receptor (sFlt-1), and soluble endoglin are factors in the angiogenesis pathway which have been implicated in the development of PPA and eclampsia [11–13]. The resulting vessel injury causes cerebral autoregulatory dysfunction and segmental alterations in vessel tone with variable areas of arterial narrowing and dilatation [10, 14, 15].

Aggressive blood pressure reduction is accepted as the treatment of hypertension in the RCVS syndromes including PPA and eclampsia [16, 17]. There are no clinical trials that have assessed treatment thresholds in these settings. There is a general consensus to lower blood pressures to less than 160/110 mmHg in patients with pre-eclampsia or eclampsia [18]. However, these recommendations are based on expert opinion and not guided by data from clinical trials. There are no clear treatment guidelines directing blood pressure management in patients with other cerebral vasoconstriction syndromes; however we routinely strive for normotensive blood pressure goals. The current American Heart Association/American Stroke Association guidelines for the management of blood pressure in acute stroke recommend permissive hypertension [19]. There seems to be no clear solution to the management of blood pressure in patients with RCVS and acute infarcts as these accepted treatments are antagonistic. In this setting, additional diagnostic studies that provide perfusion information, such as Xe-CT, CT perfusion, or MRI perfusion, can be helpful to guide management.

This is the first reported case of an intracranial vertebrobasilar dissection causing ischemic stroke in a patient with PPA and eclampsia. This is significant because of the uniqueness of the case and the uncertainty about blood pressure management. A flow-limiting intracranial dissection may alter the optimal target blood pressure. Blood pressure management tailored to the individual patient's cerebral hemodynamic needs is likely the best solution to optimizing CBF to areas of relative ischemia while avoiding excessive elevations in perfusion pressure which can exacerbate RCVS. Xe-CT has been utilized to determine CBF in acute stroke, differentiate between normal, ischemic, and irreversibly infarcted tissue, and optimize hemodynamic treatment parameters [20–22]. It has also previously been reported to show changes in regional CBF in a patient with eclampsia [23]. Xe-CT was used in our case to help direct our blood pressure management by presumably increasing CBF to areas of relative ischemia, while minimizing the perfusion pressure needed to accomplish this goal.

## 3. Conclusion

Intracranial vertebrobasilar dissection is a rare postpartum complication and likely occurs in vessels with endothelial damage from associated underlying conditions such as eclampsia and PPA. Antihypertensive therapy to treat these diseases may exacerbate ischemia in patients with concurrent cerebral infarction. Individualized therapy, utilizing methods to quantify CBF, may allow clinicians to optimize treatment of their patients and warrants further study.

## References

[1] C.-H. Kim, Y.-J. Son, S. H. Paek, et al., "Clinical analysis of vertebrobasilar dissection," *Acta Neurochirurgica*, vol. 148, no. 4, pp. 395–404, 2006.

[2] T. Hosoya, M. Adachi, K. Yamaguchi, T. Haku, T. Kayama, and T. Kato, "Clinical and neuroradiological features of intracranial vertebrobasilar artery dissection," *Stroke*, vol. 30, no. 5, pp. 1083–1090, 1999.

[3] E. Van de Kelft, J. Kunnen, L. Truyen, and L. Heytens, "Postpartum dissecting aneurysm of the basilar artery," *Stroke*, vol. 23, no. 1, pp. 114–116, 1992.

[4] J. Abisaab, N. Nevadunsky, and N. Flomenbaum, "Emergency department presentation of bilateral carotid artery dissections in a postpartum patient," *Annals of Emergency Medicine*, vol. 44, no. 5, pp. 484–489, 2004.

[5] T. Inoue, S. Nishimura, N. Hayashi, Y. Numagami, H. Takazawa, and M. Nishijima, "Postpartum dissecting aneurysm of the posterior cerebral artery," *Journal of Clinical Neuroscience*, vol. 14, no. 6, pp. 576–581, 2007.

[6] J. M. Waidelich, A. S. Bullough, and J. M. Mhyre, "Internal carotid artery dissection: an unusual cause of postpartum headache," *International Journal of Obstetric Anesthesia*, vol. 17, no. 1, pp. 61–65, 2008.

[7] M. Arnold, M. Camus-Jacqmin, C. Stapf, et al., "Postpartum cervicocephalic artery dissection," *Stroke*, vol. 39, no. 8, pp. 2377–2379, 2008.

[8] W. I. Schievink, B. Mokri, and J. P. Whisnant, "Internal carotid artery dissection in a community: Rochester, Minnesota, 1987–1992," *Stroke*, vol. 24, no. 11, pp. 1678–1680, 1993.

[9] T. Sharshar, C. Lamy, and J. L. Mas, "Incidence and causes of strokes associated with pregnancy and puerperium: a study in public hospitals of Ile de France," *Stroke*, vol. 26, no. 6, pp. 930–936, 1995.

[10] A. B. Singhal, "Postpartum angiopathy with reversible posterior leukoencephalopathy," *Archives of Neurology*, vol. 61, no. 3, pp. 411–416, 2004.

[11] R. J. Levine, S. E. Maynard, C. Qian, et al., "Circulating angiogenic factors and the risk of preeclampsia," *The New England Journal of Medicine*, vol. 350, no. 7, pp. 672–683, 2004.

[12] R. J. Levine, C. Lam, C. Qian, et al., "Soluble endoglin and other circulating antiangiogenic factors in preeclampsia," *The New England Journal of Medicine*, vol. 355, no. 10, pp. 992–1005, 2006.

[13] A. B. Singhal, W. T. Kimberly, P. W. Schaefer, and E. T. Hedley-Whyte, "Case 8-2009: a 36-year-old woman with headache, hypertension, and seizure 2 weeks post partum," *The New England Journal of Medicine*, vol. 360, no. 11, pp. 1126–1137, 2009.

[14] J. Hinchey, C. Chaves, B. Appignani, et al., "A reversible posterior leukoencephalopathy syndrome," *The New England Journal of Medicine*, vol. 334, no. 8, pp. 494–500, 1996.

[15] M. C. Morriss, D. M. Twickler, M. R. Hatab, G. D. Clarke, R. M. Peshock, and F. G. Cunningham, "Cerebral blood flow and cranial magnetic resonance imaging in eclampsia and severe preeclampsia," *Obstetrics and Gynecology*, vol. 89, no. 4, pp. 561–568, 1997.

[16] G. G. Zeeman, "Obstetric critical care: a blueprint for improved outcomes," *Critical Care Medicine*, vol. 34, supplement 9, pp. S208–S214, 2006.

[17] A. Ducros, M. Boukobza, R. Porcher, M. Sarov, D. Valade, and M.-G. Bousser, "The clinical and radiological spectrum of reversible cerebral vasoconstriction syndrome. A prospective series of 67 patients," *Brain*, vol. 130, no. 12, pp. 3091–3101, 2007.

[18] "Report of the National High Blood Pressure Education Program Working Group on High Blood Pressure in Pregnancy," *American Journal of Obstetrics and Gynecology*, vol. 183, no. 1, pp. S1–S22, 2000.

[19] H. P. Adams Jr., G. del Zoppo, M. J. Alberts, et al., "Guidelines for the early management of adults with ischemic stroke: a guideline from the American Heart Association/American Stroke Association Stroke Council, Clinical Cardiology Council, Cardiovascular Radiology and Intervention Council, and the Atherosclerotic Peripheral Vascular Disease and Quality of Care Outcomes in Research Interdisciplinary Working Groups: The American Academy of Neurology affirms the value of this guideline as an educational tool for neurologists," *Circulation*, vol. 115, no. 20, pp. e478–e534, 2007.

[20] R. R. Pindzola and H. Yonas, "The xenon-enhanced computed tomography cerebral blood flow method," *Neurosurgery*, vol. 43, no. 6, pp. 1488–1492, 1998.

[21] A. M. Kaufmann, A. D. Firlik, M. B. Fukui, L. R. Wechsler, C. A. Jungries, and H. Yonas, "Ischemic core and penumbra in human stroke," *Stroke*, vol. 30, no. 1, pp. 93–99, 1999.

[22] M. M. Kilpatrick, H. Yonas, S. Goldstein, et al., "CT-based assessment of acute stroke: CT,CT angiography, and xenon-enhanced CT cerebral blood flow," *Stroke*, vol. 32, no. 11, pp. 2543–2549, 2001.

[23] K. Yamaguchi, Y. Fukuuchi, S. Nogawa, T. Dembo, Y. Tomita, and K. Tanaka, "Recovery of decreased local cerebral blood flow detected by the xenon/CT CBF method in a patient with eclampsia," *The Keio Journal of Medicine*, vol. 49, supplement 1, pp. A71–A74, 2000.

19

# Intraoperative and Histological Visualization of Disrupted Vulnerable Plaques following Diagnostic Angiography of Moderate Carotid Stenosis

**Tatsushi Mutoh,[1,2] Tatsuya Ishikawa,[2] Akifumi Suzuki,[1] and Nobuyuki Yasui[2]**

[1] *Department of Stroke Science, Research Institute for Brain and Blood Vessels-Akita, Akita 010-0874, Japan*
[2] *Department of Surgical Neurology, Research Institute for Brain and Blood Vessels-Akita, Akita 010-0874, Japan*

Correspondence should be addressed to Tatsushi Mutoh, tmutoh@tiara.ocn.ne.jp

Academic Editor: Turgut Tatlisumak

*Background.* Digital subtraction angiography (DSA) remains an important tool for diagnosis of carotid stenosis but is associated with risk for periprocedural complications. This is the first report of direct intraoperative and histolopathologic visualization of DSA-related carotid plaque disruption. *Case.* A 64-year-old man diagnosed to have a 60% right carotid stenosis received diagnostic DSA for therapeutic decision-making. He developed transient left hand numbness and weakness immediately after the procedure. Intraoperative imaging during carotid endarterectomy revealed a fragile plaque with sharp surface laceration and intraplaque hemorrhage at the bifurcation. Microscopy of the specimen demonstrated a large atheromatous plaque with fibrous hypertrophy and intraplaque hemorrhage filled with recent hemorrhagic debris. *Conclusion.* The visualized carotid lesion was more serious than expected, warning the danger of embolization or occlusion associated with the catheter maneuvers. Thus the highest level of practitioner training and technical expertise that ensures precise assessment of plaque characteristics should be encouraged.

## 1. Introduction

Despite recent advances in minimally invasive imaging techniques for carotid vessels like Doppler ultrasonography (US), MR angiography (MRA), and CT angiography (CTA), digital subtraction angiography (DSA) provides the highest spatial resolution and still remains the "gold standard" for diagnosis of carotid artery stenosis, but it is associated with risk for procedure-related neurologic complications. In fact, therapeutic decisions in large clinical trials [1–4] have been based on maximal internal carotid artery (ICA) stenosis depicted with conventional DSA.

It is well known that vulnerable carotid plaque is an atheromatous plaque that is particularly prone to disruption, fracture, or fissuring with a higher risk for embolization, occlusion, and consequent ischemic neurological events [5]. Although disruption of such unstable plaques has been commonly implicated as a risk for procedure-related neurological complications in patients undergoing DSA, most resultant stroke events are clinically silent or transient [6, 7], and there are few descriptions of the affected vessel walls.

We report a case of direct visualization and histolopathologic examination of carotid plaque disruption associated with the diagnostic DSA for therapeutic consideration of asymptomatic moderate-grade carotid stenosis, which was incidentally detected later during carotid endarterectomy (CEA).

## 2. Case Report

A 64-year-old man with past medical history of hypertension, type 2 diabetes mellitus, hypercholesterolemia, and symptomatic ischemic stroke in the territory of the thalamoperforate artery diagnosed to have an asymptomatic moderate (approximately 50%) right ICA stenosis that was observed on MRA was referred to our center for consideration of surgical intervention. Carotid Doppler ultrasonography demonstrated hypoechoic plaques with an irregular surface at the carotid bifurcation extending to the proximal ICA with stenosis of 83% (by area method) and peak systolic flow velocity at 1.89 m/s (Figures 1(a) and 1(b)). Resting single photon emission CT (SPECT) showed severe hypoperfusion in the right ICA territory (Figure 1(c)), presumably due to less prevalence of collateral flow via the anterior or posterior communicating artery (Figures 1(d) and 1(e)) [8].

For therapeutic decision-making, diagnostic carotid angiography was then performed via a femoral approach. It was difficult to cannulate a 5-Fr. JB-2 catheter (Cook, Bloomington, IN) over an angled 0.035 inch Radifocus guidewire (Terumo, Tokyo, Japan) selectively advanced into the right common carotid artery (CCA). The procedure was repeated with a 5-Fr. Simmons II catheter (Cook, Bloomington, IN) but failed to engage in the CCA due to severe vascular elongation. Therefore, the guidewire was advanced carefully, with special attention not to cross the stenotic lesion at the proximal ICA, into the lingual branch of the external carotid artery (ECA) for support, and the catheter was successfully advanced to the CCA. The DSA revealed a 60% stenosis of the proximal right ICA with wall irregularities (Figure 2(a)), calculated according to the North American Symptomatic Carotid Endarterectomy Trial (NASCET) method [2]. The contralateral carotid angiogram demonstrated a mild stenosis in the posterior wall of the ICA. Vertebral angiography was discontinued as it was difficult to probe the bilateral vessels due to elongation.

The patient developed numbness and mild weakness of the left hand immediately after the procedure. Diffusion-weighted MR imaging showed multiple, small hyperintense lesions in the distal ICA territory of the right front-parietal lobe indicative of an embolic origin from the carotid plaques (Figure 2(c)). The symptoms were transient and resolved within 24 hours of the procedure with supplemental intravenous fluids followed by oral clopidogrel (Plavix, Sanofi Pharmaceuticals, New York, NY) 75 mg once daily. Based on the results of the Asymptomatic Carotid Atherosclerosis Study (ACAS) [1] and the Medical Council Asymptomatic Carotid Surgery Trial (ACST) [4], the patient is considered to be a good candidate for elective surgery and given informed consent about CEA.

Two weeks later, the patient underwent successful right CEA. Fragile atherosclerotic plaque with sharp surface laceration, somewhat different from atheromatous plaque rupture, accompanied by intraplaque hemorrhage was observed at the proximal ICA close to the bifurcation (Figures 3(a) and 3(b)). There was no evidence of perforation outside the wall. Microscopic examination of the endarterectomy specimen revealed a large atheromatous plaque with fibrous hypertrophy and intraplaque hemorrhage filled with recent hemorrhagic debris that stained red to brown with Elastica-Masson stain, cholesterol crystal formation, and speckled calcification (Figure 3(c)). The postoperative course was uneventful and the stenosis had improved significantly on follow-up MRA (Figure 2(b)) with no apparent distal embolization (Figure 2(d)). The patient was asymptomatic at his neurological baseline without any postoperative complications and was discharged on postoperative day 10.

## 3. Discussion

Although minimally invasive MRA and CTA have partially replaced conventional DSA in clinical routine, it is still not a standardized method for detection and grading of carotid artery stenosis, especially for asymptomatic patients with moderate carotid stenosis (50%–69%) where the quantification of stenosis can seriously impact on clinical decision-making.

According to the current United States guidelines from the American Academy of Neurology, surgical treatment of asymptomatic patients with carotid stenosis 60%–99% in patients with a 5-year life expectancy are recommended if the operator has a perioperative complication rate of <3% (level A) [9]. By contrast, there is no treatment recommendation for asymptomatic patients with stenosis 50%–59%. This patient has already diagnosed as 50% moderate stenosis on MRA, and thus confirmatory imaging was required for therapeutic decision-making. Although multidetector CT had initially been taken into consideration for assessment of carotid stenosis; however, conventional DSA was chosen after all because we were worried about misclassification of patients within the surgical range associated with greater underestimation with CTA in moderate grades of stenosis [10].

It should be noted that the high diagnostic accuracy of DSA before deciding on carotid intervention must be balanced against the risk of neurological complications. The neurologic complications are more common when indication for DSA is carotid stenosis or ischemic stroke (1.8%) [11]. Furthermore, it has also been pointed out that such clinically overt neurological symptoms are only the "tip of the iceberg" since the rates of DSA-related silent microemboli detected by diffusion-weighted MR abnormalities are considerably higher [7, 12, 13]. Although it remains a matter of debate, the level of operator experience (procedural and fluoroscopy time, multiple catheters use, and aortography) and the nature of the underlying disease are thought to be predictors of the occurrence of cerebral ischemic events following diagnostic DSA [7, 11]. At the authors' institution, diagnostic cerebral angiographies are generally performed by neurosurgical fellows who had already performed at least 250 cerebral angiographies and allowed to perform the procedures on their own, with an acceptable neurologic complication rate (0.8%) compatible to those of recent data [7, 11, 14].

We postulate that the periprocedural manipulation could have resulted in the symptomatic neurological event. This might be related to the difficulties in probing the vessels, the presence of vulnerable atherosclerotic plaque located at the carotid bifurcation that might be impinged and scraped off the vessel wall presumably during the guidewire maneuver in the ECA, and the instability of fresh thrombus in exulcerating plaques that might embolize during the procedure. Unfortunately, the surface morphology of the excised carotid plaque corresponding to the affected intimal lesion could not be well characterized in this case because of artifacts introduced during the removal of the lesion, and nor could we distinguish the hemorrhagic lesion caused

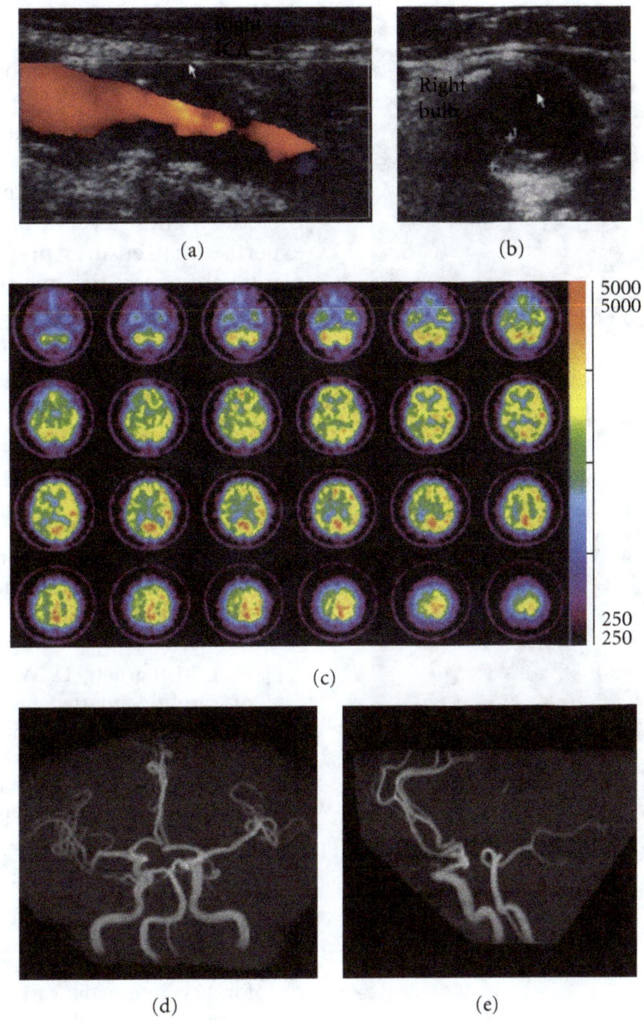


FIGURE 1: (a) B-mode ultrasound with color flow Doppler image on the longitudinal display of the carotid plaque with irregular surface. (b) The transverse display of the plaque at the carotid bifurcation. (c) $^{123}$I-IMP SPECT transaxial slices of a patient with right ICA stenosis. MR angiography ((d) submental vertical projection; (e) lateral projection) with a hypoplastic or absent anterior and posterior communicating arteries.

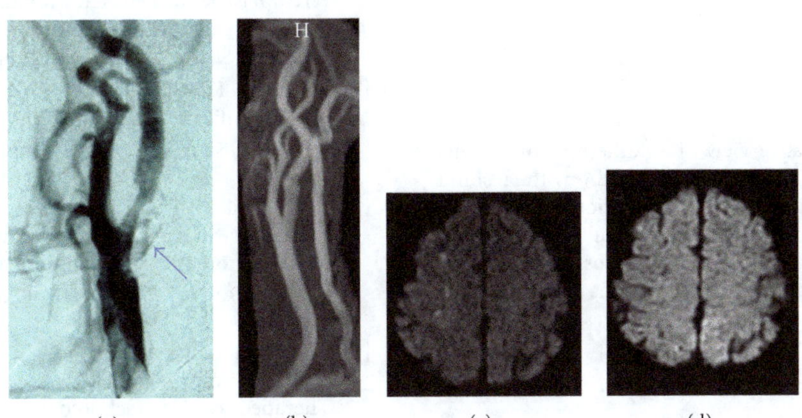


FIGURE 2: (a) Peroperative common carotid angiogram (lateral projection) of a 64-year-old asymptomatic patient with a 60% stenosis of the right ICA by NASCET criteria (*arrow*). (b) Postoperative MR angiography confirmed disappearance of the stenosis. (c) Axial diffusion-weighted MR imaging of the brain immediately after the occurrence of neurologic events following the DSA. Ipsilateral hyperintense lesions are appreciable at the cortical-subcortical junction of right front-parietal lobes. (d) Postoperative diffusion-weighted imaging indicative of no ischemic lesions associated with CEA. Postoperative MR imagings ((b) and (d)) were performed on the next day after CEA.

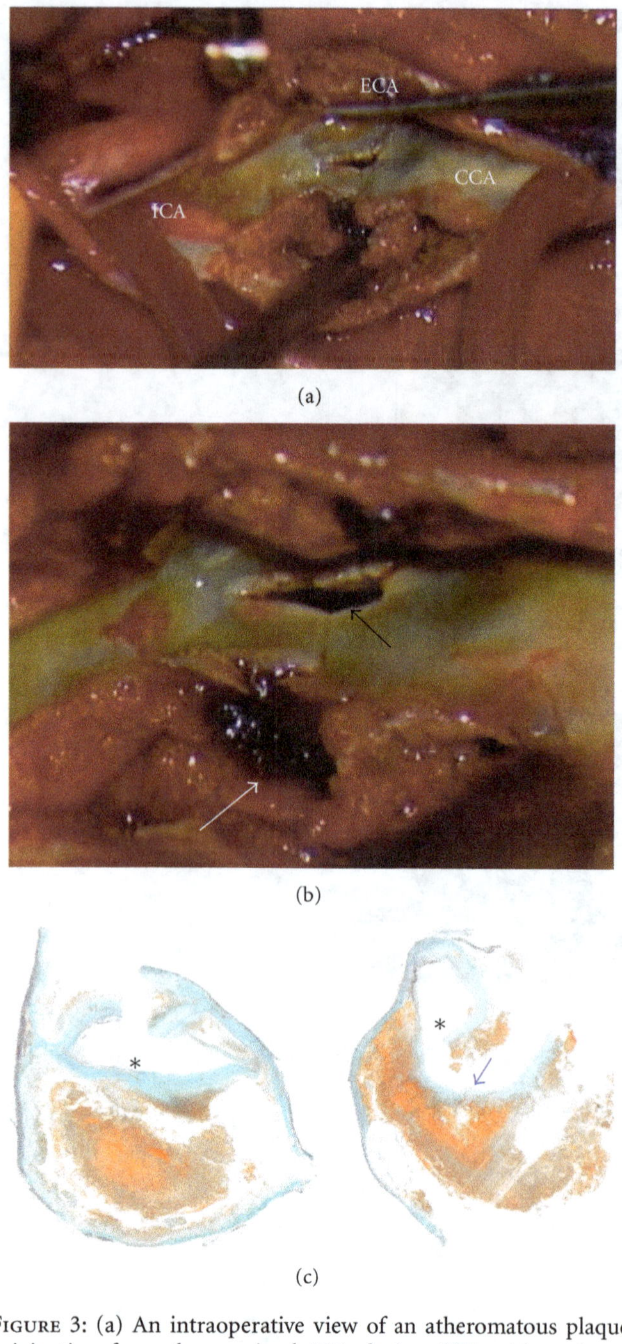


FIGURE 3: (a) An intraoperative view of an atheromatous plaque originating from the proximal ICA during CEA with a shunt. (b) Magnified image revealing the sharp laceration of the plaque surface (*black arrow*) and intraplaque hemorrhage (*white arrow*). (c) Elastica-Masson stain matching histology cross section of the carotid plaque showing a large lateralized atheroma and intraplaque hemorrhage. A ditch shown in *blue arrow* suggests a part of the lacerating injury. Asterisks indicate the lumen.

directly by the angiographical procedure and/or by its natural course of bleeding. During CEA, the full thickness of the plaque was incised, thereby disrupting the luminal surface of the lesion. However, the disrupted plaque showed sharp laceration (Figure 2(b)) that cannot be explained simply by atheromatous plaque rupture.

## 4. Conclusion

This is, to the authors' knowledge, the first report of direct visualization and histolopathologic examination of DSA-related carotid plaque disruption. The impact of the invasive diagnostic carotid angiography on vessel wall injuries warns the danger of serious procedure-related complications, and thus the highest level of practitioner training and technical expertise that ensures precise preprocedural assessment of plaque characteristics by multimodal methods (e.g., ulcerations, surface irregularities, number of plaques, echolucent plaques, plaque distribution along the carotid bifurcation, intraplaque hemorrhage, and lipid-rich necrotic core) [5, 15, 16] should be encouraged in the patient subgroup where the DSA remains necessary.

## References

[1] J. F. Toole, "Endarterectomy for asymptomatic carotid artery stenosis: Executive Committee for Asymptomatic Carotid Atherosclerosis Study," *Journal of the American Medical Association*, vol. 273, no. 18, pp. 1421–1428, 1995.

[2] H. J. M. Barnett, D. W. Taylor, M. Eliasziw, et al., "Benefit of carotid endarterectomy in patients with symptomatic moderate or severe stenosis. North American Symptomatic Carotid Endarterectomy Trial Collaborators," *The New England Journal of Medicine*, vol. 339, no. 20, pp. 1415–1425, 1998.

[3] C. Warlow, B. Farrell, A. Fraser, P. Sandercock, and J. Slattery, "Randomised trial of endarterectomy for recently symptomatic carotid stenosis: final results of the MRC European Carotid Surgery Trial (ECST)," *The Lancet*, vol. 351, no. 9113, pp. 1379–1387, 1998.

[4] P. M. Rothwell and L. B. Goldstein, "Carotid endarterectomy for asymptomatic carotid stenosis: asymptomatic carotid surgery trial," *Stroke*, vol. 35, no. 10, pp. 2425–2427, 2004.

[5] N. Nighoghossian, L. Derex, and P. Douek, "The vulnerable carotid artery plaque: current imaging methods and new perspectives," *Stroke*, vol. 36, no. 12, pp. 2764–2772, 2005.

[6] M. Cosottini, M. C. Michelassi, M. Puglioli, et al., "Silent cerebral ischemia detected with diffusion-weighted imaging in patients treated with protected and unprotected carotid artery stenting," *Stroke*, vol. 36, no. 11, pp. 2389–2393, 2005.

[7] T. Krings, K. Willmes, R. Becker, et al., "Silent microemboli related to diagnostic cerebral angiography: a matter of operator's experience and patient's disease," *Neuroradiology*, vol. 48, no. 6, pp. 387–393, 2006.

[8] J. Hendrikse, B. C. Eikelboom, and J. van der Grond, "Magnetic resonance angiography of collateral compensation in asymptomatic and symptomatic internal carotid artery stenosis," *Journal of Vascular Surgery*, vol. 36, no. 4, pp. 799–805, 2002.

[9] S. Chaturvedi, A. Bruno, T. Feasby, et al., "Carotid endarterectomy—an evidence-based review: report of the Therapeutics and Technology Assessment Subcommittee of the American Academy of Neurology," *Neurology*, vol. 65, no. 6, pp. 794–801, 2005.

[10] H. Silvennoinen, S. Ikonen, L. Soinne, M. Railo, and L. Valanne, "CT angiographic analysis of carotid artery stenosis: comparison of manual assessment, semiautomatic vessel analysis, and digital subtraction angiography," *American Journal of Neuroradiology*, vol. 28, no. 1, pp. 97–103, 2007.

[11] R. A. Willinsky, S. M. Taylor, K. TerBrugge, R. I. Farb, G. Tomlinson, and W. Montanera, "Neurologic complications of cerebral angiography: prospective analysis of 2,899 procedures and review of the literature," *Radiology*, vol. 227, no. 2, pp. 522–528, 2003.

[12] K. Kato, N. Tomura, S. Takahasi, I. Sakuma, and J. Watarai, "Ischemic lesions related to cerebral angiography: evaluation by diffusion weighted MR imaging," *Neuroradiology*, vol. 45, no. 1, pp. 39–43, 2003.

[13] T. J. Kaufmann, J. Huston III, J. N. Mandrekar, C. D. Schleck, K. R. Thielen, and D. F. Kallmes, "Complications of diagnostic cerebral angiography: evaluation of 19 826 consecutive patients," *Radiology*, vol. 243, no. 3, pp. 812–819, 2007.

[14] J. J. Connors III, D. Sacks, A. J. Furlan, et al., "Training, competency, and credentialing standards for diagnostic cervicocerebral angiography, carotid stenting, and cerebrovascular intervention: a joint statement from the American Academy of Neurology, the American Association of Neurological Surgeons, the American Society of Interventional and Therapeutic Neuroradiology, the American Society of Neuroradiology, the Congress of Neurological Surgeons, the AANS/CNS Cerebrovascular Section, and the Society of Interventional Radiology," *Neurology*, vol. 64, no. 2, pp. 190–198, 2005.

[15] N. Takaya, C. Yuan, B. Chu, et al., "Association between carotid plaque characteristics and subsequent ischemic cerebrovascular events: a prospective assessment with MRI—initial results," *Stroke*, vol. 37, no. 3, pp. 818–823, 2006.

[16] S. Prabhakaran, T. Rundek, R. Ramas, et al., "Carotid plaque surface irregularity predicts ischemic stroke: the northern Manhattan study," *Stroke*, vol. 37, no. 11, pp. 2696–2701, 2006.

20

# Bipolar Disorder after Stroke in an Elderly Patient

**Raquel Calvão de Melo,[1] Rui Lopes,[2] and José Carlos Alves[1]**

[1] *Department of Psychiatry, Divino Espírito Santo Hospital, 9500-370 Ponta Delgada, Portugal*
[2] *Clinic of Psychiatry and Mental Health, São João Hospital, 4200-319 Porto, Portugal*

Correspondence should be addressed to Raquel Calvão de Melo; rsmcmelo@gmail.com

Academic Editor: Liliana Dell'Osso

The onset of bipolar disorder (BD) secondary to a stroke event is a rare clinical entity. Although it may be related to specific regions of the brain, several other factors have been linked to its expression such as subcortical atrophy or chronic vascular burden. While precise locations and cerebral circuits involved in the bipolarity expression after stroke still need to be determined, their investigation represents an opportunity to study brain function and BD etiopathogenesis. We present a BD secondary to multiple subcortical biparietal lacunar infarctions, a lacunar infarction in left putamen and an ischemic lesion at the cerebral trunk evolving the right median portion, in a 65-year-old male patient who experienced manic, hypomanic, and depressive episodes, after 6, 10, and 16 months, respectively, of the cerebrovascular events.

## 1. Introduction

Bipolar disorder (BD) is a severe chronic mood disorder whose onset is commonly associated with early adult life. Among older people in the community, it has been demonstrated in a recent meta-analysis to have a low prevalence of 0.53% [1]; however, it represents approximately 20% of mood disorders [2] and may account for around 8–10% of psychiatric admissions in the elderly [3]. Secondary mania as described by Krauthammer and Klerman [4] has been documented in 17–43% of manic cases in the elderly and has been associated with higher prevalence of cerebral organic disorders [5, 6] such as cerebrovascular disease [7], dementia [8, 9], space occupying lesions, infections, and head injury [10].

Despite the fact that vascular incidents are very high in older people, mania remains a rare clinical entity in this age group [11, 12]. The most relevant imagiological findings in late onset mania are silent cerebral infarctions and also subcortical lesions [11, 13]. These findings, however, need to be considered in the evidence of higher cerebrovascular risk factors in patients with late onset BD that may predict a poor prognosis compared to early onset BD patients [14]. Vascular factors, metabolic abnormalities, and systemic inflammation have been proposed to play an important role in the development of late onset BD [14–16]. But, the question whether a single or multiple lesions are essential for the establishment of secondary BD after stroke is still intriguing investigators, trying to find the exact mechanisms involved. Moreover, whether infarctions lesions could contribute as an allostatic load factor [17] or to accelerate neuroprogression of BD [18] still remains an important field for investigation.

## 2. Case Report

We present the case of a 65-year-old Caucasian man without previous psychiatric history that presented to our outpatient clinic due to elevated mood, reduced need of sleep, pressured speech, thoughts race, elevated energy, and disinhibition with a month of evolution. The worsening of the symptoms led his niece and brother-in-law to make an appointment in our outpatient psychiatry services. According to his family, the patient also started money overspending and abuse of alcoholic drinks and had frequent conflicts with the rest of the family, especially with his son with whom he had an emotional break-up just after the beginning of the symptoms. There was no previous history of manic or depressive symptoms.

The patient is the older of two sons, in a family of middle socioeconomic status. He had a eutocic birth and had normal psychomotor development with no relevant health problems. At 6 years of age he was enrolled in primary school. He was a sociable child and his adolescence had no relevant issues. At 18 years he went to college and took a degree in economics. During that time he met his future wife with whom he would marry after he began working as an economist in a private company at the age of 24, and they had one son. His marriage lasted until 13 years ago when he got divorced and started living alone and after 3 years he also retired from his work.

Six months before the beginning of symptoms the patient had a stroke and was admitted at the neurology inpatient service. Computed tomography (CT) scan and brain magnetic resonance imaging (MRI) revealed generalized cerebral atrophy with multiple subcortical biparietal lacunar infarctions (Figure 1), a lacunar infarction in left putamen (Figure 2) and an ischemic lesion at the cerebral trunk evolving the right median portion (Figure 3).

At the neurology inpatient service, he started taking acetylsalicylic acid 100 mg/day and irbesartan/hydrochlorothiazide 150/12.5 mg/day for a diagnosed hypertension. He was already taking simvastatin 20 mg/day for dyslipidaemia. His medical history also revealed that he had been smoking about 30 cigarettes per day for the last years but no illicit drugs consumption.

The patient was resistant to receiving treatment in our inpatient facilities so he was admitted to our day hospital for psychopathological compensation. On the mental examination at admission he presented with good appearance, was alert, cooperative, oriented in time and space, attention procurable but difficult to maintain, and easily irritable, and had elevated mood. He was unable to stay sited and gesticulated more than usual when talking, according to his niece.

The patient had pressure of speech and thoughts race with megalomaniac ideas of grandiosity. There was no hallucinatory activity and patient had no insight or critical appraisal for his clinical situation. Neurological examination revealed a stooped, stiff posture with the head and neck bent forward, dysarthric speech, and discrete hemiparesis in the right hemibody.

We ran a brief test battery to exclude other organic causes, including blood chemistry, thyroid function, folic acid, vitamin B12, C-reactive protein, summary analysis of urine type II, coagulation studies, illicit drugs on urine and alcohol in blood, EEG, chest radiography, HIV, HCV, and HBV viral markers, and syphilis serology, which revealed no significant alterations. He also had a brief screening neuropsychological assessment, scoring 29 points in the Saint Louis University mental status examination (SLUMS), demonstrating apparently normal cognitive functioning (normal score range for high school education patient between 27 and 30) [19, 20].

The patient started pharmacological therapy with diazepam 10 mg/day, olanzapine 10 mg/day, and sodium valproate 1000 mg/day. After a month of inpatient he was asymptomatic, with therapeutic plasmatic levels of sodium valproate (70 mg/L), was discharged, and maintained regular observations in our outpatient clinic.

After 4 months he presented with hypomanic symptoms, so we made adjustments in pharmacotherapy to olanzapine 15 mg/day and diazepam 15 mg/day, maintaining sodium valproate 1000 mg/day that resulted in remission of the symptoms after one week. He remained euthymic in the next 6 months of follow-up till he progressively presented with psychomotor inhibition, terminal insomnia, anhedonia, depressed mood, despair, asthenia, and death thoughts as "a relief from this situation." We proceeded to another pharmacotherapy adjustment adding bupropion 150 mg once a day and olanzapine and diazepam were slowly reduced each to 5 mg/day. After one month with this therapy he maintained depressive mood; however, the rest of the clinical picture improved and two months later he was asymptomatic.

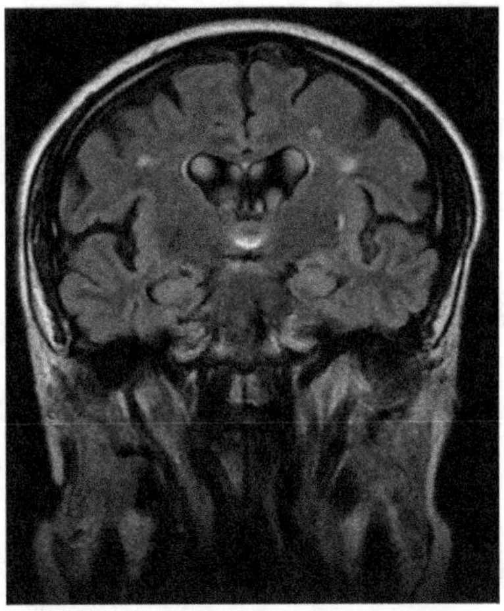

FIGURE 1: MRI Flair—multiple subcortical biparietal lacunar infarctions.

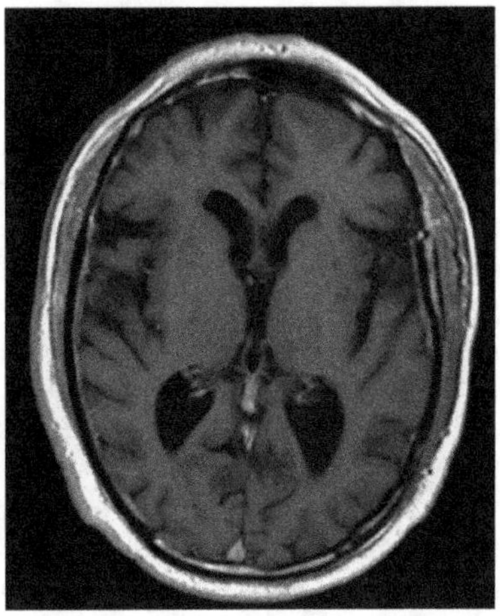

FIGURE 2: MRI T1—lacunar infarction in left putamen.

## 3. Discussion

The "organic hypothesis" of late onset BD implies that patients develop symptoms of mania or hypomania for the first time after having brain lesions [21]. The diagnosis of BD due to another medical condition according to DSM-5 requires a prominent and persistent period of abnormally elevated, expansive, or irritable mood and increased activity or energy

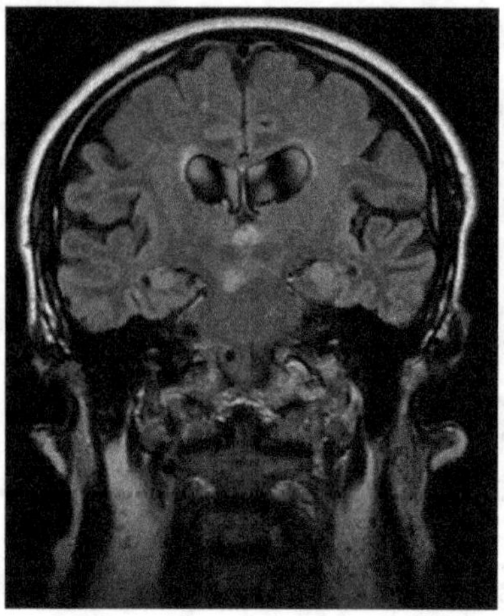

FIGURE 3: MRI Flair—ischemic lesion at the cerebral trunk evolving the right median portion.

predominating in the clinical picture that is attributable to the direct pathophysiological consequence of another medical condition. The manic/hypomanic symptoms usually have acute or subacute onset related to the beginning of the associated medical condition, are not better explained by another mental disorder, and do not occur exclusively during a course of delirium [22].

Our patient presented elevated mood, reduced need of sleep, pressured speech, thoughts race, elevated energy, and disinhibition with a month of evolution and these symptoms appeared 6 months after he suffered a stroke. Before the onset of the stroke our patient was asymptomatic, without a previous psychiatric history. Also, according to DSM-5 diagnostic criteria the disturbance must cause clinically significant distress or impairment in social, occupational, or other important areas of functioning. In our case the patient underwent money overspending and abuse of alcoholic drinks, had frequent conflicts with his family, also needed hospitalization to prevent harm to self or others, and also had psychotic symptoms [22].

The plausibility and probability of causal relationship of the patient's development of BD secondary to the multiple subcortical biparietal lacunar infarctions, a lacunar infarction in left putamen and an ischemic lesion at the cerebral trunk evolving the right median portion, are based on temporal sequence and clinical evidence. Usually, the manic/hypomanic picture due to another medical condition may appear within weeks [22, 23] or a few months [23]. Also, there is absence of evidence to suggest an alternative cause of the mental syndrome, such as a strong family history or precipitating stress [23]. Moreover, patient neuroimaging studies showed generalized cerebral atrophy, which has also been recognized as a vulnerability increasing factor to mania after stroke [24].

Secondary mania and BD after stroke result mostly from focal and solitary lesions, however literature describes correlation between this pathology and lesions with various locations [25]. Although the majority of the studies reporting secondary mania and BD after stroke allocate lesions to the right hemisphere [26–28], a putative effect for laterality on its etiopathogenesis remains under discussion [29–31]. A mechanism implying the activation or release of left hemisphere influence after a right hemisphere contralesion has been proposed [30]. Corroborating this hypothesis, it has been recently demonstrated by comparison of pre- and poststroke single-photon emission computed tomography (SPECT) scans, a left frontotemporal hyperperfusion, and extensive right frontal hypoperfusion in a patient with poststroke mania after right infarction in the territory of the middle cerebral artery [29]. Interestingly, this proposed release of left hemisphere also seems to be present in the manic pole of bipolar syndrome (not postlesion) [32, 33]. We cannot ascertain in our patient that this left hemisphere release phenomenon is the determining factor for the bipolarity expression as the patient presents with lesions on several locations. In fact, it may probably comprise the alternatively proposed hypothesis of the involvement of lesions located on several cortical and subcortical circuits. Starkstein et al. have documented that the majority of patients with right cortical lesions had poststroke mania, oppositely to patients experiencing mania and depression after stroke in right hemisphere subcortical areas [25]. Accordingly, our patient has experienced both mania and depression, as lesions comprised both cortical and subcortical areas.

Moreover, as the localization of lesions was reported on frontal lobe (including orbitofrontal cortex), temporal lobe, basal ganglia (head of caudate nucleus), and thalamus [29, 34, 35], it has been suggested that dysfunction of the frontolimbic circuits could negatively influence mood modulation resulting in the expression of bipolarity through manic symptoms. Due to the involvement of cerebellar-pontine lesions in these circuits [36, 37], the involvement of rostral brainstem dopaminergic nuclei damage and its ascending dopaminergic projections to the frontal-subcortical circuit components in the cases of poststroke mania located in pontomesencephalic area has also been hypothesized [38, 39]. Accordingly, the ischemic lesion at the cerebral trunk evolving the right median portion in our patient could involve also these ascending dopaminergic projections.

BD with late onset is a relatively rare condition and its management must take into account several organic comorbidities. The treatment includes a mood stabilizer (such as sodium valproate or carbamazepine) and a special care should be taken when introducing antidepressants, and also lithium should be used carefully [40]. Due to association of expression of BD in later life with higher cerebrovascular risk, additional research is needed to better understand the interrelationship between the expression of bipolarity and vascular brain lesions and also to determine clinical biomarkers and preventable measures of progression and treatment of BD poststroke. Neuroimaging may play an important role in identifying and staging these risk factors.

## Conflict of Interests

The authors declare that there is no conflict of interests regarding the publication of this paper.

## References


[1] J. Volkert, H. Schulz, M. Härter, O. Wlodarczyk, and S. Andreas, "The prevalence of mental disorders in older people in Western countries—a meta-analysis," *Ageing Research Reviews*, vol. 12, no. 1, pp. 339–353, 2013.

[2] O. P. Almeida and S. Fenner, "Bipolar disorder: similarities and differences between patients with illness onset before and after 65 years of age," *International Psychogeriatrics*, vol. 14, no. 3, pp. 311–322, 2002.

[3] C. A. Depp and D. V. Jeste, "Bipolar disorder in older adults: a critical review," *Bipolar Disorders*, vol. 6, no. 5, pp. 343–367, 2004.

[4] C. Krauthammer and G. L. Klerman, "Secondary mania. Manic syndromes associated with antecedent physical illness or drugs," *Archives of General Psychiatry*, vol. 35, no. 11, pp. 1333–1338, 1978.

[5] J. L. Cummings and M. F. Mendez, "Secondary mania with focal cerebrovascular lesions," *The American Journal of Psychiatry*, vol. 141, no. 9, pp. 1084–1087, 1984.

[6] R. C. Young, "Geriatric mania," *Clinics in Geriatric Medicine*, vol. 8, no. 2, pp. 387–399, 1992.

[7] H. C. Lin, S. Y. Tsai, and H. C. Lee, "Increased risk of developing stroke among patients with bipolar disorder after an acute mood episode: a six-year follow-up study," *Journal of Affective Disorders*, vol. 100, no. 1–3, pp. 49–54, 2007.

[8] R. Lopes and L. Fernandes, "Bipolar disorder: clinical perspectives and implications with cognitive dysfunction and dementia," *Depression Research and Treatment*, vol. 2012, Article ID 275957, 11 pages, 2012.

[9] R. Lopes and L. Fernandes, "Perturbação afectiva bipolar, disfunção cognitiva e demência," *Arquivos de Medicina*, vol. 26, no. 5, pp. 202–210, 2012.

[10] M. W. van Gerpen, J. E. Johnson, and D. K. Winstead, "Mania in the geriatric patient population," *The American Journal of Geriatric Psychiatry*, vol. 7, no. 3, pp. 188–202, 1999.

[11] T. Fujikawa, S. Yamawaki, and Y. Touhouda, "Silent cerebral infarctions in patients with late-onset mania," *Stroke*, vol. 26, no. 6, pp. 946–949, 1995.

[12] F. E. de Leeuw, J. C. de Groot, and M. Oudkerk, "A follow-up study of blood pressure and cerebral white matter lesions," *Annals of Neurology*, vol. 46, no. 6, pp. 827–833, 1999.

[13] W. M. McDonald, K. R. R. Krishnan, P. M. Doraiswamy, and D. G. Blazer, "Occurrence of subcortical hyperintensities elderly subjects with mania," *Psychiatry Research—Neuroimaging*, vol. 40, no. 4, pp. 211–220, 1991.

[14] H. Subramaniam, M. S. Dennis, and E. J. Byrne, "The role of vascular risk factors in late onset bipolar disorder," *International Journal of Geriatric Psychiatry*, vol. 22, no. 8, pp. 733–737, 2007.

[15] S. H. Huang, K. H. Chung, J. L. Hsu, J. Y. Wu, Y. L. Huang, and S. Y. Tsai, "The risk factors for elderly patients with bipolar disorder having cerebral infarction," *Journal of Geriatric Psychiatry and Neurology*, vol. 25, no. 1, pp. 15–19, 2012.

[16] C. Wijeratne and G. S. Malhi, "Vascular mania: an old concept in danger of sclerosing? A clinical overview," *Acta Psychiatrica Scandinavica*, vol. 116, no. 434, pp. 35–40, 2007.

[17] F. Kapczinski, E. Vieta, A. C. Andreazza et al., "Allostatic load in bipolar disorder: implications for pathophysiology and treatment," *Neuroscience and Biobehavioral Reviews*, vol. 32, no. 4, pp. 675–692, 2008.

[18] M. Berk, F. Kapczinski, A. C. Andreazza et al., "Pathways underlying neuroprogression in bipolar disorder: focus on inflammation, oxidative stress and neurotrophic factors," *Neuroscience and Biobehavioral Reviews*, vol. 35, no. 3, pp. 804–817, 2011.

[19] A. C. Pinto, "O teste SLUMS: apresentação, tradução e normas de cotação," *Psicologia, Educação e Cultura*, vol. 11, no. 2, pp. 393–403, 2007.

[20] S. H. Tariq, N. Tumosa, J. T. Chibnall, M. H. Perry III, and J. E. Morley, "Comparison of the Saint Louis University Mental Status examination and the Mini-Mental State Examination for detecting dementia and mild neurocognitive disorder—a pilot study," *The American Journal of Geriatric Psychiatry*, vol. 14, no. 11, pp. 900–910, 2006.

[21] K. Shulman and F. Post, "Bipolar affective disorder in old age," *British Journal of Psychiatry*, vol. 136, no. 1, pp. 26–32, 1980.

[22] American Psychiatric Association, *Diagnostic and Statistical Manual of Mental Disorders: DSM-5*, American Psychiatric Association, Washington, DC, USA, 5th edition, 2013.

[23] World Health Organization, *The ICD-10 Classification of Mental and Behavioral Disorders*, World Health Organization, Geneva, Switzerland, 1992.

[24] F. F. da Rocha, H. Correa, and A. L. Teixeira, "A successful outcome with valproic acid in a case of mania secondary to stroke of the right frontal lobe," *Progress in Neuro-Psychopharmacology and Biological Psychiatry*, vol. 32, no. 2, pp. 587–588, 2008.

[25] S. E. Starkstein, P. Fedoroff, M. L. Berthier, and R. G. Robinson, "Manic-depressive and pure manic states after brain lesions," *Biological Psychiatry*, vol. 29, no. 2, pp. 149–158, 1991.

[26] R. G. Robinson, J. D. Boston, S. E. Starkstein, and T. R. Price, "Comparison of mania and depression after brain injury: causal factors," *The American Journal of Psychiatry*, vol. 145, no. 2, pp. 172–178, 1988.

[27] M. A. Carran, C. G. Kohler, M. J. O'Connor, W. B. Bilker, and M. R. Sperling, "Mania following temporal lobectomy," *Neurology*, vol. 61, no. 6, pp. 770–774, 2003.

[28] C. M. J. Braun, C. Larocque, S. Daigneault, and I. Montour-Proulx, "Mania, pseudomania, depression, and pseudodepression resulting from focal unilateral cortical lesions," *Neuropsychiatry, Neuropsychology and Behavioral Neurology*, vol. 12, no. 1, pp. 35–51, 1999.

[29] M. Mimura, K. Nakagome, N. Hirashima et al., "Left frontotemporal hyperperfusion in a patient with post-stroke mania," *Psychiatry Research—Neuroimaging*, vol. 139, no. 3, pp. 263–267, 2005.

[30] S. E. Starkstein and R. G. Robinson, "Mechanism of disinhibition after brain lesions," *Journal of Nervous and Mental Disease*, vol. 185, no. 2, pp. 108–114, 1997.

[31] C. M. J. Braun, R. Daigneault, S. Gaudelet, and A. Guimond, "Diagnostic and Statistical Manual of Mental Disorders, Fourth Edition symptoms of mania: which one(s) result(s) more often from right than left hemisphere lesions?" *Comprehensive Psychiatry*, vol. 49, no. 5, pp. 441–459, 2008.

[32] R. Migliorelli, S. E. Starkstein, A. Teson et al., "SPECT findings in patients with primary mania," *Journal of Neuropsychiatry and Clinical Neurosciences*, vol. 5, no. 4, pp. 379–383, 1993.

[33] H. P. Blumberg, E. Stern, D. Martinez et al., "Increased anterior cingulate and caudate activity in bipolar mania," *Biological Psychiatry*, vol. 48, no. 11, pp. 1045–1052, 2000.

[34] S. Kumar, R. R. Jacobson, and K. Sathananthan, "Seasonal cyclothymia to seasonal bipolar affective disorder: a double switch after stroke," *Journal of Neurology Neurosurgery and Psychiatry*, vol. 63, no. 6, pp. 796–797, 1997.

[35] S. E. Starkstein and R. G. Robinson, "Affective disorders and cerebral vascular disease," *British Journal of Psychiatry*, vol. 154, pp. 170–182, 1989.

[36] Y. Amino, S.-I. Kyuhou, R. Matsuzaki, and H. Gemba, "Cerebello-thalamo-cortical projections to the posterior parietal cortex in the macaque monkey," *Neuroscience Letters*, vol. 309, no. 1, pp. 29–32, 2001.

[37] S. Nagao, "Pontine nuclei-mediated cerebello-cerebral interactions and its functional role," *Cerebellum*, vol. 3, no. 1, pp. 11–15, 2004.

[38] Y. W. Yeh and G. S. Peng, "Post-stroke mania precipitated by withdrawal of antidepressant in an elderly patient with chronic major depression," *General Hospital Psychiatry*, vol. 33, no. 3, pp. 301–e15, 2011.

[39] Y. Nishio, K. Ishii, H. Kazui, Y. Hosokai, and E. Mori, "Frontal-lobe syndrome and psychosis after damage to the brainstem dopaminergic nuclei," *Journal of the Neurological Sciences*, vol. 260, no. 1-2, pp. 271–274, 2007.

[40] K. I. Shulman, "Bipolar disorder in old age," *Canadian Family Physician*, vol. 45, pp. 1229–1237, 1999.

# 21

# Fatal Heat Stroke in a Schizophrenic Patient

**María Jesús Gómez Ramos,[1] Francisco Miguel González Valverde,[2] Carmen Sánchez Álvarez,[1] Lisa Ortin Katnich,[1] and Francisco Pastor Quirante[3]**

[1] *Department of ICU, Reina Sofía General University Hospital, University of Murcia, 30.003 Murcia, Spain*
[2] *Department of Surgery, Reina Sofía General University Hospital, University of Murcia, 30.003 Murcia, Spain*
[3] *Department of Pathology, Reina Sofía General University Hospital, University of Murcia, 30.003 Murcia, Spain*

Correspondence should be addressed to F. Miguel González Valverde, migova@terra.es

Academic Editors: M. Egi, A. Grippo, H. Kern, and J. Starkopf

*Objective.* The case of a patient who developed a fatal post-exertional heat stroke is reported. *Case Report.* A 20-year-old man with a history of morbid obesity, hypertension, and schizophrenia was admitted to our intensive care unit because of multiorgan failure due to severe heat stroke. He had been working under the sun. Treatment included aggressive body cooling but, in spite of the best supportive care, the patient succumbed in a few hours. We concluded that the adverse event was possibly associated with his obesity and the use of antipsychotics. Histological evaluation revealed lesions consistent with severe hyperthermia and shock. *Conclusions.* Heat stroke is an uncommon clinical entity characterized by systemic heat and loss of the body's normal mechanisms for dealing with heat stress, such as sweating and temperature control. When heat stroke is diagnosed early and supportive care begins promptly the prognosis is optimal but it becomes a life-threatening disease when treatment is delayed. Lack of physical acclimatization and the use of certain medications that interfere with salt and water balance can impair thermoregulation under conditions of high environmental temperature. Health professionals must be adequately prepared to prevent, recognise, and treat them urgently.

## 1. Introduction

Heat stroke (HS) is a potentially life-threatening disease characterized by an extreme elevation of core body temperature and neurologic disorders resulting in delirium, convulsion, or coma [1]. It is usually the result of exposure to high environmental temperature and strenuous exercise. Although treatable and preventable, a substantial number of people die from extreme heat in Europe each year.

The most frequent cause of death directly attributable to heat is HS but heat conditions are known to aggravate chronic disorders and leads to increased all-cause mortality, specially circulatory and respiratory mortality. So, the reported incidence of heat-related mortality is imprecise and grossly underdiagnosed in specific risk groups as the elderly, those with chronic medical diseases or morbid obesity, and the socially isolated [2].

## 2. Case Report

In late May 2008, a man aged 20 years was working in a field in Murcia (south-eastern Spain) for 4 hours in 30°C heat. He had a history of arterial hypertension, morbid obesity, and schizophrenia. His medications included risperidone 6 mg, biperiden hydrochloride, and enalapril 20 mg daily. At 4 pm he complained of dizziness and headache. After about 10 minutes he came running out in a highly agitated state and suddenly collapsed. The patient stayed under direct sunlight during approximately 2 hours until emergencies arrived and found him moaning and unresponsive (Glasgow Coma Scale 7: E2, V2, M3), with eye deviation, and breathless. His skin felt very hot and dry, blood pressure was 80/25 mmHg, pulse rate 176 bpm, and his axillary temperature—which underestimates core temperature—39.6°C. The patient was given intravenous fluids, intubated, rapidly cooled, and transported to our hospital, 50 minutes away.

On arrival to the ICU the patient was deeply sedated and still hypotensive (50/20 mm Hg). At this time his rectal temperature was 41.8°C. Electrocardiogram revealed sinus tachycardia with diffuse subendocardial lesion in ST; serum levels of myocardial markers were remarkably high and diffuse hypokinesis was observed on the echocardiogram. Chest X-ray was compatible with an early pulmonary edema. The cerebral CT scan did not reveal any pathology and, to exclude an infectious origin, a lumbar puncture was performed yielding normal cerebrospinal fluid.

Laboratory results revealed severe acidosis (pH 7.11, PCO2 70 mmHg, HCO3 17) and abnormal serum levels: creatinine (2.6 mg/dL) as well as blood urea nitrogen (BUN: 30 mg/dL) were elevated indicating the beginning of renal failure. Sodium was 138 mmol/L, potassium 4.6 mmol/L and chloride 115 mmol/L. Haematology analysis presented low platelet count (41.000) and severe alteration of coagulation levels (prothrombin time 13%, partial thromboplastin time >200 sec, INR 737, and fibrinogen 70). Hematocrit was 52.9%, hemoglobin 189 g/L, and leukocyte count 28400 (58% neutrophils and 12% band cells).

During the first hours, temperature control methods were continued with intravenous cold fluid infusion, vitamin K, sodium bicarbonate 1 molar, platelet, and fresh frozen plasma therapy. Conventional external cooling devices such as cooling blankets, cold compresses, and fans, warm water sprayed, and a gastric irrigation with cold water did not lead to any significant decrease in body temperature.

One hour of intensive care later, core body temperature was 39°C. The patient started bleeding by venous access and gastrointestinal tube. Because of subsequent deterioration of the patient's condition and insufficient temperature control, use of vasopressors (noradrenaline) and hemodynamic monitoring with pulmonary artery catheter was required. Despite aggressive therapy, multiorgan dysfunction syndrome with anuria and disseminated intravascular coagulopathy developed and the patient died 9 hours after his access to ICU.

In the autopsy, severe superficial skin burns with epidermal loss were observed on groin, neck, trunk, axillae, and other non-exposure areas (Figure 1). The lungs, the larynx, and the high respiratory airways were heavily congested and hemorrhagic (Figure 2). Histological study also revealed moderate brain edema, necrosis of the renal tubules, subendocardial necrosis (Figure 3), numerous petechial haemorrhages, and generalized visceral congestion. The underlying cause of death was heat stroke.

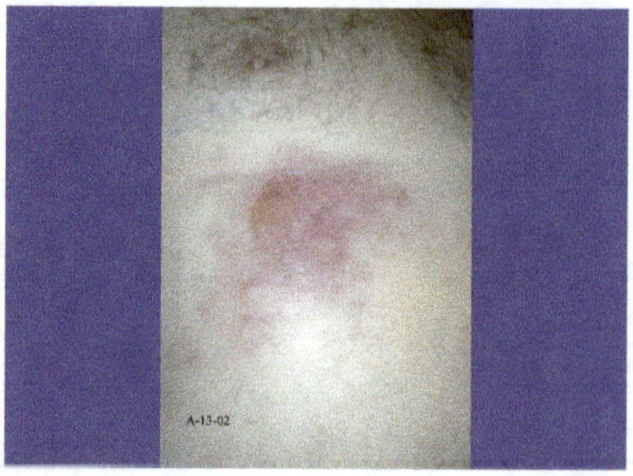

FIGURE 1: Superficial burn blisters with epidermal loss on non-exposure areas.

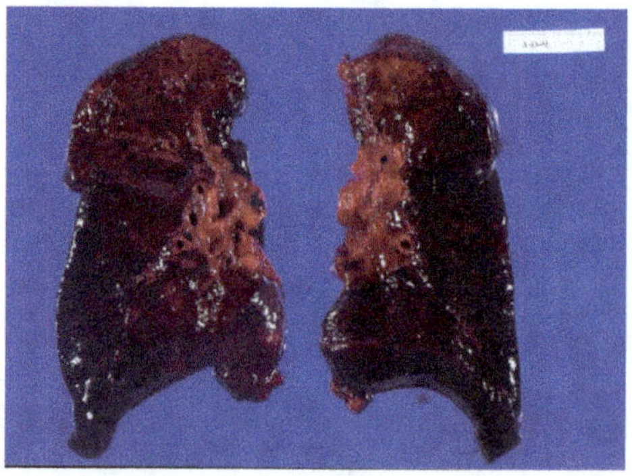

FIGURE 2: The lungs were heavily congested and hemorrhagic.

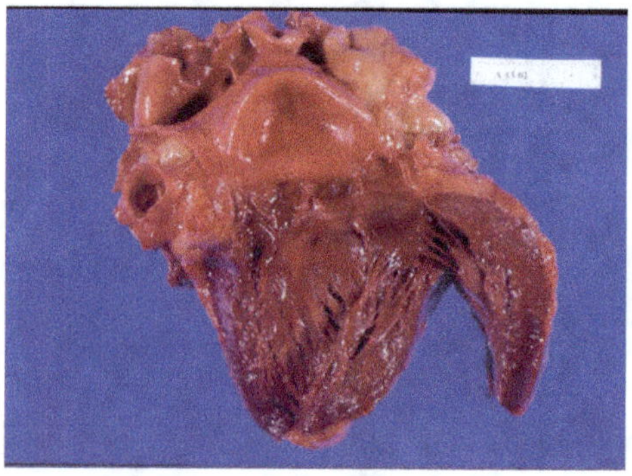

FIGURE 3: Heart specimen showing acute subendocardial-myocardial infarction.

## 3. Discussion

The incidence of heat-related disorders is higher during the summer but it can also occur in moderate conditions, depending on environmental factors, age, and the use of several drugs (Table 1). The continuum of classic heat-related illnesses includes mild disease (heat edema, rash, cramps, syncope), heat exhaustion, and the most severe form, heat stroke. The last two situations are commonly treated in critical care units because of the highest risk of morbid-mortality. Clinically HS is distinguished from heat exhaustion by disturbances of the central nervous system, usually prolonged unconsciousness and coma often preceded by confusion, delirium, ataxia, or convulsions [3, 4].

Although HS has been classically documented as a medical condition, a universally accepted definition is lacking because its pathophysiology is not fully understood. It must be considered in anyone who presents with hyperthermia (exceeding 40°C) and altered mental status. Despite adequate hypothermia or other care-therapy, permanent neurological damage occurs in approximately 20% of patients and the mortality rate may be as high as 10 to 80% [1, 4–6].

TABLE 1: Conditons contributing to the risk of heat illness.

| | Risk factors | Mechanism |
|---|---|---|
| Physical conditions | Prolonged exertion | |
| | Fever | |
| | Dehydration | |
| Medications | Drugs of abuse: amphetamines, heroine, cocaine, LSD, ethanol. | Increase endogenous heat production |
| | Anticholinergic: tricyclic antidepressants, antispasmodics and phenothiazides. | Disrupt hypothalamic function and reduce sweating |
| | Beta-adrenergic and Calcium channel blockers | Inhibit the compensatory increase in cardiac output |
| | Diuretics | Produce a relative state of dehydration that affects central thermoregulation and sweating |
| | Others: antiparkinsonian agents, antihistamines | |
| Chronic illness | Cardiac conditions | |
| | Cystic fibrosis | |
| | Extensive skin disease | |
| | Hyperthyroidism | |
| | Psychiatric conditions | |
| Older age | | |

TABLE 2

| Characteristic | Classic | Exertional |
|---|---|---|
| Health condition | Predisposing factors | Healthy |
| Age | Elderly | Younger |
| Conditions | High environmental temp | Occurs sporadically |
| Sweating | Usually absent | Present |
| Activity | Sedentary | Strenuous |
| Disseminated intravascular coagulation | Mild | Marked |
| Acute renal failure | <5% patients | 25–30% patients |
| Lactic acidosis | Rare | Common |
| Hyperuricemia | Moderate | Severe |
| Hypocalcemia | Rare | Common |
| Hypoglycaemia | Rare | Common |
| Hypokalemia | Rare | Common |
| Rhabdomyolysis | Rare | Common |
| CPK | Mildly elevated | Marked elevated |
| Mechanism | Poor dissipation of environmental heat | Excessive endogenous heat production |

Information from [3, 8].

Hyperpyrexia and neurologic dysfunction are necessary but not sufficient to diagnose HS. Associated clinical manifestations such as extreme fatigue and flu-like symptoms; hot dry skin or heavy perspiration; nausea; vomiting; diarrhea; disorientation; dizziness; uncoordinated movements; reddened face are frequently observed (Table 2). Clinical signs of dehydration and salt depletion are almost always present in the form of tachycardia, hypotension, and diaphoresis. Potential complications related to severe HS are acute renal failure, disseminated intravascular coagulation, rhabdomyolysis, acute respiratory distress syndrome, acid-base disorders, and electrolyte disturbances [4, 7, 8]. Above 42.4°C, thermal damage becomes critical, oxidative phosphorylation becomes uncoupled, proteins denature inducing changes in

Table 3: Heat illness.

| | Edema | Cramps | Tetany | Syncope | Exhaustion | Stroke |
|---|---|---|---|---|---|---|
| Symptoms | Minimal clinical significance but important interstitial fluid accumulation | Cramps | Cramps, carpopedal spasm, and perioral and distal paresthesias | Nausea, sighing, yawning, restlessness, and orthostatic syncope | Flulike | Flulike |
| Central nervous system symptoms | NO | NO | NO | NO | NO | Present |
| Temperature | <41°C | <41°C | <41°C | <41°C | <41°C | >41°C |
| Sweating | Present | Present | Present | Present | Present | Absent |
| Mechanism | Unacclimatisation, peripheral vasodilatation | Unacclimatisation and negative sodium balance | Unacclimatisation and severe negative sodium balance | Unacclimatisation, dehydration and inadequate cardiac output | Excess sweating in a hot humid environment causing volume depletion | Heat production exceeds dissipation |
| Treatment | Periodic exercise, elevation of the legs, or diuretic medication | Oral sodium replacement | Oral or parenteral sodium replacement | Placing supine position, and replacing water deficit | Cool area to rest, placing supine position and replacing water deficit | Emergency treatment |

the membrane fluidity, and enzyme systems are affected [4]. HS resembles sepsis in many aspects, and endotoxemia and cytokines may be implicated in its pathogenesis [1, 9, 10].

Two forms of HS are recognized (Table 3): classic (no exertional), usually occurring in elderly persons with chronic illnesses, children, the obese, and those receiving medications such as diuretics, antipsychotics, antihypertensives, and antidepressants; exertional HS, more common in physically active individuals who develop a strenuous and exceptional exercise [3, 6, 8–10].

In our case the patient was a morbidly obese subject that intook antipsychotics and antihypertensives, practising a strenuous activity at sunshine, and accompanied by inadequate fluid intake. Clinical manifestation was sudden and concurrent with exertional type but he had no sweating and hypoglycaemia, presenting several characteristics of the classic type. Certain drugs may induce or worsen heat-related illnesses. Drugs with anticholinergic effects can inhibit sweating and reduce heat elimination. Neuroleptics and tranquillizers, such as phenothiazines, have combined anticholinergic and central thermoregulatory effects. The set point of the temperature regulation centre can be elevated by the antidopaminergic effect of antipsychotics, such as phenothiazines and thioxanthenes [11–13].

The diagnosis of HS is suspected in the presence of a markedly elevated temperature and changes in mental status following heat exposure. Medical work-up include chest X-ray, electrocardiogram, and lab work with a complete blood count, electrolytes, BUN and creatinine, liver enzymes, creatine kinase, prothrombin time and partial thromboplastin time, arterial blood gasses, and urinalysis. The differential diagnosis includes hyperthyroid storm, pheochromocytoma, central nervous system injury, infection, anticholinergic poisoning, drug ingestion, and neuroleptic malignant syndrome [3].

In autopsy, edema of the brain, leptomeninges, petechial haemorrhages, and neuronal degeneration may be observed. The cardiovascular system may show right heart dilatation, pericardial effusion, edema, degeneration, and necrosis of myocardial fibres. Pulmonary infarction and high airways submucosal haemorrhages have also been described. The kidneys are enlarged with numerous petechial haemorrhages as well as the gastrointestinal submucosa. The liver may be congestive but structural injuries are infrequently found. Skin scalds with different depth degree on non-exposure areas and rigid and contracted muscles with necrosis of fibres are possible [14–16].

Assuming that HS is an acute life threatening emergency, the prognosis can be greatly improved if the symptoms are recognised early and emergency measures are instituted promptly. The prognosis is poorest when treatment is delayed >2 hours [10, 17, 18]. Early management should include the use of cold water or watersoaked towels, support of organ-system function, fluid resuscitation and electrolyte replacement if possible, and immediate transfer to a hospital. Aggressive cooling measures should be continued until the core temperature reaches 39°C. There is controversy regarding which cooling techniques are most effective. A combination of cold-water immersion and evaporative methods (spraying the body with atomised 15°C water and warmed air) is the best option for treatment [19, 20]. Other methods include ice packs placed over the axilla, groin, and neck. Disadvantages include peripheral vasoconstriction that retard heat loss; induced shivering, resulting in increased internal heat generation. If shivering does occur, medications as meperidine and diazepam can inhibit it; extreme discomfort to patients and medical attendants; difficulty in monitoring and resuscitating vital signs of patient [8, 20]. Internal methods for cooling as cold water irrigation to the stomach or rectum may be used but only in addition to external cooling methods [20]. Peritoneal lavage and cardiopulmonary bypass in severe cases have been advocated but their clinic efficacy is debated.

The use of pharmacological agents as antipyretics or steroids is not helpful in the treatment of HS. The hypothalamic setpoint is not elevated as it is in fever so that aspirin and acetaminophen are ineffective; furthermore aspirin is contraindicated for its effect on platelets and clotting [1, 4, 8]. Supportive cares are necessary and respiratory, neurologic, and cardiac status must be specially monitored [21]. In a comatose patient, a cuffed endotracheal tube should be placed to protect the airway as respiratory assistance is indicated. Invariably a venous access to replace fluids is required even if the patient is not hypotensive. Furthermore hemodynamic monitoring with pulmonary artery catheter may be indicated. This technique helps us for fluidotherapy management and vasopressors drugs if hypotension is not controlled well. Other aspects of monitoring include urine output measurement as indicator of acute renal failure.

Due to the risk and the prognosis, the best treatment is prevention. It requires awareness of risk factors and appropriate hydration.

## 4. Conclusions

Heat stroke is a true medical emergency requiring immediate admission to an intensive care unit. Early recognition and management with aggressive measures to lower the body temperature with other supportive therapies can substantially reduce the mortality. Emergency departments and public health agencies should be adequately prepared to prevent, suspect, and manage heat-related illnesses, especially during heat waves.

## Abbreviations

HS: Heat stroke
pm: Post meridiem
bpm: Beats per minute.

## References

[1] A. Bouchama and J. P. Knochel, "Medical progress: heat stroke," *The New England Journal of Medicine*, vol. 346, no. 25, pp. 1978–1988, 2002.

[2] G. M. Varghese, G. John, K. Thomas, O. C. Abraham, and D. Mathai, "Predictors of multi-organ dysfunction in heatstroke," *Emergency Medicine Journal*, vol. 22, no. 3, pp. 185–187, 2005.

[3] M. W. Barrow and K. A. Clark, "Heat-related illnesses," *American Family Physician*, vol. 58, no. 3, pp. 749–756, 1998.

[4] T. A. Waters, "Heat illness: tips for recognition and treatment," *Cleveland Clinic Journal of Medicine*, vol. 68, no. 8, pp. 685–687, 2001.

[5] Centers for Disease Control, "Heat-related illness and deaths—United States, 1994-1995," *Morbidity and Mortality Weekly Report (MMWR)*, vol. 44, pp. 465–468.

[6] J. E. Dematte, K. O'Mara, J. Buescher et al., "Near-fatal heat stroke during the 1995 heat wave in Chicago," *Annals of Internal Medicine*, vol. 129, no. 3, pp. 173–181, 1998.

[7] A. S. Howe and B. P. Boden, "Heat-related illness in athletes," *American Journal of Sports Medicine*, vol. 35, no. 8, pp. 1384–1395, 2007.

[8] R. Khosla and K. K. Guntupalli, "Heat-related illnesses," *Critical Care Clinics*, vol. 15, no. 2, pp. 251–262, 1999.

[9] K. C. Lu, J. Y. Wang, S. H. Lin, P. Chu, and Y. F. Lin, "Role of circulating cytokines and chemokines in exertional heatstroke," *Critical Care Medicine*, vol. 32, no. 2, pp. 399–403, 2004.

[10] H. Grogan and P. M. Hopkins, "Heat stroke: implications for critical care and anaesthesia," *British Journal of Anaesthesia*, vol. 88, no. 5, pp. 700–707, 2002.

[11] J. S. S. Kwok and T. Y. K. Chan, "Recurrent heat-related illnesses during antipsychotic treatment," *Annals of Pharmacotherapy*, vol. 39, no. 11, pp. 1940–1942, 2005.

[12] K. Martin-Latry, M. P. Goumy, P. Latry et al., "Psychotropic drugs use and risk of heat-related hospitalisation," *European Psychiatry*, vol. 22, no. 6, pp. 335–338, 2007.

[13] T. H. Reilly and M. A. Kirk, "Atypical antipsychotics and newer antidepressants," *Emergency Medicine Clinics of North America*, vol. 25, no. 2, pp. 477–497, 2007.

[14] J. P. Knochel, W. R. Beisel, E. G. Herndon, E. S. Gerard, and K. G. Barry, "The renal, cardiovascular, hematologic and serum electrolyte abnormalities of heat stroke," *The American Journal of Medicine*, vol. 30, no. 2, pp. 299–309, 1961.

[15] M. Rav-Acha, E. Hadad, Y. Epstein, Y. Heled, and D. S. Moran, "Fatal exertional heart stroke: a case series," *American Journal of the Medical Sciences*, vol. 328, no. 2, pp. 84–87, 2004.

[16] K. Niizato, K. Tsuchiya, K. Oshima et al., "An autopsied case of schizophrenic patient who died from heat stroke," *No To Shinkei*, vol. 58, no. 5, pp. 418–424, 2006.

[17] J. L. Glazer, "Management of heatstroke and heat exhaustion," *American Family Physician*, vol. 71, no. 11, pp. 2133–2140, 2005.

[18] T. P. Yeo, "Heat stroke: a comprehensive review," *AACN Clinical Issues*, vol. 15, no. 2, pp. 280–293, 2004.

[19] J. S. Weiner and M. Khogali, "A physiological body-cooling unit for treatment of heat stroke," *The Lancet*, vol. 1, no. 8167, pp. 507–509, 1980.

[20] T. L. Lee-Chiong and J. T. Stitt, "Heatstroke and other heat-related illnesses: the maladies of summer," *Postgraduate Medicine*, vol. 98, no. 1, pp. 26–36, 1995.

[21] S. H. Chen, F. M. Chang, H. K. Chang, W. C. Chen, K. F. Huang, and M. T. Lin, "Human umbilical cord blood-derived CD34+ cells cause attenuation of multiorgan dysfunction during experimental heatstroke," *Shock*, vol. 27, no. 6, pp. 663–671, 2007.

22

# Case of "Slow" Stroke from Carotid Artery Occlusion Treated by Delayed but Cautious Endovascular Intervention

**Kachi Illoh,[1] Emilio Supsupin,[2] Hashem M. Shaltoni,[3] and Edwin D. Cacayorin[2]**

[1] *Division of Neurology Products, Center for Drug Evaluation and Research, U. S. Food and Drug Administration, Building 22, Room 5402, 10903 New Hampshire Avenue, Silver Spring, MD 20993, USA*
[2] *Department of Diagnostic and Interventional Imaging, The University of Texas Medical School at Houston, 6431 Fannin Street, MSB 2.130B, Houston, TX 77030, USA*
[3] *Department of Radiology, Baylor College of Medicine, One Baylor Plaza, Mail Stop BCM360, Houston, TX 77030, USA*

Correspondence should be addressed to Kachi Illoh, kachikwu.illoh@fda.hhs.gov

Academic Editor: Osama O. Zaidat

In a challenging case of carotid occlusion with slowly evolving stroke, we used brain imaging to facilitate endovascular revascularization resulting in the relief of the patient's symptoms. Patients with carotid occlusion and continued neurological worsening or fluctuations present enormous treatment challenges. These patients may present "slow" strokes with subacute infarcts that present significant challenges and risks during attempts at revascularization of the occluded artery. We present such a case in which we used multimodal imaging techniques, including MR-perfusion, to facilitate endovascular revascularization. Our approach of delayed but cautious intra-arterial thrombolytic therapy, guided by brain imaging, and followed by stent placement across the residual stenosis, enabled revascularization of the occluded artery without overt in-hospital complications.

## 1. Introduction

The management of ischemic stroke patients with acute carotid artery occlusion who experience neurological worsening is challenging and may require innovative approaches. The coexistence of carotid artery occlusion and evolving stroke symptoms poses major treatment challenges because of the presence of recent brain infarcts. Aggressive interventions with an aim of revascularization of the carotid artery are put on hold to avoid complications of reperfusion injury at the infarct sites. One such intervention, intra-arterial thrombolysis, is offered within six hours of onset in anterior circulation ischemic stroke [1]. Treatment beyond the 6-hour window is associated with high risks of complications with limited chances of neurological improvement. In this report, we present an unusual case of a patient with acute carotid occlusion who developed neurological worsening and fluctuations ("slow" stroke) that required complex management decisions. Our approach was to perform delayed, but closely monitored, intra-arterial thrombolysis four days from initial stroke presentation. Our goal in presenting this case is to raise awareness of management challenges in the subacute phase of an ischemic stroke and highlight an interventional approach that may improve the patient's outcome. We show that delayed intra-arterial thrombolysis is achievable with improvement in the patient's condition and without untoward consequences.

## 2. Clinical Summary

The patient is a 66-year-old African American female who presented with repeated clinical events of brain ischemia and imaging confirmation of an infarct. She had a history of hypertension, type 2 diabetes mellitus, and hyperlipidemia. Initially, she presented to an outside hospital with a sudden-onset of slurred speech that lasted 2 hours. She was diagnosed with transient ischemic attack (TIA) before discharge home on oral antiplatelet therapy. The following day, she developed another episode of slurred speech associated with left-sided weakness involving the face, arm, and leg. On presentation to the same outside facility, brain imaging revealed a right basal ganglia infarct with distal right internal carotid artery

(ICA) stenosis. She was started on heparin infusion for possible dissection of the distal right ICA and transferred to our facility for a higher level of care. Her home medications included lisinopril, atorvastatin, long-acting insulin, rosiglitazone, and glyburide. Family history indicated her grandmother had a stroke of unclear cause. She did not smoke, drink alcohol, or use illicit drugs. Clearly, her hospital transfer indicated a deteriorating ischemic process of the brain that was referable to carotid artery pathology.

The patient's subsequent hospitalization was marked by episodes of neurological worsening. On transfer to our facility three days from her initial TIA symptoms, her blood pressure was 155/81 mmHg and heart rate was105 beats per minute (bpm). Neurological examination revealed a mild left facial droop with an NIH stroke scale (NIHSS) score of 1; other aspects of neurological and systemic examination were unremarkable. A head CT scan showed the right basal ganglia infarct, and CT angiography confirmed the ICA stenosis. She was started on antiplatelet therapy (clopidogrel) and discontinued heparin treatment. Within 10 hours of transfer, she developed the first neurological worsening in our facility. She had a partial right gaze preference, partial left visual field cut, more prominent left facial droop, and left arm drift (NIHSS 4). Her vital signs at this time indicated a drop in blood pressure to 115/55 mmHg, with a pulse rate of 79 bpm. She received additional normal saline infusion and was started on eptifibatide infusion. Seven hours from onset of worsening, she improved to the point of having no neurological deficits (NIHSS 0). Her blood pressure at that time was 145/75 mmHg with pulse rate of 77 bpm. The next day (four days from initial TIA symptoms), we performed a cerebral angiogram to better define her vasculature and identified a right carotid terminus (carotid T) occlusion. The right anterior cerebral artery (ACA) was perfused from the anterior communicating (A-Comm) artery while the right middle cerebral artery (MCA) territory was perfused by leptomeningeal collaterals and right posterior cerebral artery (PCA). No evidence of carotid artery dissection was found. No interventional revascularization procedure was attempted at this point given recent infarct and potential risks of reperfusion injury. Following the arteriography, she continued to have neurological fluctuations despite attempts to keep her blood pressure elevated. Each time she sat up for up to 15 minutes, she developed a left-face and arm weakness typically with a drop in systolic blood pressure to below 114 mmHg. Notably, she was remarkably frustrated (she felt miserable, saying she would rather die than continue to have these episodes) though her NIHSS score only worsened to a score of 4. For this patient, her level of psychological distress especially with inability to sit up was a major disability, a feature not captured by the severity scale of NIHSS.

An MRI showed extensive perfusion defects suggesting considerable risk of imminent brain damage, which prompted our subsequent endovascular intervention. We obtained additional investigative studies including electroencephalogram (EEG) and echocardiography (both transthoracic and transesophageal); the results of these were unremarkable. However, an MRI of the brain showed the right basal ganglia infarct with extensive perfusion defect in the right MCA territory (Figure 1) and no evidence of hemorrhagic transformation of infarct. These findings, in addition to the patient's clinical condition, prompted our endovascular intervention five days from her initial TIA event. With the patient under conscious sedation and being monitored for neurological status, we slowly infused urokinase through a microcatheter at site of occlusion (Figure 2(a)). After the intra-arterial infusion of 107,000 units of urokinase, the patency of the right ICA and MCA were reestablished; perfusion of the lateral lenticulostriate arteries became evident. However, an underlying severe stenosis remained at the distal right ICA bifurcation (Figure 2(b)). Again, due to concerns of reperfusion injury, it was elected to proceed with treatment of the residual stenosis at a later date. She remained free of neurological fluctuations following the procedure. Twelve days from her initial symptoms, a balloon-mounted, drug-eluting 2.5 × 8 mm Cypher Stent (Cordis, Miami Lakes, Florida) was successfully deployed at the stenotic segment of the right supraclinoid ICA bifurcation. Complete recanalization was achieved with the procedure, enabling an improvement in ICA luminal diameter from 1 mm to 2.5 mm as shown in Figure 3. Following the procedure, she was maintained on an antiplatelet regimen of clopidogrel and aspirin to maintain stent patency and measures to keep her systolic blood pressure below 140 mmHg to prevent hyperperfusion injury. The patient was discharged home the following day without neurological deficits or further episodes of worsening.

## 3. Discussion

This case is striking because it highlights the use of slowly delivered intra-arterial thrombolysis to revascularize an occluded carotid artery terminus in the subacute ischemic stroke period, followed by stenting of the residual stenosis. This management approach was necessitated by the continued neurological fluctuations despite conservative medical measures. Also, there was imaging suggestive of additional brain tissue at risk of further damage. This imaging information provided the basis for our interventional approach. The clinical presentation of our patient is unusual in that she had an acute large vessel occlusion at the carotid T and slowly developed very minimal neurological deficits accentuated with intermittent fluctuations. Acute carotid T occlusions are typically devastating with poor clinical outcomes. The manner of our patient's presentation, termed "slow" stroke, is invariably difficult to treat because of the risk of reperfusion injury. Therefore, our therapeutic approach was facilitated largely by serial brain imaging besides the clinical fluctuations exhibited by the patient. We used MR imaging to delineate the infarct and brain tissue at risk of dying (penumbra). The penumbra that persisted many days from onset of initial insult presented a window of opportunity for intervention. The presence of perfusion defect or penumbra as estimated on MRI appears to be a useful marker in identifying patients that could be treated beyond the hyperacute period [2–5]. However, these studies evaluated imaging markers of penumbra in patients within

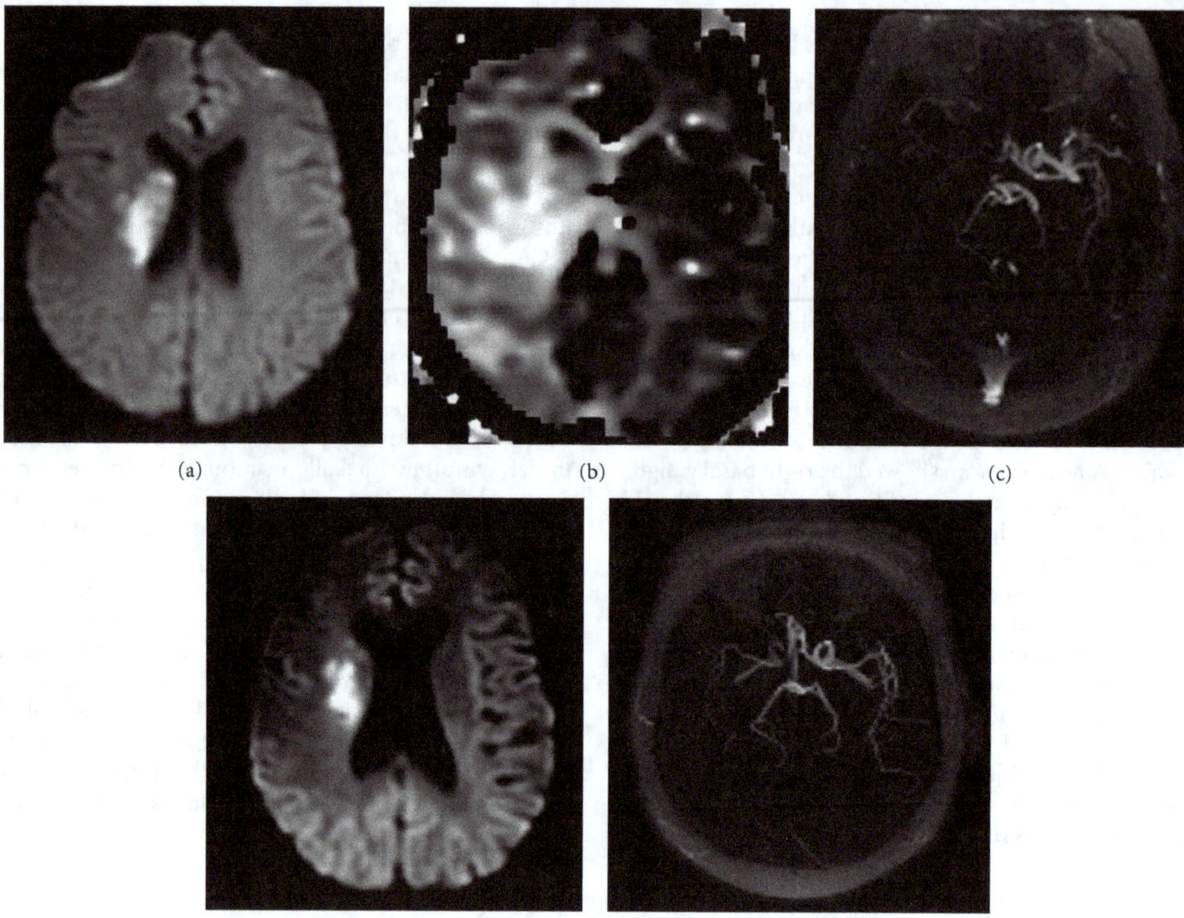

(a) (b) (c) (d) (e)

FIGURE 1: Magnetic resonance imaging of the brain, (a) prethrombolysis diffusion-weighted image (DWI) shows brain infarct in the right MCA territory, (b) prethrombolysis Perfusion-weighted image (PWI) shows right brain hemisphere with perfusion defect, (c) prethrombolysis Magnetic resonance Angiography (MRA) shows absence of blood flow in the right MCA, (d) postthrombolysis DWI shows no significant interval changes in brain parenchyma, and (e) postthrombolysis MRA with patent right MCA.

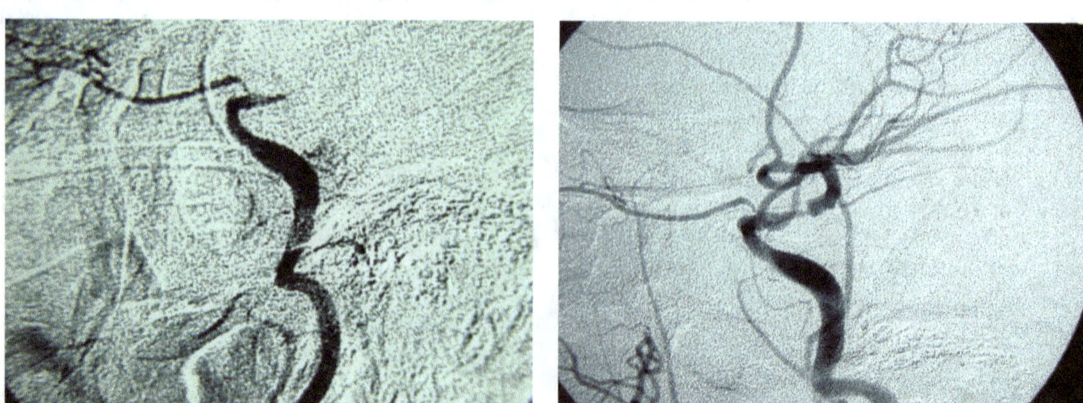

(a) (b)

FIGURE 2: (a) Slow injection of dilute urokinase with microcatheter at site of occlusion; (b) recanalization of the right MCA with residual carotid stenosis.

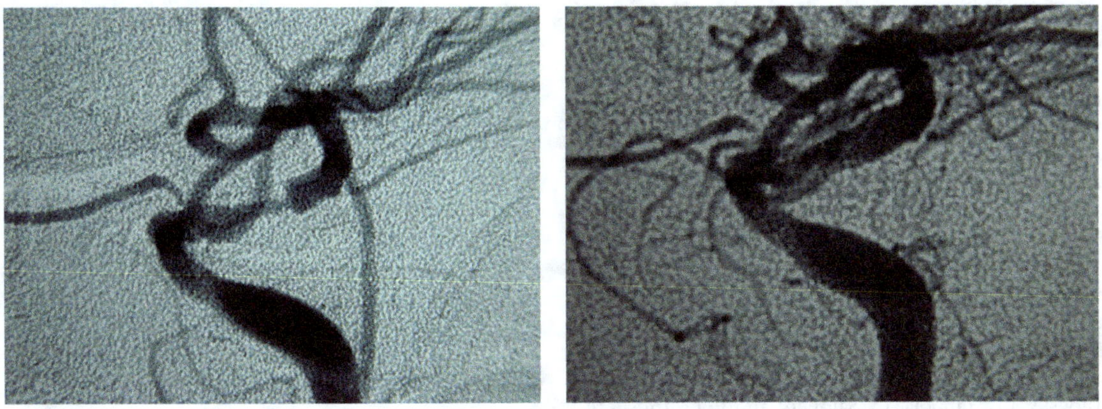

(a) (b)

FIGURE 3: (a) Prestenting cerebral arteriography shows occluded terminal carotid artery; (b) Poststenting arteriography shows complete carotid recanalization.

6 hours of stroke onset and not days after as in our patient's case.

Our approach differs from those of others who have employed various means such as induction of hypertension. Medically induced hypertension improves brain perfusion and has been shown to ameliorate stroke symptoms beyond the thrombolysis window [6, 7]. We were unable to stabilize our patient's condition with such conservative measures. Also, it is possible that medically induced hypertension using vasopressors on the long term could pose a risk of damage in other vascular beds given a patient's vascular risk factors [1]. Even so, keeping her hypertensive in hospital was difficult suggesting that continuation of such therapy as an outpatient would be impracticable. Had carotid dissection been confirmed on initial angiography, anticoagulation could have been an option of medical therapy. Nonetheless, we were unable to achieve neurological stability with medical therapy that consisted of antiplatelet therapy and attempts at keeping the patient hypertensive. Revascularization of acute carotid occlusion with thrombolysis and device-assisted approaches is promising in the acute stroke setting [8]. Complications of such revascularization (procedures and thrombolysis) and lack of palpable benefit limit the use of this therapeutic approach beyond the acute stroke period. Typically, it is unlikely that our patient would be a candidate for aggressive interventions to reopen the occluded carotid artery given her presentation with initial negligible deficits. No doubt, her development of neurological worsening despite conservative measures helped direct our therapeutic approach. With the risk of hemorrhage from thrombolysis, we considered mechanical thrombectomy as an alternative method of intervention. However, we wanted to avoid abrupt recanalization of the occluded artery that could precipitate reperfusion injury especially in the setting of a subacute infarct. Therefore, we decided on urokinase infusion with the goal of slow carotid recanalization. Although recent reports highlight the feasibility of delayed reperfusion modalities [9, 10], it remains to be determined whether our approach was the optimum in the clinical setting. A systematic evaluation of the approach, including long-term clinical outcomes, is needed before it can be recommended.

Other treatment options appeared to be of limited value in addressing the patient's misery from neurological fluctuations. Arterial bypass surgery would be unlikely to ameliorate the symptoms that early after the stroke. Moreover, its benefits in stroke patients remain unclear. Though not common, carotid endarterectomy (CEA) has been reportedly successful in some patients with acutely occluded ICA [11]. In our patient, the location of the carotid occlusion made such surgical revascularization untenable. In such tenuous vascular locations, revascularization using stent placement can be successfully achieved in patients with acute carotid occlusion and subacute infarcts [12]. In conclusion, we demonstrate that delayed and closely monitored intra-arterial therapy followed by stenting of residual atherosclerotic stenosis is achievable in a patient presenting with a subacute ischemic stroke and neurological fluctuations. In such a case, brain imaging showing evidence of substantial brain tissue at risk with absence of hemorrhagic transformation is useful in facilitating management decisions.

## Disclosure

The views expressed in this paper are those of the authors and do not necessarily represent the official position of their employers, including the U.S. Food and Drug Administration.

## References

[1] H. P. Adams, G. Del Zoppo, M. J. Alberts et al., "Guidelines for the early management of adults with ischemic stroke," *Stroke*, vol. 38, no. 5, pp. 1655–1711, 2007.

[2] J. J. Legos, S. C. Lenhard, R. E. Haimbach et al., "SB 234551 selective ET receptor antagonism: perfusion/Diffusion MRI used to define treatable stroke model, time to treatment and mechanism of protection," *Experimental Neurology*, vol. 212, no. 1, pp. 53–62, 2008.

[3] S. M. Davis, G. A. Donnan, M. W. Parsons et al., "Effects of alteplase beyond 3 h after stroke in the Echoplanar Imaging Thrombolytic Evaluation Trial (EPITHET): a placebo-controlled randomised trial," *The Lancet Neurology*, vol. 7, no. 4, pp. 299–309, 2008.
[4] M. Köhrmann, E. Jüttler, H. B. Huttner, T. Nowe, and P. D. Schellinger, "Acute stroke imaging for thrombolytic therapy—an update," *Cerebrovascular Diseases*, vol. 24, no. 2-3, pp. 161–169, 2007.
[5] G. W. Albers, V. N. Thijs, L. Wechsler et al., "Magnetic resonance imaging profiles predict clinical response to early reperfusion: the diffusion and perfusion imaging evaluation for understanding stroke evolution (DEFUSE) study," *Annals of Neurology*, vol. 60, no. 5, pp. 508–517, 2006.
[6] T. Bogoslovsky, O. Häppölä, O. Salonen, and P. J. Lindsberg, "Induced hypertension for the treatment of acute MCA occlusion beyond the thrombolysis window: case report," *BMC Neurology*, vol. 6, article 46, 2006.
[7] A. E. Hillis, R. J. Wityk, N. J. Beauchamp, J. A. Ulatowski, M. A. Jacobs, and P. B. Barker, "Perfusion-weighted MRI as a marker of response to treatment in acute and subacute stroke," *Neuroradiology*, vol. 46, no. 1, pp. 31–39, 2004.
[8] T. Tomsick, J. Broderick, J. Carrozella et al., "Revascularization results in the interventional management of stroke II trial," *American Journal of Neuroradiology*, vol. 29, no. 3, pp. 582–587, 2008.
[9] C. A. Molina and J. L. Saver, "Extending reperfusion therapy for acute ischemic stroke: emerging pharmacological, mechanical, and imaging strategies," *Stroke*, vol. 36, no. 10, pp. 2311–2320, 2005.
[10] A. Abou-Chebl, "Endovascular treatment of acute ischemic stroke may be safely performed with no time window limit in appropriately selected patients," *Stroke*, vol. 41, no. 9, pp. 1996–2000, 2010.
[11] B. T. Weis-Müller, R. Huber, A. Spivak-Dats, B. Turowski, M. Siebler, and W. Sandmann, "Symptomatic acute occlusion of the internal carotid artery: reappraisal of urgent vascular reconstruction based on current stroke imaging," *Journal of Vascular Surgery*, vol. 47, no. 4, pp. 752–759, 2008.
[12] K. Imai, T. Mori, H. Izumoto et al., "Successful stenting seven days after atherothrombotic occlusion of the intracranial internal carotid artery," *Journal of Endovascular Therapy*, vol. 13, no. 2, pp. 254–259, 2006.

# Ischemic Stroke in Confederation with Trivial Head Trauma

**Archana Balachandran, Siddarameshwar Kalyanshettar, Shankargouda Patil, and Vijaykumar Shegji**

*Department of Pediatrics, Shri. B.M. Patil Medical College Hospital and Research Centre, BLDE University, Vijayapur, Karnataka 586103, India*

Correspondence should be addressed to Siddarameshwar Kalyanshettar; ssk_dr@yahoo.co.in

Academic Editor: Piero Pavone

Minor head injuries in children are common, resulting in brain concussion, and these injuries mostly end up without complications. Usually head trauma results in hemorrhagic stroke. Here we present a case of ischemic stroke following a trivial head trauma. A 10-month-old girl presented with posttraumatic right sided hemiparesis with right sided facial palsy. MRI brain revealed an area of acute infarct in the left capsuloganglionic region. The child was initially managed conservatively, as the hematological parameters were normal, and was started on anticoagulant therapy. An improvement in the clinical condition was achieved in 12 hrs of treatment with gain in power and resolution of weakness in 10 days. The specific cause for hemiparesis in the child is not elicited; possibility of genetic and environmental factors can be attributable.

## 1. Introduction

Trivial head injuries are the most common accidents in childhood. They most often present with normal neurological findings. The severity of the head trauma correlates with the clinical symptoms. Cranial trauma in young children can cause ischemic infarct [1]. Incidence of cerebrovascular disease in children in India is 13–33/100,000 per year [2]. Head trauma in children mostly results in hemorrhagic stroke and ischemic stroke, of which ischemic cause is of lesser frequency. Hemorrhagic strokes are usually common in preceding vascular or coagulation anomaly [3]. Ischemic stroke constitutes slightly more than 50% of childhood and 80–85% of adult stroke cases [4]. Head trauma appears to act as a trigger for arterial strokes and dehydration for venous strokes [5]. The occurrence of ischemic lesion in the basal ganglia is a rarely described event following a minor head trauma with an incidence of less than 2% of all ischemic strokes in childhood [3]. The occurrence of ischemic lesions confined to the subcortical region is uncommon [6], and despite several case reports and descriptions a complete analysis of this illness in childhood is not available. Usually, mild pediatric stroke cases will have a good prognosis and complete recovery by proper management.

Here we report a case with neurological deficit following a minor head injury probably due to postbleed thrombosis resulting in ischemia of small vessel territories.

## 2. Case Report

A 10-month-old girl born of nonconsanguineous marriage with normal developmental history, with no prior medical problems, was brought to our emergency room with history of fall on the head when the child was trying to walk on her own. She cried for a brief period and there was no loss of consciousness. There was no vomiting or convulsions following the head injury. Next day morning, about 12 hours after the injury, child developed weakness involving right side of the face, right arm, and the right leg. Child was unable to sit or stand. On examination child was conscious and active showing decreased movements in the right half of the body with muscle power 2/5 in both right upper and lower extremity along with right sided UMN type of facial palsy, with a positive Babinski sign on the same side. There were no signs of raised intracranial pressure or meningeal irritation. Other neurological examinations were normal. Child did not have any signs suggestive of nonaccidental injury and did not have any external signs of trauma to the head or elsewhere on

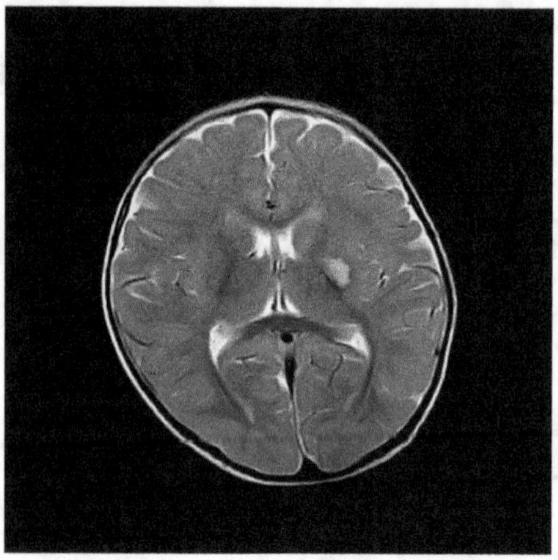

Figure 1: T2 weighted imaging of brain showing acute infarct of left capsuloganglionic region.

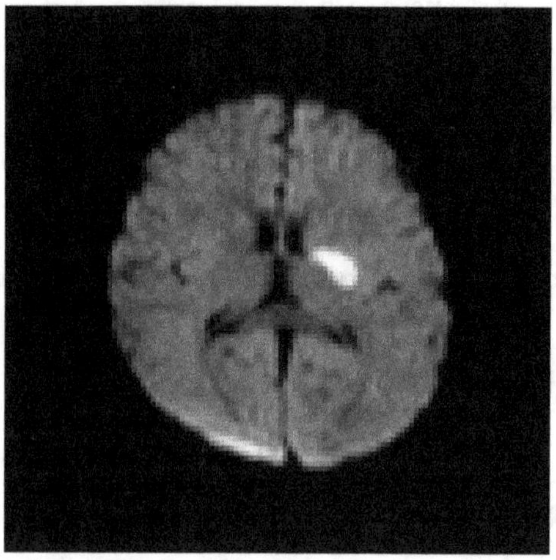

Figure 2: Restricted diffusion on DWI noted in left capsuloganglionic region suggestive of acute infarct.

the body. Child had no clinical history suggestive of varicella, measles, or ear discharge in the past. There was no history of feeding difficulty which suggests that there was no lower cranial nerve involvement. Perinatal history was uneventful. There were no significant family history suggestive of thromboembolic disorders and no history of recent vaccination. Investigations like routine blood count, peripheral smear, serum electrolytes, bleeding, and coagulation profile were done and found to be within normal limits. MRI brain suggested acute infarct involving the left capsuloganglionic region (Figures 1 and 2). Child was managed conservatively with osmotic diuretics to reduce perilesional oedema and also was started on anticoagulant therapy subcutaneously. Low molecular weight heparin was given for a total of 5 days and was stopped without any continuation of oral antiplatelet therapy. Parents could not afford other relevant investigations including MRA, Doppler evaluation of the vessels, lipoprotein A and homocysteine estimation, protein C and S, antithrombin III, and antiphospholipid antibody. The child started moving her right leg with gain in power after 12 hrs of anticoagulant therapy. The facial paralysis and the hemiparesis improved following 5 days of treatment and the child was discharged with advice of physiotherapy. Neurological evaluation on follow-up after 10 days of treatment showed good clinical resolution, with power 5/5 in both right upper and lower limbs with normal reflexes and no residual facial weakness.

## 3. Discussion

Minor head injuries are very common during childhood and are rarely complicated. Acute ischemic stroke most often presents as a focal neurologic deficit. Hemiplegia is the most common focal manifestation, occurring in up to 94% of stroke cases [7, 8]. Hemorrhagic strokes most commonly present as headaches or altered level of consciousness and are more likely to cause vomiting than in ischemic stroke [7–9]. In children, ischemic stroke following trivial head trauma is exceedingly rare and should be considered after systematic exclusion of other causes. The plausibility of an insult preexisting and resulting head injury may be difficult to discriminate. In our case, the child had a history of neurological signs after a fall witnessed by her parents. It is unlikely to be nonaccidental injury since there is no other supporting clinical or radiological evidence. The child presented with neurological deficits after 12 hours of a minor head injury. Kieslich et al. observed a latency of 15 min–16 days for the evolution of basal ganglia lesion following minor head injury [10].

The presentation of hemiplegia with UMN type facial palsy with no cortical signs suggests the probable location of the lesion above the level of pons in the subcortical region.

The pathophysiology of this case can be explained by the peculiarity of the blood vessels arrangement in the brain of a child compared to that of an adult. The basal ganglia and the internal capsule are supplied by the lenticulostriate arteries which are functional end arteries. They originate from the middle cerebral artery at acute angle (the angle is more acute in children) after which it follows a recurrent course and then pierces the anterior perforated substance. Therefore any motion of the brain due to head injury may disrupt these perforating branches leading to vessel damage and thereby causes a decrease in the blood flow or intimal trauma resulting in subsequent thrombosis or spasm [11]. Brain vasculature of children is more susceptible to shearing and conductive and other biomechanical forces than that of adults.

A hypothesis suggests that an injury to the middle cerebral artery leads to its spasm and associated reduction in PCO2 due to crying, resulting in narrowing of the blood vessel, thereby decreasing the blood supply and increasing the chances of thrombosis [3]. The relative delay in the occurrence of symptoms in this case may be explained on the basis of intimal injury followed by thrombus formation. Another possibility being, with an impact from a head injury the brain parenchyma moves in opposite direction, resulting in shearing and other effects on the vessels. As the angle at the origin of blood vessels from the MCA varies with age [12]

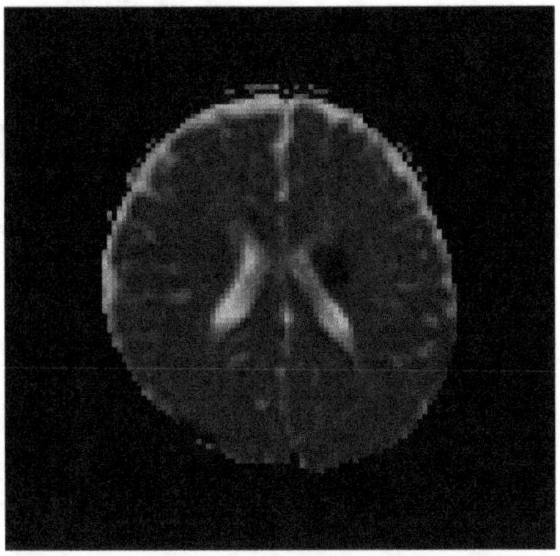

Figure 3: MRI brain (ADC) low signals noted in the left capsule-ganglionic region suggestive of acute infarct.

children are more susceptible to ischemic stroke. This can also be the cause in this case. Similar concerns are assumed by Kieslich et al. [10].

In this child, MRI brain showed acute infarct in the left capsuloganglionic region (Figure 3). This explains the clinical features that are seen.

Other acquired metabolic causes as well as genetic causes leading to thrombosis should have been ruled out. Acquired prothrombotic disorders secondary to deficiencies in protein C and S may occur in children with renal and liver disease, including nephrotic syndrome with loss of coagulation factors [4, 13]. Protein C deficiency has also been reported in children taking valproate [14]. Hemorrhagic strokes can arise from both factor VII and factor VIII deficiency [15, 16]. Iron deficiency anemia has been reported in children with both ischemic stroke and venous thrombosis with no other apparent etiology [5, 17, 18].

Among viral infections varicella is known to cause secondary vasculopathy, thus increasing the susceptibility to develop arterial thrombosis or spasm after minor head injury [19]. Varicella zoster virus reactivation is one of the potential causes of cerebral vasculopathy; for this reason, it must be considered in the differential diagnosis of pediatric transient ischemic attack and/or stroke, even when the rash is temporally remote from the acute event. However, there was no history suggestive of varicella in our case.

A genetic predisposition may also be attributed for the severity in manifestation of minor head injuries, resulting in the unfavourable outcome such as malignant syndrome which is characterized by delayed cerebral oedema and coma. A genetic mutation in the CANA1A calcium channel subunit genes was believed to be responsible for it [20].

Stroke in childhood is multifactorial. It is very important to exclude other causes of ischemic stroke in children. The common conditions predisposing to ischemic stroke include embolism due to congenital or acquired heart disease, thrombophilia and acute traumatic arterial dissections, dehydration, meningitis, acquired immunodeficiency syndrome, hemolytic uremic syndrome, homocystinuria, and syndromes like Down's syndrome and Williams syndrome [21, 22]. Other causes include sickle cell disease, which is a very common cause of pediatric stroke, occurring in 285 cases per 100,000 affected children [7]. Strokes may occur as early as 18 months of age, but most children present after five years of age [23]. Venous sinus thrombosis can present in all ages with fever and lethargy; an older child would likely present with more slowly progressing signs, such as vomiting, headache, or any other signs of increased intracranial pressure [24].

Here, the case showed no abnormality with the routine blood investigations. There are no features of anemia, high counts, and abnormal cells, thereby excluding the causes discussed above. There are no features and investigations suggestive of other organ involvement. This helped in narrowing the possibility of the cause, to be traumatic etiology.

Usually the prognosis of pediatric stroke is good. Our child showed good progress with anticoagulant therapy and had complete improvement in 10 days.

Many authors mentioned such cases in the literature like Rana et al. who presented 7 cases of ischemic stroke in minor head injury in children [25].

The clinical manifestations and the radiological features following a minor head injury, with exclusion of other causes with relevant available investigations, suggest a confederation among ischemic stroke and trivial head injuries by the aforementioned assumed mechanisms.

An elaborated history, with multidisciplinary approach in evaluation of ischemic strokes in pediatric patients with head injury, makes way for the future to prove the expected association.

## Consent

A written informed consent was taken from the parent of the child for the publication of this case report and accompanying images.

## Competing Interests

The authors declare that they have no competing interests.

## References

[1] A. N. Williams, "Running around in circles following ischemic stroke," *Archives of Disease in Childhood*, vol. 88, no. 8, article 743, 2003.

[2] V. Kalra, *Practical Paediatric Neurology*, Arya Publication, New Delhi, India, 1st edition, 1999.

[3] L. Shaffer, P. M. Rich, K. R. E. Pohl, and V. Ganesan, "Can mild head injury cause ischaemic stroke?" *Archives of Disease in Childhood*, vol. 88, no. 3, pp. 267–269, 2003.

[4] K. S. Carvalho and B. P. Garg, "Arterial strokes in children," *Neurologic Clinics*, vol. 20, no. 4, pp. 1079–1100, 2002.

[5] V. Ganesan, M. Prengler, M. A. McShane, A. M. Wade, and F. J. Kirkham, "Investigation of risk factors in children with arterial ischemic stroke," *Annals of Neurology*, vol. 53, no. 2, pp. 167–173, 2003.

[6] L. J. Kappelle, J. Willemse, L. M. P. Ramos, and J. Van Gijn, "Ischaemic stroke in the basal ganglia and internal capsule in childhood," *Brain and Development*, vol. 11, no. 5, pp. 283–292, 1989.

[7] C. J. Earley, S. J. Kittner, B. R. Feeser et al., "Stroke in children and sickle-cell disease: Baltimore-Washington cooperative young stroke study," *Neurology*, vol. 51, no. 1, pp. 169–176, 1998.

[8] O. Eeg Olofsson and Y. Ringheim, "Stroke in children. Clinical characteristics and prognosis," *Acta Paediatrica Scandinavica*, vol. 72, no. 3, pp. 391–395, 1983.

[9] W. Zenz, Z. Bodó, J. Plotho et al., "Factor V Leiden and prothrombin gene G 20210 a variant in children with ischemic stroke," *Thrombosis and Haemostasis*, vol. 80, no. 5, pp. 763–766, 1998.

[10] M. Kieslich, A. Fiedler, C. Heller, W. Kreuz, and G. Jacobi, "Minor head injury as cause and co-factor in the aetiology of stroke in childhood: a report of eight cases," *Journal of Neurology Neurosurgery and Psychiatry*, vol. 73, no. 1, pp. 13–16, 2002.

[11] S. R. Dharker, R. S. Mittal, N. Bhargava, L. F. Marshall, and H. M. Eisenberg, "Ischemic lesions in basal ganglia in children after minor head injury," *Neurosurgery*, vol. 33, no. 5, pp. 863–865, 1993.

[12] K. K. Jain, "Some observations of anatomy of the middle cerebral artery," *Canadian Journal of Surgery*, vol. 7, pp. 134–139, 1964.

[13] N. Schlegel, "Thromboembolic risks and complications in nephrotic children," *Seminars in Thrombosis and Hemostasis*, vol. 23, no. 3, pp. 271–280, 1997.

[14] R. Gruppo, A. DeGrauw, H. Fogelson, T. Glauser, V. Balasa, and P. Gartside, "Protein C deficiency related to valproic acid therapy: a possible association with childhood stroke," *The Journal of Pediatrics*, vol. 137, no. 5, pp. 714–718, 2000.

[15] G. L. Bray and N. L. C. Luban, "Hemophilia presenting with intracranial hemorrhage. An approach to the infant with intracranial bleeding and coagulopathy," *American Journal of Diseases of Children*, vol. 141, no. 11, pp. 1215–1217, 1987.

[16] M. Ries, D. Wölfel, and B. Maier-Brandt, "Severe intracranial hemorrhage in a newborn infant with transplacental transfer of an acquired factor VIII:C inhibitor," *The Journal of Pediatrics*, vol. 127, no. 4, pp. 649–650, 1995.

[17] D. S. Hartfield, N. J. Lowry, D. L. Keene, and J. Y. Yager, "Iron deficiency: a cause of stroke in infants and children," *Pediatric Neurology*, vol. 16, no. 1, pp. 50–53, 1997.

[18] J. L. Maguire, G. Deveber, and P. C. Parkin, "Association between iron-deficiency anemia and stroke in young children," *Pediatrics*, vol. 120, no. 5, pp. 1053–1057, 2007.

[19] J. B. Bodensteiner, M. R. Hille, and J. E. Riggs, "Clinical features of vasculopathy associated with primary varicella infection," *The American Journal of Diseases of Children*, vol. 146, article 100, 1992.

[20] E. E. Kors, G. M. Terwindt, F. L. M. G. Vermeulen et al., "Delayed cerebral edema and fatal coma after minor head trauma: role of the CACNA1A calcium channel subunit gene and relationship with familial hemiplegic migraine," *Annals of Neurology*, vol. 49, no. 6, pp. 753–760, 2001.

[21] F. J. Kirkham, "Stroke in children," *Archives of Disease in Childhood*, vol. 81, no. 1, pp. 85–89, 1999.

[22] F. J. Kirkham, M. Prengler, D. K. M. Hewes, and V. Ganesan, "Risk factors for arterial ischemic stroke in children," *Journal of Child Neurology*, vol. 15, no. 5, pp. 299–307, 2000.

[23] W. S. Ball Jr., "Cerebrovascular occlusive disease in childhood," *Neuroimaging Clinics of North America*, vol. 4, no. 2, pp. 393–421, 1994.

[24] K. S. Carvalho, J. B. Bodensteiner, P. J. Connolly, and B. P. Garg, "Cerebral venous thrombosis in children," *Journal of Child Neurology*, vol. 16, no. 8, pp. 574–580, 2001.

[25] K. S. Rana, M. K. Behera, and K. M. Adhikari, "Ischemic stroke following mild head injury: is it the cause?" *Indian Pediatrics*, vol. 43, no. 11, pp. 994–997, 2006.

# A Rare Case of Carotid Web Presenting with Ischemic Stroke in a Young Woman and a Brief Review of the Literature

**Kyaw Kyaw**,[1] **Htun Latt**,[2] **Sammy San Myint Aung**,[1] **Jay Babu**,[3] **and Rajesh Rangaswamy**[4]

[1]*Institute for Heart and Vascular Health, Renown Regional Medical Center, 1500 E. 2nd St. No. 302, Reno, NV 89502, USA*
[2]*Department of Internal Medicine, University of Nevada, Reno School of Medicine, 1155 Mill St. No. W11, Reno, NV 89502, USA*
[3]*Department of Biology, University of Nevada, Reno, 1664 N. Virginia Street, Reno, NV 89557, USA*
[4]*Department of Radiology, Renown Regional Medical Center, 1155 Mill St., Reno, NV 89502, USA*

Correspondence should be addressed to Kyaw Kyaw; drkyawkyawmd@gmail.com

Academic Editor: Simon Ching-Shun Kao

Carotid web is a radiological description of a shelf-like intraluminal filling defect in the carotid bulb. It is histologically defined as atypical fibromuscular dysplasia (FMD), with abnormal fibrosis and smooth muscle cell hyperplasia in the *tunica intima*. The spur-like intraluminal protrusion can serve as a nidus for thrombus formation, which could cause systemic embolism and ischemic strokes. We report a case of a 20-year-old female patient presenting with acute ischemic stroke in the ipsilateral middle cerebral artery (MCA) territory. We also discuss the incidence, the prevalence, the pathophysiology, the treatment, and the recurrence of carotid web based on the currently available literature.

## 1. Introduction

Carotid web is a radiological description of a shelf-like intraluminal filling defect in the carotid bulb [1–4]. The word "web" was firstly used by Momose and New to analyze the causes of nonatheromatous stenosis in the internal carotid artery (ICA) in 1973 [5]. Because of the extreme rarity and unfamiliarity of the disease, the carotid web was variously described in the literature as carotid bulb web, carotid bulb diaphragm, carotid bulb septa, pseudovalvular folds, atypical fibromuscular dysplasia, and atypical fibromuscular hyperplasia [6]. Carotid web is a very rare cause of ischemic stroke in young patients (age < 60 years old) with suspected stroke [1–4]. Here, we report a case of a 20-year-old female patient with left carotid web, who presented with acute ischemic stroke in ipsilateral middle cerebral artery (MCA) territory.

## 2. Case Description

A 20-year-old Caucasian female with no known medical problem was transferred to our facility for left MCA stroke 8 hours after the new onset of aphasia. She initially presented to outside facility where magnetic resonance imaging of the brain (MRI brain) without contrast showed acute ischemic infarct involving the distribution of left MCA, approximately 9 cm in the area of left temporoparietal lobe (Figure 1). MR angiogram (MRA) showed total occlusion of M1 segment of left MCA (Figure 2). Her only medication was oral contraceptive pill, and she was a nonsmoker.

At our facility, vital signs were stable. On examination, expressive aphasia and slight right-sided facial droop were noted. Other cranial nerves including facial sensation were intact. Gross motor and sensory functions, deep tendon reflexes, and Babinski reflexes were normal. NIH Stroke Scale/Score (NIHSS) was 6 (1B +2, aphasic; 1C +2, unable to perform tasks for blink eyes and squeeze hands; 10 +2, severe dysarthria). Neurology was immediately consulted. Aspirin suppository 300 mg was given rectally and shortly afterwards, and atorvastatin 80 mg was given through a nasogastric tube. However, no tissue plasminogen activator (tPA) was given since she was outside therapeutic window. Computed tomography angiogram (CTA) neck showed a short segment of partially recanalized vessel between M1

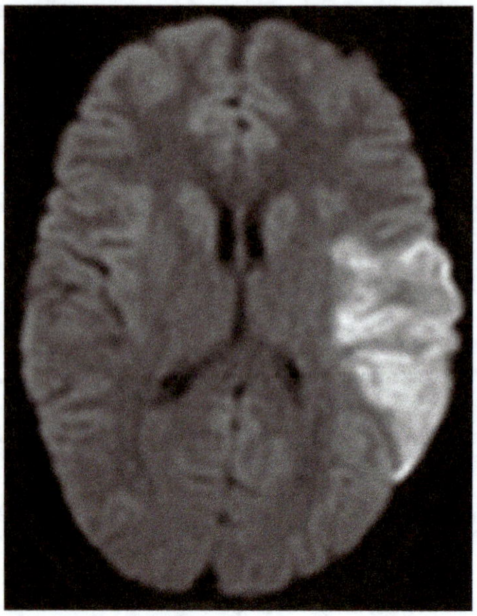

FIGURE 1: MRI brain without contrast (DWI—diffusion-weighted image) showing acute ischemic infarct in left temporoparietal lobe in the distribution of left MCA.

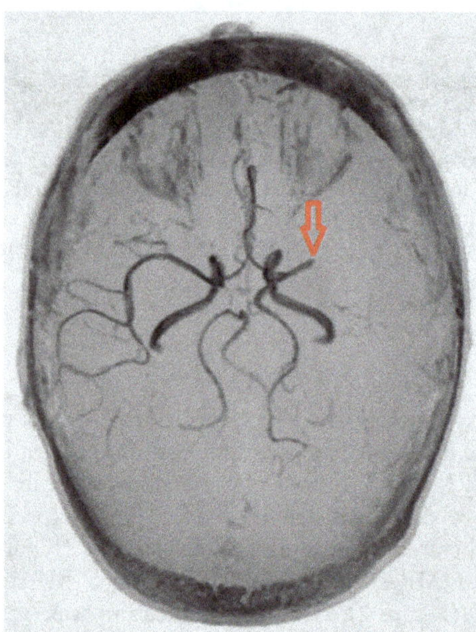

FIGURE 2: MRA brain showing total occlusion of M1 segment of left MCA (red arrow) and normal circle of Willis.

and M2 segments of left MCA (Figure 3). Also CTA neck revealed a short segment of linear filling defect in proximal left ICA, most consistent with a carotid web (Figure 4). Neurointerventionist and vascular surgeon were consulted, and both consultants deferred any invasive procedure because of acute cerebrovascular accident (CVA), large area of infarct, and partial recanalization of the previously thrombosed vessel as evidenced in CTA. No anticoagulation was given, but clopidogrel was added. She was conservatively treated with permissive hypertension. Twelve-lead resting electrocardiogram showed normal sinus rhythm.

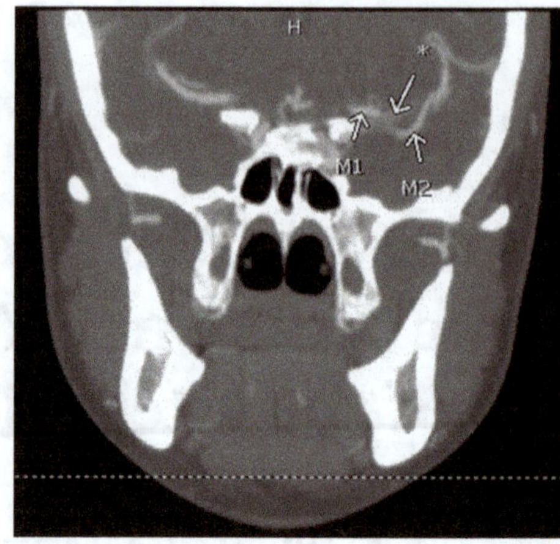


FIGURE 3: CTA neck showing a short segment of partially recanalized vessel (∗) between M1 and M2 segments of left MCA.

Later, workup for hypercoagulability and vasculitis was done. Blood tests showed normal protein C and S and antithrombin III levels. Factor V Leiden, C-reactive protein, antinuclear antibody, pregnancy test, and lupus anticoagulant were negative. Transthoracic echocardiogram with saline (bubble) study was performed and showed no evidence of right to left shunt by agitated saline challenge. MR venogram was normal. She continued to have severe dysphagia, requiring feeding gastrostomy tube. No new or recurrent events were noted during the hospital stay. No abnormal rhythm was reported on cardiac monitor. She was discharged on conservative medical therapy with aspirin, clopidogrel, and atorvastatin.

## 3. Discussion

Carotid web is identified in angiogram as a linear spur-like intraluminal projection along the posterior wall of proximal internal carotid artery (ICA) on oblique sagittal section and as a septum on axial section [1, 2]. It recently has been referred as an atypical variant of fibromuscular dysplasia (FMD), with histological feature of abnormal fibrosis and smooth muscle cell hyperplasia in the tunica intima [3, 7–11]. Typical FMD has abnormal cell growth within the tunica media. Furthermore, typical FMD usually occurs in renal and carotid arteries of middle-age white women but is rarely symptomatic [7, 10, 11]. In contrast, the atypical FMD with abnormal intimal cell growth in the carotid web tends to extend into the arterial lumen and creates turbulent flow [1]. It serves as a nidus of thrombus formation and may cause ischemic stroke via arterial embolism [1–4].

Limited data are available for the epidemiology of carotid webs. We reviewed and summarized 4 recent case-control studies regarding the incidence and prevalence of carotid web. Joux et al. reported the incidence of carotid web with ipsilateral stroke was 3.8 (4.3 in women and 3.2 in men) per 100,000 person-year in young Afro-Caribbean population [2]. Choi et al. and Coutinho et al. estimated that the prevalence of carotid web was 1.0–1.2% in patients who were suspected of strokes and underwent CTA [1, 4]. And Sajedi

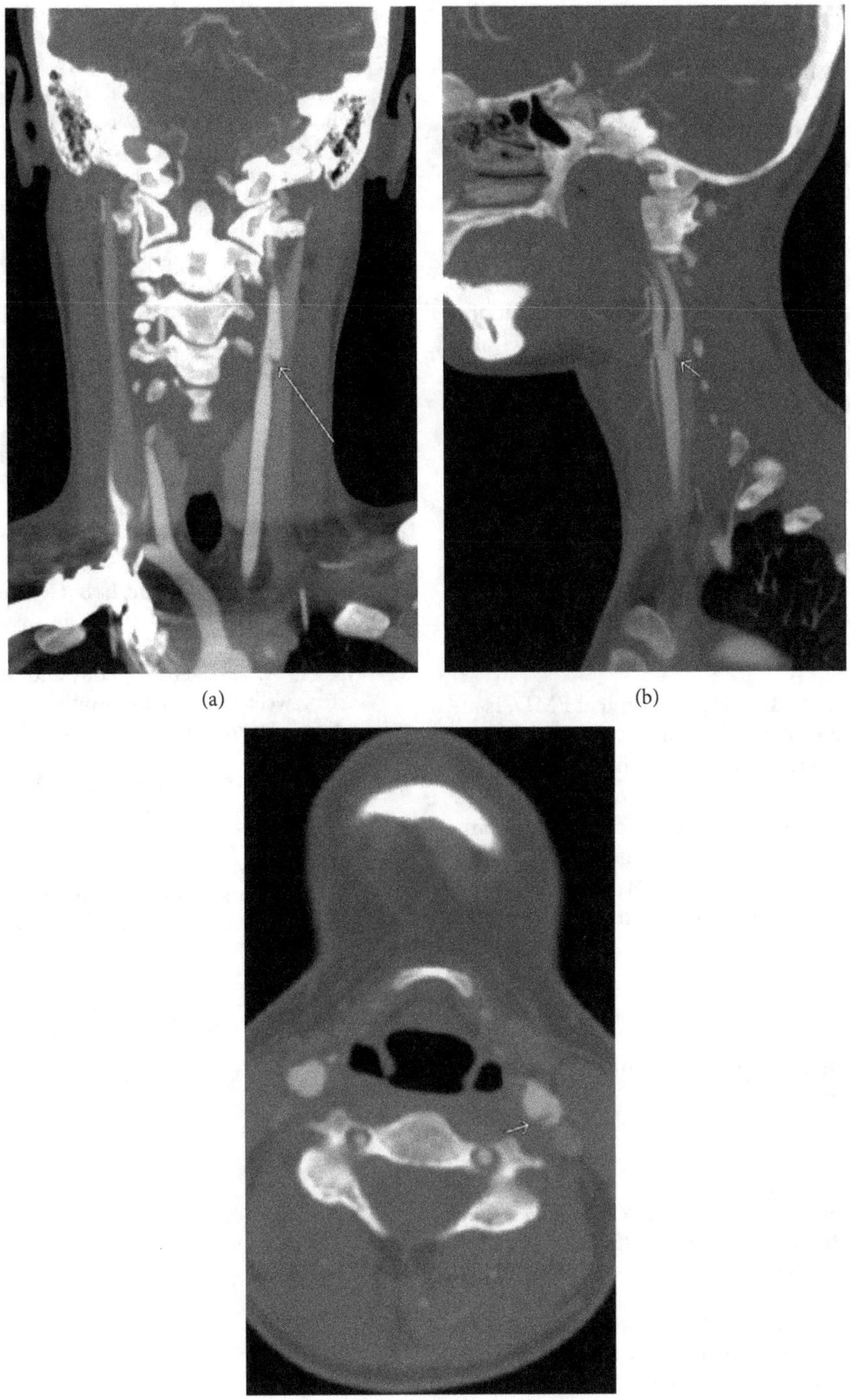

(a) (b) (c)

FIGURE 4: CTA neck showing carotid web in the left internal carotid artery (arrows).

et al. outlined that the prevalence of carotid web was 9.4–37% in stroke patients without identifiable cause as against 1–7% in nonstroke patients [2–4]. The mean age of symptomatic carotid web was 38.3–46.7 years old [2, 3]. Generally, the carotid web is more common in young women with strokes of unknown origin [1–4].

The etiology of carotid web is unknown. Some possible explanations are genetic propensity, chronic vascular injury, hormonal factors, and vasa vasorum abnormalities [9]. Oral contraceptive (OC) pills may cause arterial intimal hyperplasia in young women and could be a possible cause of carotid web [12, 13]. Carotid web may present with ischemic stroke in ipsilateral MCA territory. It is often diagnosed by CTA though it can be detected in sonogram or MRI [14–16]. Digital subtraction angiography (DSA) is the gold standard test for carotid web. The current treatment of carotid web includes carotid endarterectomy (CEA), endovascular stenting, and conservative medical therapy with antiplatelet or anticoagulant. In 2014, Joux et al. published 30% recurrent symptoms of carotid web in patients with antiplatelet therapy and no recurrent symptoms of carotid web in patients with surgical therapy [17]. To date, no large studies have reported the recurrent rate among the patients treated with endovascular stenting or anticoagulant therapy. CEA or endovascular stenting is preferred to prevent recurrence of stroke [3, 6, 8, 17].

Our 20-year-old Caucasian female patient initially presented with left MCA infarct as evidenced in MRI and MRA brain. Subsequently, a proximal left ICA carotid web was discovered in carotid CTA. Workup was negative for vasculitis, hypercoagulability, and right to left intracardiac shunt. And MRV of the brain was unremarkable. Because of the acute CVA, large infarct size, and partial recanalization of the previously thrombosed MCA as evidenced in CTA, no intervention was performed during this admission. Follow-up is planned in next 4 weeks for further management.

## 4. Conclusion

Carotid web, a radiological entity and an atypical FMD, is an exceptionally rare cause of acute ischemic stroke in young patients. Since its first description in 1973, the knowledge of the rare disease has been expanded. However, more studies are demanded for a better understanding of the epidemiology, pathophysiology, treatment, and prognosis of carotid web. Our case highlights the awareness of carotid web in young patients, who have ischemic stroke in MCA territory without any identifiable cause.

## Conflicts of Interest

The authors declare that there are no conflicts of interest regarding the publication of this paper.

## References


[1] P. M. C. Choi, D. Singh, A. Trivedi et al., "Carotid webs and recurrent ischemic strokes in the era of CT angiography," *American Journal of Neuroradiology*, vol. 36, no. 11, pp. 2134–2139, 2015.

[2] J. Joux, M. Boulanger, S. Jeannin et al., "Association between carotid bulb diaphragm and ischemic stroke in young Afro-Caribbean patients," *Stroke*, vol. 47, no. 10, pp. 2641–2644, 2016.

[3] P. I. Sajedi, J. N. Gonzalez, C. A. Cronin et al., "Carotid bulb webs as a cause of "cryptogenic" ischemic stroke," *American Journal of Neuroradiology*, vol. 38, no. 7, pp. 1399–1404, 2017.

[4] J. M. Coutinho, S. Derkatch, A. R. Potvin et al., "Carotid artery web and ischemic stroke: a case-control study," *Neurology*, vol. 88, no. 1, pp. 65–69, 2017.

[5] K. J. Momose and P. F. New, "Non-atheromatous stenosis and occlusion of the internal carotid artery and its main branches," *American Journal of Roentgenology*, vol. 118, no. 3, pp. 550–566, 1973.

[6] A. H. Elmokadem, S. A. Ansari, R. Sangha, S. Prabhakaran, A. Shaibani, and MC. Hurley, "Neurointerventional management of carotid webs associated with recurrent and acute cerebral ischemic syndromes," *Interventional Neuroradiology*, vol. 22, no. 4, pp. 432–437, 2016.

[7] A. G. Osborn and R. E. Anderson, "Angiographic spectrum of cervical and intracranial fibromuscular dysplasia," *Stroke*, vol. 8, no. 5, pp. 617–626, 1977.

[8] D. Verscheure, D. Fabre, D. Smadja, and E. Fadel, "Symptomatic carotid-bulb atypical fibromuscular dysplasia," *Annals of Vascular Surgery*, vol. 43, pp. 310.e1–310.e3, 2017.

[9] F. P. Wirth, W. A. Miller, and A. P. Russell, "Atypical fibromuscular hyperplasia: report of two cases," *Journal of Neurosurgery*, vol. 54, no. 5, pp. 685–689, 1981.

[10] S. Watanabe, K. Tanaka, T. Nakayama, and M. Kaneko, "Fibromuscular dysplasia at the internal carotid origin: a case of carotid web," *No shinkei Geka. Neurological Surgery*, vol. 21, no. 5, pp. 449–452, 1993.

[11] E. Touzé, C. Oppenheim, D. Trystram et al., "Fibromuscular dysplasia of cervical and intracranial arteries," *International Journal of Stroke*, vol. 5, no. 4, pp. 296–305, 2010.

[12] N. S. Irey, H. A. McAllister, and J. M. Henry, "Oral contraceptives and stroke in young women: a clinicopathologic correlation," *Neurology*, vol. 28, no. 12, p. 1216, 1978.

[13] J. C. Morgenlander and L. B. Goldstein, "Recurrent transient ischemic attacks and stroke in association with an internal carotid artery web," *Stroke*, vol. 22, no. 1, pp. 94–98, 1991.

[14] W. Fu, A. Crockett, G. Low, and V. Patel, "Internal carotid artery web: Doppler ultrasound with CT angiography correlation," *Journal of Radiology Case Reports*, vol. 9, no. 5, p. 1, 2015.

[15] M. E. Boesen, P. V. Eswaradass, D. Singh et al., "MR imaging of carotid webs," *Neuroradiology*, vol. 59, no. 4, pp. 361–365, 2017.

[16] J. Joux, M. Mejdoubi, J. B. Quere et al., "MRI characteristics of carotid bulb atypical fibromuscular dysplasia in black stroke patients," *Journal of Neuroradiology*, vol. 43, no. 3, pp. 214–217, 2016.

[17] J. Joux, N. Chausson, S. Jeannin et al., "Carotid-bulb atypical fibromuscular dysplasia in young Afro-Caribbean patients with stroke," *Stroke*, vol. 45, no. 12, pp. 3711–3713, 2014.

# 25

# The Presence of a Large Chiari Network in a Patient with Atrial Fibrillation and Stroke

**Nneka Schwimmer-Okike,[1] Johannes Niebuhr,[1] Grit Gesine Ruth Schramek,[2] Stefan Frantz,[3] and Heike Kielstein[1]**

[1]*Department of Anatomy and Cell Biology, Faculty of Medicine, Martin Luther University Halle-Wittenberg, 06108 Halle (Saale), Germany*
[2]*Institute for Pathology, University Hospital Halle, 06108 Halle (Saale), Germany*
[3]*Department of Internal Medicine III, University Hospital Halle, 06120 Halle (Saale), Germany*

Correspondence should be addressed to Heike Kielstein; heike.kielstein@medizin.uni-halle.de

Academic Editor: Assad Movahed

The Chiari network is an embryological remnant found in the right atrium, mostly without any significant pathophysiological consequences. However, several cardiac associations are reported in the literature including supraventricular tachyarrhythmias. We present a case of a 96-year-old body donor with a stroke episode and intermittent atrial fibrillations. The dissection of the heart revealed the presence of an immense Chiari network with a large central thrombus. The role of a Chiari network in the pathogenesis of stroke and pulmonary embolism is discussed.

## 1. Introduction

While the fetal heart is developing the venous confluence in the right atrium has two valves, called Eustachii and Thebesii. Both valves are secured in the right atrium by the septum spurium. Later in the development these valves and the septum spurium usually regress. However, in some cases the regression remains incomplete resulting in a cor triatriatum. In cases of a partial regression, a fenestrated membrane remains, the so-called Chiari network [1]. While Carl von Rokitansky is believed to be the first describing this anatomical remnant in a single case, it was named after Hans Chiari who described it in a review of 11 cases [2]. In the beginning the Chiari network was believed to be clinically silent, but several publications showed a possible link to cardiac diseases like embolism [3], infective endocarditis [4], or supraventricular tachyarrhythmias [5]. In the vast majority of published cases the Chiari network was diagnosed and illustrated by echocardiography. Here, we report a case of a Chiari network with prior atrial fibrillation and stroke. The immense Chiari network is shown in the dissected heart of the patient.

## 2. Case Report

A 96-year-old man was hospitalized because of a neurological failure. The patient showed a flaccid paralysis of the right arm and leg, an incomplete facial paresis on the right, dysphagia, global aphasia, and unilateral neglect, suggesting a stroke. The cranial CT showed no signs of bleeding and no middle line shift. Electrocardiography revealed a tachyarrhythmia caused by an atrial fibrillation with a rate of 100–140 beats/min. Patients' medical record showed intermitted atrial fibrillations and a thrombectomy due to a TIA (transient ischemic attack) six years ahead of the current event. A treated prostate cancer and nontreated squamous cell cancer were further diagnoses of the patient. One month later and still under observation and treatment the patient died in the hospital.

According to his living will the deceased became a body donor for the dissection course at our Institute for Anatomy. During the examination and dissection of the heart the students discovered a net-like structure with a large central thrombus inside the right atrium in close proximity to the inferior vena cava. Figure 1 shows the orifice of the inferior vena cava with view to the thrombus. After the removal of

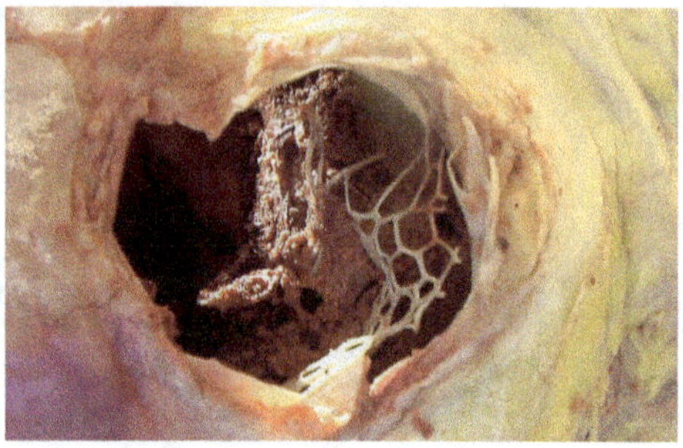

FIGURE 1: Large thrombus in the center of the Chiari network within the right atrium of the heart.

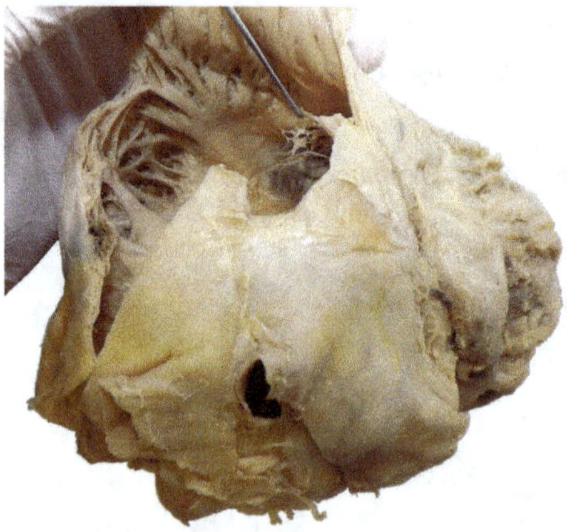

FIGURE 2: Opened right atrium of the heart and an overview of the Chiari network.

the thrombus a careful examination of the net structure was performed showing its fixation in the inner surface of the right atrium. The histological examination of the resected net structure showed mainly fibrous connective tissue and no cardiomyocytes. The microscopic and macroscopic aspects are consistent with the Chiari network. Figures 2 and 3 show an overview and the opened right atrium and the immense size of the net (4.0 × 2.5 cm). Because of the stiffness of the tissue caused by the fixation procedure of the body donor we neither could confirm nor ruled out further heart malformations like a patent foramen ovale.

## 3. Discussion

The Chiari network is an anomaly of the heart with a prevalence ranging from 1.3 to 4.0% [6]. However, more recent studies show prevalence rates up to 10.5% [7]. This anatomic variation and embryologic remnant is believed to be mostly clinical inapparent. Nevertheless, several cases have been described showing relevant pathophysiological consequences. Chang described a case of tricuspid valve regurgitation caused by a Chiari network [8] and Goedde and coworkers showed a case of supraventricular fibrillations demanding the surgical removal of the Chiari network [9].

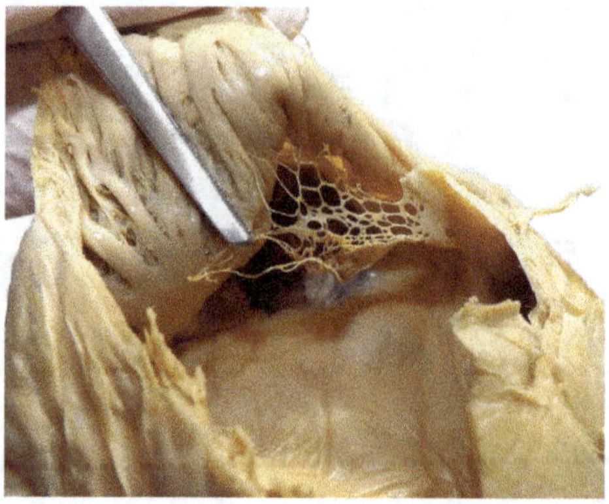

FIGURE 3: Fixed Chiari network in proximity to the inferior vena cava after removal of the thrombus.

Atrial fibrillation and tricuspid valve regurgitation are relevant diseases and therefore the presence of a Chiari network has to be taken seriously.

The case described by Goedde and coworkers has various similarities with the case presented here: both patients had a Chiari network with a thrombus enmeshed in between. The medical records of both patients showed atrial fibrillations and atrial embolism. While the patient in the case report from Goedde and coworkers suffered from a pulmonary embolism, the patient in the present case had a stroke.

The presence of a patent foramen ovale is a prerequisite to cause a paradoxical embolism, leading to a stroke or pulmonary embolism. Schneider and coworkers demonstrated significantly higher prevalence rates for a patent foramen ovale in patients with a Chiari network and herewith a serious risk for the development of an atrial embolism [10]. However, other studies showed a rather minor role of the presence of a patent foramen ovale in the pathogenesis of paradoxical embolism [11]. Various cases of patients suffering a paradoxical embolism without patent foramen ovale have been published [12, 13].

To date, only few photographs of a Chiari network have been published. Here we show an immense Chiari network as the possible cause for the longtime intermittent atrial fibrillation, a TIA, and a stroke, finally leading to the death of the patient. In conclusion, the possibility of the presence of a Chiari network with or without a patent foramen ovale should be taken into consideration as a possible (additional) diagnosis for a patient suffering from embolism, infective endocarditis, or supraventricular arrthythmias.

## Competing Interests

The authors declare that they have no competing interests.

## References

[1] D. Franck, "Über atypische Diaphragmen und Sehnenfäden des menschlichen Herzens," *Virchows Archiv*, vol. 349, no. 2, pp. 152–162, 1970.

[2] H. Chiari, "Über netzbildungen im rechten vorhofe des herzens," *Virchows Archiv*, vol. 22, pp. 1–10, 1897.

[3] P. Edwards, M. Wozniak, M. Corretti, and T. R. Price, "Cardiac Chiari network as an etiology for embolic stroke," *Journal of Stroke and Cerebrovascular Diseases*, vol. 4, no. 4, pp. 238–241, 1994.

[4] N. Mousavi, K. Bhagirath, V. Ariyarajah et al., "Chiari network endocarditis: not just an innocent bystander," *Echocardiography*, vol. 25, no. 6, pp. 642–645, 2008.

[5] D. Dregoesc, M. Rejent, A. Zhang, and R. Abousy, "Incidental discovery of Chiari network in a patient with new onset of atrial fibrillation," *Journal of Clinical Case Reports*, vol. 4, no. 2, article 331, pp. 1–2, 2013.

[6] W. M. Yater, "The paradox of Chiari's network: review and report of a case of Chiari's network ensnaring a large embolus," *American Heart Journal*, vol. 11, no. 5, pp. 542–553, 1936.

[7] K. P. Bhatnagar, G. S. Nettleton, F. R. Campbell, C. E. Wagner, N. Kuwabara, and H. Muresian, "Chiari anomalies in the human right atrium," *Clinical Anatomy*, vol. 19, no. 6, pp. 510–516, 2006.

[8] J.-P. Chang, "Tricuspid regurgitation as a result of Chiari network attachment," *Journal of Thoracic and Cardiovascular Surgery*, vol. 143, no. 1, p. 235, 2012.

[9] T. A. Goedde, D. Conetta, and J. D. Rumisek, "Chiari network entrapment of thromboemboli: congenital inferior vena cava filter," *The Annals of Thoracic Surgery*, vol. 49, no. 2, pp. 317–318, 1990.

[10] B. Schneider, T. Hofmann, M. H. Justen, and T. Meinertz, "Chiari's network: normal anatomic variant or risk factor for arterial embolic events?" *Journal of the American College of Cardiology*, vol. 26, no. 1, pp. 203–210, 1995.

[11] B. Meier, "Patent foramen ovale, guilty but only as a gang member and for a lesser crime," *Journal of the American College of Cardiology*, vol. 47, no. 2, pp. 446–448, 2006.

[12] A. C. Pearson, D. Nagelhout, R. Castello, C. R. Gomez, and A. J. Labovitz, "Atrial septal aneurysm and stroke: a transesophageal echocardiographic study," *Journal of the American College of Cardiology*, vol. 18, no. 5, pp. 1223–1229, 1991.

[13] L. S. Ralston and W. A. Wasdahl, "Chiari's network," *The American Journal of Medicine*, vol. 25, no. 5, pp. 810–813, 1958.

# 26

# A Rare Case of Fatal Hemorrhagic Stroke in a Young Female with Early Mixed Connective Tissue Disease

**James R. Agapoff IV**

*Department of Psychiatry, University of Hawai'i at Mānoa, John A. Burns School of Medicine, Honolulu, HI, USA*

Correspondence should be addressed to James R. Agapoff IV; nubis13@gmail.com

Academic Editor: Gregory J. Tsay

Mixed connective tissue disease (MCTD) often presents as a slow progressive illness with low morbidity and mortality. Serious central nervous system disease is uncommon, and fatal outcomes are rarely seen. Here, we report a rare case of fatal hemorrhagic stroke in a 43-year-old female with a rapidly progressive MCTD. She presented to primary care with a history of headaches, visual disturbances, and unprovoked lower extremity swelling and pain. A rheumatological workup showed positive antinuclear (ANA) and ribonucleoprotein (RNP) antibodies. Magnetic resonance imaging (MRI) found a 12 mm hemorrhage along a cortical sulcus of the right frontal lobe, and a follow-up magnetic resonance angiography (MRA) and ophthalmological exam showed no definitive signs of vasculitis. Over the course of her workup, she developed swollen hands, Raynaud's syndrome, myalgias, and synovitis characteristic of evolving MCTD. The patient then began to experience severe headaches over one month. Repeat MRI was ordered, but never completed, and the patient presented to the emergency department (ED) with a severe, right-sided headache, and left-sided visual disturbance. In the ED, she began to display evidence of delirium and seizure activity and became unresponsive. A computerized tomography scan (CT) of the brain showed a right parietal lobe intraparenchymal hemorrhage approximately $5 \times 3 \times 5$ cm in size with secondary mass effect including mid- and hind-brain herniation. Computerized tomography angiography (CTA) of the brain showed signs of large vessel vasculitis. A craniectomy was performed; however, the patient never regained consciousness and died several days later. Vasculitis, while rare in connective tissue diseases, should be aggressively assessed for and managed in patients with any early signs and symptoms of cerebrovascular involvement to prevent fatal outcomes.

## 1. Introduction

Mixed connective tissue disease (MCTD) is an autoimmune condition characterized by overlapping features of several connective tissue diseases including polymyositis, rheumatoid arthritis, systemic lupus erythematosus, and systemic sclerosis in the presence of high levels of RNP antibodies [1]. Of the diagnostic algorithms available, the Alarcon–Segovia's and Kahn's criteria are considered to have highest sensitivity and specificity [2].

MCTD is a rare disease with incidence rates between 0.2 and 2.1 per 100,000 person-years based on several studies [1, 3, 4]. In one nationwide sample, the prevalence of MCTD was 3.8 (95% CI 3.2 to 4.4) per 100,000 adults, the average age was 37.9 years (95% CI: 35.3 to 40.4 years), and the diagnostic ratio of females to males was 3.3 [3].

Compared to other connective tissue diseases, MCTD is generally considered to have lower morbidity and mortality. In one study, mortality to MCTD did not differ from the general population sampled with a mortality ratio of 1.1 (95% CI, 0.4–2.6) [1]. In another study, 15-year survival rates from diagnosis were 88% [5]. Survival rates may be better considering that it often takes a median time of 3.6 years to make the diagnosis from the onset of first symptoms.

Neurological symptoms are uncommon in MCTD; headache, seizure, encephalopathy, aseptic meningitis, and neuropathy are seen in 10–20% of patients. Reports of immune-mediated central nervous system (CNS) vasculitis seen as the initial presentation of MCTD are uncommon [6–8].

Here, we report on the case of a 43-year-old, healthy Caucasian female, with rapidly progressive MCTD who developed neurological symptoms and later died of hemorrhagic stroke associated with probable CNS vasculitis.

## 2. Case Presentation

A 43-year-old healthy Caucasian female presented to primary care with short (7–10 days), recurrent flares of lower extremity tenderness, swelling, and redness over several months. She also reported myalgias in the upper back and neck, and a one-year history of headache with transient, reoccurring curtain-like visual disturbances in her right eye that ophthalmology diagnosed as ocular migraines. A rheumatologic workup was initiated. Labs were positive for an elevated sedimentation rate (ESR) 31 mm/H (normal 0–20 mmH), positive antinuclear antibodies (ANA), and an elevated ribonucleoprotein antibodies (RNP) 2.4 AI (reference <1.0 AI). Double-stranded (DS) DNA 1 IU/mL (<4 = Neg), antichromatin (AC), anti-Smith (SM), SM/RNP, and lyme disease antibodies were negative. Based on these results, the patient received a presumptive diagnosis of undifferentiated connective tissue disease (UCTD), started 20 mg of oral prednisone as needed for flares, and referred to rheumatology.

Two months after her initial evaluation, the patient continued to experience episodes or erythema nodosum of the lower extremities. She also began to experience early signs of Raynaud's phenomenon, chest pain, and visual disturbances concerning for amaurosis fugax. A personal symptom journal kept by the patient indicated transient episodes of fatigue and painful hand/finger swelling with petechiae and purpura. Magnetic resonance imaging (MRI) of the brain was ordered, and repeat labs done by rheumatology showed an elevated ESR, 39 mm/H; RNP, 1.8 AI; CRP, 3.7 (normal <0.8 mg/dL); and a negative anti-neutrophil cytoplasmic antibody (ANCA), myeloperoxidase antibodies, proteinase-3 antibodies, and ANA. Complement C3, 118 mg/dL (normal 90–180 mg/dL), and C4, 29 mg/dL (normal 16–47 mg/dL), were within normal limits. The patient was referred for further evaluation at an academic medical center.

The MRI showed a 6 mm lacunar infarct within the left cerebellum and a 12 mm hemorrhage along a cortical sulcus of the right frontal lobe. The findings were noted to be "abnormal" for a woman in her early forties, and a further work was recommended for vasculitis and/or connective tissue disease via magnetic resonance angiography (MRA). The MRA and ophthalmological assessment were unremarkable, and cardiology found no evidence of vascular disease on carotid ultrasound and no evidence of exercise-induced myocardial ischemia on stress echocardiogram.

A second rheumatological consult was completed where concern for possible evolving MCTD was raised; however, the diagnosis of UCTD was retained due to the negative ANA. Seven months following her initial presentation, the patient saw neurology where she reported worsening lightheadedness and 6-7/10 bifrontal/apical headaches lasting hours to days over the previous month. Despite the history of arthralgias/myalgias, purpura, chest pain, evidence of cerebral hemorrhage, and initial labs showing nonspecific inflammation and markers of autoimmunity, vasculitis was considered low on the differential due to a lack of a clear prodromal history and changes in cognition. Similarly, neuro-ophthalmology found no definite retinal vasculitis and believed her homonymous right visual field defect to be associated with the brain lesion previously appreciated on MRI and not amaurosis fugax. A non-emergent repeat MRI with contrast and an MR venogram of the brain were ordered by neurology to rule out thrombosis and evaluate for new lesions.

Approximately two months after her neurology appointment, the patient presented to the emergency room with a severe, right-sided headache with a left-sided visual disturbance. Shortly after arrival, the patient became delirious and exhibited seizure-like activity. A computerized tomography scan (CT) of the brain was conducted that showed a right parietal lobe intraparenchymal hemorrhage approximately $5 \times 3 \times 5$ cm in size with secondary mass effect including mid- and hind-brain herniation (see Figure 1). A CTA showed multifocal narrowing and an abnormal "beaded" contour of the entire cerebral arterial vasculature consistent for vasculitis. Neurosurgical assets were not available, and the patient was transferred to a sister center where craniectomy was performed to evacuate intracerebral hemorrhage and treat intracranial hypertension (see Figure 2). Postoperative prognosis was poor, and palliative measures were initiated. The patient passed away peacefully surrounded by family several days later.

## 3. Discussion

During the patient's clinical course, the diagnosis of MCTD remained in the differential; however, there was early serological and clinical evidence for this condition. The patient was initially ANA and RNP positive and would experience all of clinical criteria for MCTD, save sclerodactyly, over her clinical course including swollen hands, Raynaud's phenomenon, myalgias, and synovitis [1]. Even though the patient's ANA would later be negative, a positive RNP is often considered diagnostic for MCTD when found in isolation of other biomarkers as seen in this patient [9].

Only 10–20% of patients with MCTD experience neurological manifestations, with few case reports known where neurological symptoms were the presenting symptom [6-8]. [6, 7] Similar to the subject of this report, the patients in these studies presented with severe headaches as a prodrome to an immune-mediated CNS vasculitis. Given the progressive nature of MCTD and the short duration (less than one-year) between the onset of this patient's neurological symptoms and her rheumatologic workup, it is likely that this patient's headaches and visual disturbances were an initial manifestation of MCTD and not an isolated case of ocular migraines.

Vasculitis is rare in connective tissue disease, occurring in less than 10% of patients [10] with central nervous system involvement occurring in a much smaller subgroup [11]. In this patient, early signs of small vessel vasculitis included petechiae and purpura on the hands and lower extremities. Evidence of systemic involvement included persistently

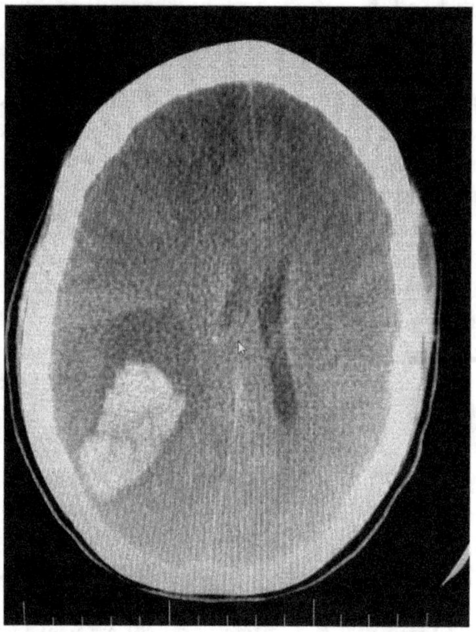

FIGURE 1: Computerized tomography (CT) axial head without contrast showing intraparenchymal hemorrhage and secondary mass effect.

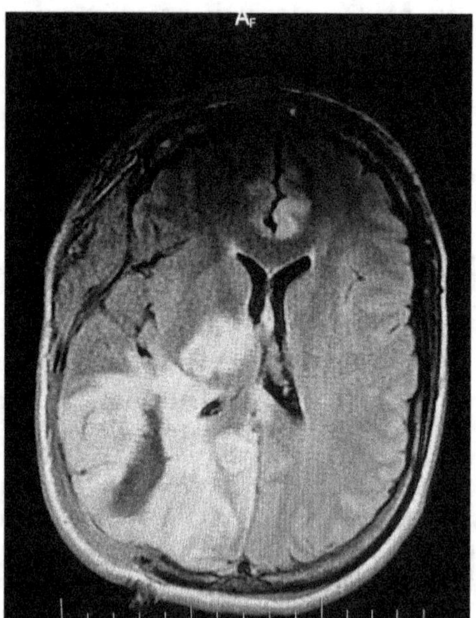

FIGURE 2: Magnetic resonance imaging (MRI) FLAIR axial head without contrast showing intraparenchymal hemorrhage status after craniectomy.

elevated inflammatory biomarkers (CRP and ESR), amaurosis fugax, and cerebrovascular hemorrhaging noted on MRI. Despite these findings, vasculitis remained low on the differential due to lack of a clear prodrome and frank cognitive deficits.

MCTD often presents as a sequential or staggered overlap of SLE, scleroderma, myositis, and rheumatoid arthritis [12]. This nonlinear presentation requires heightened curiosity of potential evolving pathologies where a clear prodrome is not apparent. Throughout her clinical course, the patient reported mental fogginess that might have been interpreted as "cognitive deficits" in a person with lower baseline intelligence and functional status. And, while the initial MRA of the brain did not show any signs of large vessel disease, it did not capture the distal mid-to-small sized vessels of the brain. This incomplete study could not rule out small dissections or other changes that may have informed clinicians about evolving pathologies including systemic vasculitis.

Had the patient's first MRA shown more definitive signs of vasculitis, her report of new and worsening headaches may have prompted her treatment team to pursue a more aggressive assessment of her symptoms. This case illustrates the importance of considering CNS vasculitis in patients with unexplained, progressive neurologic symptoms and adds support to the case reports by Awad, Matsui, and Graf showing MCTD as a possible cause of severe neurological disease [6–8]. Together, these cases illustrate the importance of rapid and assertive assessment and management of neurological symptoms in persons with suspected connective tissue diseases. Awareness of this link may aid in early diagnosis and initiation of appropriate treatments to improve positive outcomes.

## Consent

Written consent was received from the patient's next of kin for the publication of this case report.

## Disclosure

The author is an acquaintance of the patient's family.

## Conflicts of Interest

The author declares no conflicts of interest.

## Acknowledgments

The author would like to thank the family of the patient who supported the publication of the case report.

## References

[1] P. Ungprasert, C. S. Crowson, V. R. Chowdhary, F. C. Ernste, K. G. Moder, and E. L. Matteson, "Epidemiology of mixed connective tissue disease, 1985–2014: a population-based study," *Arthritis Care & Research*, vol. 68, no. 12, pp. 1843–1848, 2016.

[2] D. Alarcon-Segovia and M. H. Cardiel, "Comparison between 3 diagnostic criteria for mixed connective tissue disease. Study of 593 patients," *Journal of Rheumatology*, vol. 16, no. 3, pp. 328–334, 1989.

[3] R. Gunnarsson, Ø. Molberg, I.-M. Gilboe, and J. T. Gran, "The prevalence and incidence of mixed connective tissue disease: a national multicentre survey of Norwegian patients," *Annals of the Rheumatic Diseases*, vol. 70, no. 6, pp. 1047–1051, 2011.

[4] O. Kaipiainen-Seppänen and K. Aho, "Incidence of rare systemic rheumatic and connective tissue diseases in Finland," *Journal of Internal Medicine*, vol. 240, no. 2, pp. 81–84, 1996.

[5] A. Hajas, P. Szodoray, B. Nakken, G. Nagy, Z. Szekanecz, and E. Bodolay, "SAT0190 long-term follow-up of 280 patients with mixed connective tissue disease," *Annals of the Rheumatic Diseases*, vol. 72, no. Suppl 3, p. A645, 2013.

[6] A. M. Awad and M. Stevenson, "Isolated central nervous system vasculitis associated with antiribonuclear protein antibody," *Case Reports in Neurological Medicine*, vol. 2011, Article ID 495201, 4 pages, 2011.

[7] H. Matsui, F. Udaka, M. Oda, T. Kubori, K. Nishinaka, and M. Kameyama, "Encephalopathy and severe neuropathy due to probable systemic vasculitis as an initial manifestation of mixed connective tissue disease," *Neurology India*, vol. 54, no. 1, pp. 83–85, 2006.

[8] W. D. Graf, J. M. Milstein, and D. D. Sherry, "Stroke and mixed connective tissue disease," *Journal of Child Neurology*, vol. 8, no. 3, pp. 256–259, 1993.

[9] Mayo Clinic Laboratories, *Neurology Catalog: RNP Antibodies, IgG, Serum*, Mayo Clinic Laboratories, Rochester, MN, USA, 2021, https://neurology.testcatalog.org/show/RNP.

[10] E. Cozzani, G. Gasparini, M. Papini, M Burlando, F Drago, and A Parodi, "Vasculitis associated with connective tissue diseases," *Giornale italiano di dermatologia e venereologia: organo ufficiale Societa italiana di dermatologia e sifilografia*, vol. 150, no. 2, pp. 221–232, 2015.

[11] A. Sharma, A. Dhooria, A. Aggarwal, M. Rathi, and V. Chandran, "Connective tissue disorder-associated vasculitis," *Current Rheumatology Reports*, vol. 18, no. 6, pp. 31–41, 2016.

[12] P. H. Pepmueller, "Undifferentiated connective tissue disease, mixed connective tissue disease, and overlap syndromes in rheumatology," *Missouri Medicine*, vol. 113, no. 2, pp. 136–140, 2016.

# 27

# Successful Left Atrial Appendage Occlusion with the New Generation Amulet® Device after Late-Occurring Embolization of an Amplatzer® Cardiac Plug in a Patient with Repetitive Strokes

**Marco R. Schroeter[1] and Wolfgang Schillinger[1,2]**

[1]*Department of Cardiology and Pneumology, Heart Center, University of Göttingen, Göttingen, Germany*
[2]*Internal Medicine I, Helios Albert-Schweitzer Clinic Northeim, Northeim, Germany*

Correspondence should be addressed to Marco R. Schroeter; mschroeter@med.uni-goettingen.de

Academic Editor: Ramazan Akdemir

The Amplatzer Cardiac Plug (ACP) is one of the most commonly used devices for percutaneous left atrial appendage (LAA) closure in order to prevent a stroke in patients with atrial fibrillation and contraindication for long-term oral anticoagulation therapy. We have previously described a patient who had experienced an embolization of the ACP device about 12 months after implantation and the device could be percutaneously retrieved. A few years later, he suffered from a posterior stroke and a stroke located in the brainstem as well as a transischemic attack (TIA). In order to protect him from further cardioembolic events a reocclusion of the LAA with the new generation of ACP device, the Amplatzer Amulet, was performed. A stable position of the device within follow-up period could be confirmed and the patient was free of additional strokes/TIA or bleeding events. This case stresses the importance of proper LAA sizing in order to prevent device embolization and notes that LAA size is not static. Moreover, it demonstrates that repeated implantation of an LAA occlusion device was still possible; one should be aware of undersizing the LAA dimensions and that the modifications of new generation LAA occlusion devices may overcome limitations of first-generation devices in order to prevent a cardioembolic stroke.

## 1. Introduction

The Amplatzer Cardiac Plug (ACP; St. Jude Medical) is one of the most commonly used devices for percutaneous left atrial appendage (LAA) closure in order to prevent a stroke in patients with atrial fibrillation and contraindication for long-term oral anticoagulation therapy.

We have previously published a paper describing a 75-year-old patient who had experienced an embolization of the ACP device about 12 months after implantation [1].

Recently, a new generation of ACP device, the Amplatzer Amulet, has been made commercially available. The main concept of the Amulet device is based on the first generation of ACP with a distal lobe and a proximal disk connected by an articulating waist. The lobe has stabilizing hooks to assure retention and the disc seals the outer shape of the LAA orifice [2]. The modifications of the Amulet device include new features to facilitate device deployment and to reduce the embolization risk [3]. The experiences with the new Amulet device are limited so far [3–5].

## 2. Case Report

The above-mentioned patient was discharged at that time after ACP retrieval without an LAA device on an antiplatelet therapy with ASA. Subsequently, he suffered from a posterior stroke and a stroke located in the brainstem as well as a transischemic attack (TIA) in the area of the left cerebri media artery. The patient had been repetitively hospitalized in the stroke-unit/neurological department of our hospital. No relevant extra- or intracerebral stenosis could be detected

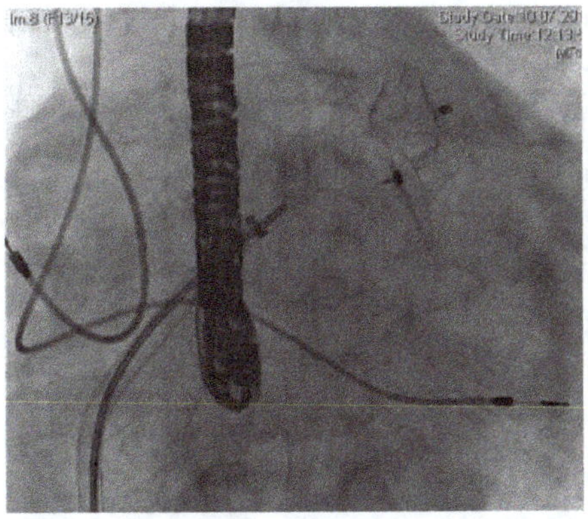

(a)

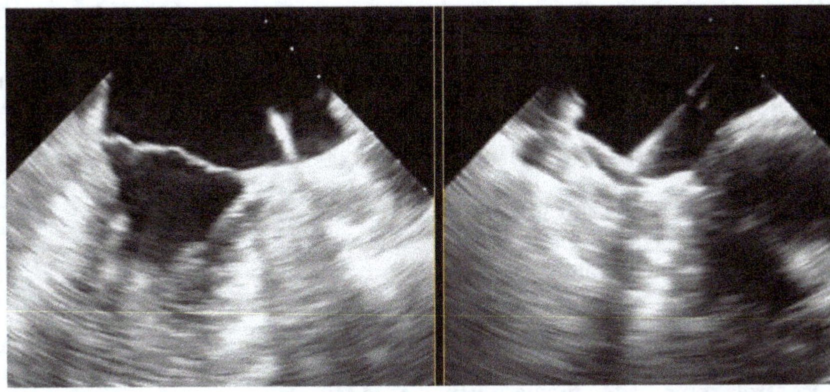

(b)

FIGURE 1: The implantation of the Amulet device was performed under fluoroscopic (a) and echocardiographic (b) guidance, similar to the Amplatzer Cardiac Plug (ACP).

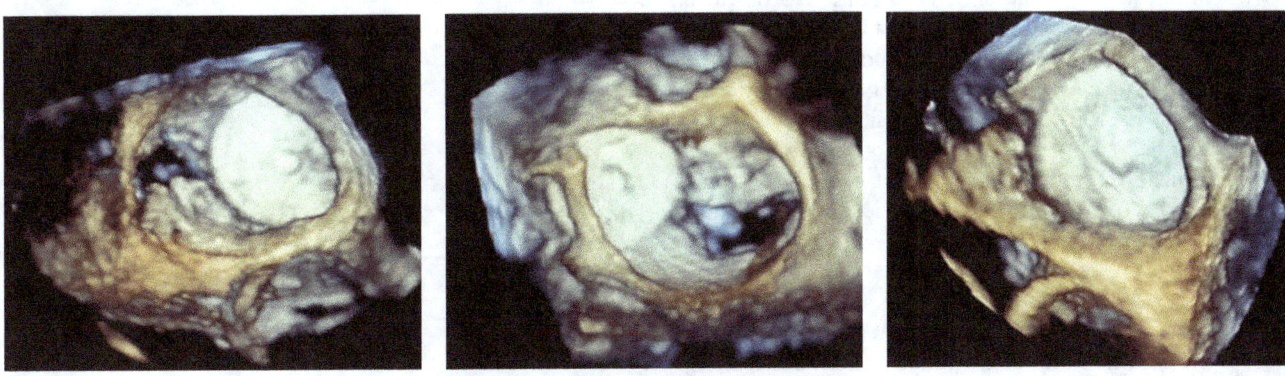

(a)

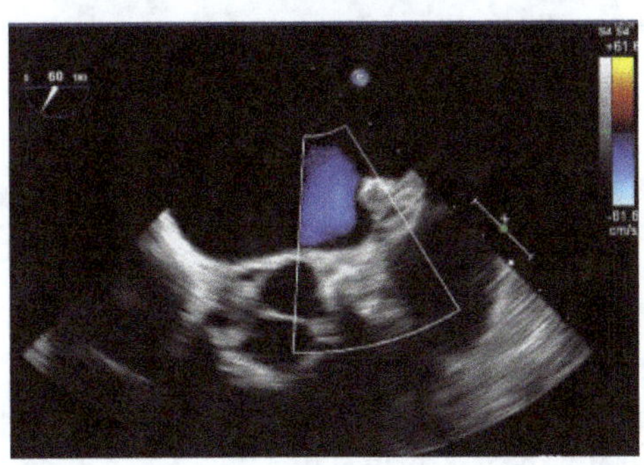

(b)

FIGURE 2: Using 3D transesophageal echocardiography, (a) a stable position of the device within follow-up period could be confirmed (*from left to right*: immediately after implantation, after 3 months and 6 months). Color Doppler TEE revealed complete device occlusion of the LAA (b).

and a cardioembolic genesis of stroke/TIA caused by atrial fibrillation was presumed. Due to the bleeding risk with the history of intracerebral bleeding, an oral anticoagulation therapy was still contraindicated. In order to protect him from further cardioembolic events we decided to perform reocclusion of the LAA.

The procedure was performed percutaneously using a transseptal approach under transesophageal echocardiography (TEE) and fluoroscopy guidance (Figure 1). The diameter of a potential "landing zone" in the LAA was unexpectedly found to be greater than during the first intervention: 23 mm (compared to 19 mm measured before) and an Amplatzer Amulet of 28 mm was successfully implanted (Figure 1). After echocardiologic and fluoroscopic control on the next day were inconspicuous, the patient was discharged on an ASA and clopidogrel therapy. Repetitive echocardiographic controls were performed at the date of implantation as well as 3 and 6 months after implantation (3D-TEE; Figure 2(a)). Color Doppler TEE revealed no signs of residual shunt between the LAA and the left atrium (Figure 2(b)). After 3 months the medication was reduced to an ASA monotherapy (100 mg SID) and the patient was free of additional strokes/TIA or bleeding events until now.

## 3. Discussion and Conclusion

The existing case reports and a recently published study with 17 patients described the implantation of the new Amulet device in the normal context of a single implanted LAA device [3–5]. In our case, it was the second device in the same patient after the embolization of the initially implanted ACP device. Subsequently, we had a longer follow-up period with TEE controls compared to previously published reports.

Moreover, this case stresses the importance of proper LAA sizing in order to prevent possible device embolization. It is of note that LAA size is not static. Changes in cardiac preload induce dynamic changes of LAA size. For this reason and with implication for the clinical operation procedure, adequate intravascular volume status must be ensured before final sizing and occluder selection. In addition, dilation of the LAA may occur over time as a result of the remodelling process associated with atrial fibrillation [6]. However, a recently published single case report hypothesizes that LAA device embolization could occur without obvious explanation, despite correct device sizing and sufficient stability tests [7].

In summary, this case demonstrates that repeated implantation of an LAA occlusion device was still possible; one should be aware of undersizing the LAA dimensions (in respect to the volume status of the patient) and modifications of new generation LAA occlusion devices may overcome limitations of first generation, even if further studies with the new devices are necessary.

## Competing Interests

M. R. Schroeter has no competing interests. W. Schillinger has received proctor and lecture fees from St. Jude Medical.

## Acknowledgments

The authors acknowledge the support from the German Research Foundation and the Open Access Publication Funds of the Göttingen University.

## References

[1] M. R. Schroeter, B. C. Danner, M. Hünlich, and W. Schillinger, "Uncommon delayed and late complications after percutaneous left atrial appendage closure with Amplatzer® Cardiac Plug," *Clinical Research in Cardiology*, vol. 103, no. 4, pp. 285–290, 2014.

[2] J. W. Park, A. Bethencourt, H. Sievert et al., "Left atrial appendage closure with Amplatzer cardiac plug in atrial fibrillation: initial European experience," *Catheterization and Cardiovascular Interventions*, vol. 77, no. 5, pp. 700–706, 2011.

[3] X. Freixa, J. L. K. Chan, A. Tzikas, P. Garceau, A. Basmadjian, and R. Ibrahim, "The Amplatzer™ cardiac plug 2 for left atrial appendage occlusion: novel features and first-in-man experience," *EuroIntervention*, vol. 8, no. 9, pp. 1094–1098, 2013.

[4] S. C. Lam, S. Bertog, S. Gafoor et al., "Left atrial appendage closure using the amulet device: an initial experience with the second generation amplatzer cardiac plug," *Catheterization and Cardiovascular Interventions*, vol. 85, no. 2, pp. 297–303, 2015.

[5] A. Tzikas, L. Karagounis, M. Bouktsi et al., "Left atrial appendage occlusion with the Amplatzer Amulet™ for stroke prevention in atrial fibrillation: the first case in Greece," *Hellenic Journal of Cardiology*, vol. 54, no. 5, pp. 408–412, 2013.

[6] R. Beigel, N. C. Wunderlich, S. Y. Ho, R. Arsanjani, and R. J. Siegel, "The left atrial appendage: anatomy, function, and noninvasive evaluation," *JACC: Cardiovascular Imaging*, vol. 7, no. 12, pp. 1251–1265, 2014.

[7] P. Mester, A. Dompnier, and L. Belle, "Asymptomatic migration of an AMPLATZER™ Amulet™ left atrial appendage occluder through the mitral valve," *Catheterization and Cardiovascular Interventions*, 2016.

# A Case Report of Thalamic Infarction after Lumbar Drain: A Unique Cause of Perioperative Stroke?

**Daniel N. Kianpour**[1], **Thomas M. Nguyen,**[1] **and Arthur M. Lam**[2]

[1]*Swedish Neuroscience Institute, Seattle, WA, USA*
[2]*University of California San Diego, USA*

Correspondence should be addressed to Daniel N. Kianpour; daniel_kianpour@urmc.rochester.edu

Academic Editor: Alparslan Apan

In the case presented, a patient has an unexplained episode of hypertension during aneurysm clipping. Following the procedure, the patient was discovered to have bilateral thalamic infarctions unrelated to the vascular location of the aneurysm. After a review of the case, it becomes apparent that intracranial hypotension caused by lumbar over drainage of cerebrospinal fluid (CSF) is the likely cause of both the episode of intraoperative hypertension and the thalamic infarcts. It is often presumed that having an open dura protects against intracranial hypotension and subsequent herniation. We present this case to suggest that opening the dura might not be protective in all cases and anesthesiologists must pay particular attention to the rate of CSF drainage. Lumbar CSF drainage is a technique frequently employed during neurological surgery and it is important for anesthesiologists to understand the signs, symptoms, and potential consequences of intracranial hypotension from rapid drainage.

## 1. Introduction

Lumbar cerebrospinal fluid drainage (CSF) drainage is a commonly used approach during cerebrovascular and skull base neurosurgical procedures to aid in brain relaxation and surgical exposure. With a closed dura, one well-known complication of lumbar drainage is the abrupt increase in an aneurysm's transmural pressure gradient caused by acute CSF drainage which can lead to catastrophic rebleeding [1]. A much less recognized complication is "brain sagging"; acute drainage of CSF can cause a rapid decrease in intracranial pressure resulting in some degree of transtentorial herniation [2]. Once the dura has been opened, rapid changes in intracranial pressure by drainage are diminished and thought to limit the brain sagging seen with a closed dura. Intraoperatively, brain sagging and herniation can manifest with Cushing's response of hypertension and bradycardia which can be underrecognized given the number of confounding variables in this setting. The case presented demonstrates an occurrence of presumed herniation syndrome from CSF drainage during elective unruptured anterior communicating artery aneurysm clipping causing significant intraoperative hypertension and subsequent bilateral thalamic infarctions. This case has been prepared following the CARE guidelines and methodology for medical case reports [3].

## 2. Case Presentation

A 64-year-old, 87 kg female presented for clipping of a 4 mm wide neck unruptured saccular anterior communicating artery aneurysm which was discovered incidentally during the evaluation of headaches and memory difficulties. Her past medical history was significant for remote breast carcinoma, hypertension, obstructive sleep apnea, and gastroesophageal reflux disease. She was a lifelong nonsmoker and notable preoperative medications included aspirin, furosemide, and propanolol. Preoperative imaging had no evidence of prior infarcts. After induction of anesthesia, a right internal jugular central venous catheter and radial arterial catheter were placed and maintenance of anesthesia was performed with a combination of 0.5 MAC sevoflurane, propofol 50 mcg/kg/min, and remifentanil 0.125 mcg/kg/min infusions. Mannitol 1 gram per kilogram for a total of 80 grams was administered. The neurosurgeon placed an 80 cm closed-tip, barium impregnated lumbar drainage catheter with a 0.7 mm inner diameter (Medtronic USA, REF 46419) at the L3-4 level prior to the start of surgery.

The surgery commenced and was progressing unremarkably. Prior to opening of the dura, 20 mL of CSF was drained over 15 minutes per neurosurgeon request. After dural opening and during dissection of the aneurysm, the surgeon requested the lumbar drain to be opened allowing further drainage of CSF. After approximately 15 minutes, the blood pressure sharply increased over the course of 1 to 2 minutes from a baseline systolic blood pressure of 130 mmHg to over 205 mmHg with an associated decrease in heart rate from 60 bpm to 50 which resolved over the course of minutes. This acute hypertension was treated with a number of interventions including 250 mg propofol and 1 mcg/kg remifentanil boluses aimed at treating light anesthesia as well as a bolus of 7.5 mg labetalol. At the time of the hypertensive event, the propofol, remifentanil, and Sevoflurane dosing had been stable and unchanged for over an hour. There was also no change in the level of surgical stimulation at this time as the dura had been incised and the neurosurgeons were using the operative microscope to expose the aneurysm. After the aneurysm was successfully clipped, the lumbar drain was closed and the surgery was completed without further episodes of hypertension. A total of 60 mL of CSF was drained via the lumbar drain during the case in addition to the losses from the surgical field.

At conclusion of the operative procedure, the patient remained comatose and unresponsive despite an hour in the operating room awaiting emergence from anesthesia. A postoperative head CT was obtained prior to transport to the intensive care unit which demonstrated mild cerebral edema and borderline inferior transtentorial herniation, but no significant hemorrhage or focal abnormalities. She was then transported to the Neurocritical Care Unit intubated and ventilated. Initial arterial blood gas analysis on arrival to the ICU did not reveal a cause to her delayed emergence (pH 7.35, pCO2 47 mmHg, pO2 323 mmHg, glucose 204 mg/dL, and sodium 137 mEq/L). She did not receive any benzodiazepines during the case, but did receive 50 mcg of fentanyl on induction and 1 gram of levetiracetam in addition to the propofol, remifentanil, and Sevoflurane maintenance. Initial neurological exam demonstrated midline and equal 4 mm pupils which were reactive to light bilaterally. She withdrew to painful stimuli in all four extremities. On postoperative day (POD) 1, her mental status continued to be depressed with a Glasgow Coma Scale of 7T (E2:V1T:M4). That day, an MRI was obtained which revealed bilateral thalamic infarctions on the diffusion weighted imaging which can be seen in Figure 1. Supportive care was continued and over the course of several days, her mental status slowly improved to GCS of 10 (E4:V1:M5) on POD 5. This allowed for safe extubation that day. She continued to improve and was alert and oriented to person, place, time, and situation with some memory and attention difficulties by POD 16. A timeline of her in-hospital recovery can be found in Table 1. She was discharged home with referrals for home physical, occupational, and speech therapy on POD 19. She continued her gradual neurological improvement and by over a year postoperatively, Neurology records indicated she was living independently and her Montreal Cognitive Assessment score had recovered to a normal 27/30.

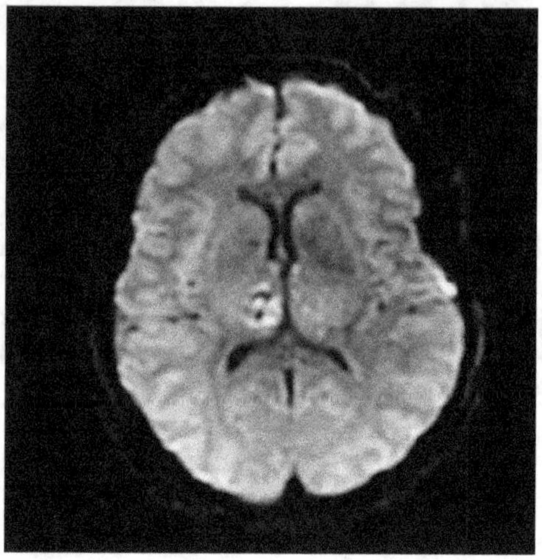

FIGURE 1: Diffusion weighted image MRI from postoperative day 1. *Note.* Increased signal intensity in right basal ganglia with punctate increases on the left indicating acute infarcts.

## 3. Discussion

The case presented describes a patient who had sudden and severe unexplained hypertension during aneurysm clipping without obvious changes in anesthetic depth or surgical stimulation, but did have an open and draining lumbar CSF catheter. Although the causality between CSF drainage and hypertension is not clear, there are two important features which argue for it as the etiology of the observations made. Firstly, this case demonstrates the phenomenon of systemic hypertension related to CSF drainage. Although not commonly seen with the relatively low flow rates of modern lumbar drainage catheters, it was well recognized with previous types of CSF drainage devices. In his 1975 letter to the editor of *Anaesthesia*, John Barker notes that with the use of an 18-gauge malleable needle, “Drainage of cerebrospinal fluid is controlled by a gate clamp in order to avoid the intense arterial pressor response and cardiac arrhythmia which can occur with free flow” [4]. With rapid drainage of CSF, the brain begins to sag, thus causing transtentorial herniation and subsequent reflexive systemic hypertension [5]. Secondly, our patient had findings of bilateral thalamic infarctions on postoperative MRI, demonstrated in Figure 1. Transtentorial herniation is known to cause compression of the posterior cerebral arteries and potentially subsequent arterial and venous infarctions in its territory which includes the thalamus [6, 7]. In one case series of 32 patients with lumbar drainage catheters, Roland describes a case of infarction caused by “kinking” of the PCA at the tentorium cerebelli [8]. In another series of patients with persistent unconsciousness and evidence of intracranial hypotension after uneventful neurological surgery, 16 of 16

Table 1: Timeline of in-hospital neurologic recovery.

| *Postoperative Day (POD)* | *0* | *1* | *2* | *3* | *5* | *10* | *15* | *19* |
|---|---|---|---|---|---|---|---|---|
| *Glasgow Coma Scale (Total)* | 7 | 8 | 9 | 10 | 11 | 14 | 14 | 15 |
| *Best Eye Response* | 2 | 3 | 3 | 4 | 4 | 4 | 4 | 4 |
| *Best Verbal Response* | 1T | 1T | 1T | 1T | 1 | 4 | 4 | 5 |
| *Best Motor Response* | 4 | 4 | 5 | 5 | 6 | 6 | 6 | 6 |
| *Wakefulness/Orientation* | Unarousable | Arousable | Arousable | Arousable | Alert Disoriented | Alert, Oriented times 2[a] | Alert, Oriented times 1[b] | Alert, Oriented times 4[c] |
| *Communication* | Unable to Assess | Unable to Assess | Unable to Assess | Unable to Assess | Expressive Aphasia | Expressive Aphasia | Nonsensical Speech | Loss of Fluency |

[a]Oriented to person and situation. [b]Oriented to person only. [c]Oriented to person, place, time, and situation.

patients displayed radiologic evidence of injury to bilateral thalamic or basal ganglia structures [9]. The combination of severe hypertension and the subsequent finding of thalamic infarction is strong evidence that intracranial hypotension from CSF drainage contributed to the findings observed.

This case illustrates an important point: dural opening may not protect against intracranial hypotension and subsequent Cushing's response as well as commonly thought. CSF over drainage should be included in the differential diagnosis of any unexplained hypertension in the presence of an open lumbar drainage catheter after other causes of hypertension such as aneurysm rupture and light anesthesia are excluded. It is also imperative to alert our neurosurgical colleagues if we notice a possible Cushing's response whether being from intracranial hypotension or other causes such as brain compression.

Although this episode of hypertension cannot be definitively linked to brain sagging and transient transtentorial herniation, the evidence strongly suggests that it is the likely etiology and anesthesiologists should be aware of this phenomenon. With the utilization of endovascular treatment for cerebral aneurysms, future anesthesiologists will continue to have decreased exposure to open surgery and the nuances associated with it. It will be increasingly important to better describe in the literature these nuances where previous generations such as that of John Barker received from clinical practice.

## Consent

Verbal consent to submit this manuscript was obtained from the patient during a follow-up phone interview.

## Disclosure

This research did not receive any specific grant from funding agencies in the public, commercial, or not-for-profit sectors. The present address of Daniel N. Kianpour is Department of Anesthesiology and Perioperative Medicine, University of Rochester, 601 Elmwood Drive, Box 604, Rochester, NY 14642. Thomas M. Nguyen's present address is US Anesthesia Partners Washington, 1229 Madison Street, Suite 1440, Seattle, WA 98104. Arthur M. Lam's present address is UC San Diego Department of Anesthesiology, 9300 Campus Point Drive #7770, La Jolla, CA 92037.

## Conflicts of Interest

The authors declare that they have no conflicts of interest.

## References

[1] H. J. Priebe, "Aneurysmal subarachnoid haemorrhage and the anaesthetist," *British Journal of Anaesthesia*, vol. 99, no. 1, pp. 102–118, 2007.

[2] R. J. Komotar, J. Mocco, E. R. Ransom et al., "Herniation secondary to critical postcraniotomy cerebrospinal fluid hypovolemia," *Neurosurgery*, vol. 57, no. 2, pp. 286–290, 2005.

[3] J. J. Gagnier, G. Kienle, D. G. Altman et al., "The CARE guidelines: consensus-based clinical case reporting guideline development," *BMJ Case Reports*, 2013.

[4] J. Barker, "Letter: an anaesthetic technique for intracranial aneurysms," *Anaesthesia*, vol. 30, no. 2, pp. 557-558, 1975.

[5] W. Fitch, D. G. McDowall, N. P. Keaney, and V. W. Pickerodt, "Systemic vascular responses to increased intracranial pressure. The 'Cushing' response in the presence of intracranial space-occupying lesions: systemic and cerebral haemodynamic studies in the dog and the baboon," *Journal of Neurology, Neurosurgery and Psychiatry*, vol. 40, no. 9, pp. 843–852, 1977.

[6] A. Bhardwaj and M. A. Mirski, *Handbook of Neurocritical Care*, Springer, New York, NY, USA, 2nd edition, 2011.

[7] J. D. Schmahmann, "Vascular syndromes of the thalamus," *Stroke*, vol. 34, no. 9, pp. 2264–2278, 2003.

[8] P. S. Roland, B. F. Marple, W. L. Meyerhoff, and B. Mickey, "Complication of lumbar spinal fluid drainage," *Otolaryngology–Head and Neck Surgery*, vol. 107, no. 4, pp. 564–569, 1992.

[9] D. R. Hadizadeh, A. Kovács, H. Tschampa, R. Kristof, J. Schramm, and H. Urbach, "Postsurgical intracranial hypotension: diagnostic and prognostic imaging findings," *American Journal of Neuroradiology*, vol. 31, no. 1, pp. 100–105, 2010.

29

# Tissue Kallikrein Activity, Detected by a Novel Method, may be a Predictor of Recurrent Stroke: A Case-Control Study

**Xiao Ran,[1] Qin Zhang,[2] and Dao Wen Wang[3]**

[1] *Department of Emergency Medicine, Tongji Hospital, Tongji Medical College, Huazhong University of Science and Technology, Jiefang Avenue No. 1095, Wuhan 430030, China*
[2] *Department of Anesthesia, Tongji Hospital, Tongji Medical College, Huazhong University of Science and Technology, Jiefang Avenue No. 1095, Wuhan 430030, China*
[3] *The Institute of Hypertension and Department of Internal Medicine, Tongji Hospital, Tongji Medical College, Huazhong University of Science and Technology, Jiefang Avenue No. 1095, Wuhan 430030, China*

Correspondence should be addressed to Qin Zhang; qin4298@sina.com

Academic Editor: Claudio Letizia

*Aim.* Tissue kallikrein (TK) protein content in plasma has been shown to be negatively associated with both incident and recurrent strokes. The aims of this study were to develop a novel method for detecting TK activity and to investigate its association with event-free survival over 5 years in Chinese first-ever stroke patients. *Methods.* We designed a case-control study with 321 stroke patients (174: ischemic stroke, 147: hemorrhagic stroke) and 323 healthy local controls. TK activity was measured by a novel assay utilizing the immunological characteristics of TK and the catalysis of benzoyl arginine ethyl ester hydrochloride (BAEE). *Results.* TK protein levels above 0.200 mg/L in plasma were not associated with urinary TK activity or the risk of stroke recurrence. TK activity was significantly lower in stroke patients compared with controls (1.583 ± 0.673 Eu/mL versus 1.934 ± 0.284 Eu/mL, $P < 0.001$). After adjusting for traditional risk factors, TK activity was negatively associated, in a dose-response manner, with the risk of overall stroke recurrence and positively associated with event-free survival during a 5-year follow-up (relative risk (RR), 0.69; 95% CI, 0.57–0.84; $P < 0.001$). *Conclusions.* Our findings suggest that urinary TK activity may be a stronger predictor of stroke recurrence than plasma TK levels.

## 1. Introduction

Stroke has become one of the leading causes of death and long-term disability in many countries and at all levels of economic development [1], with a high occurrence and recurrence rate [2, 3]. In China, 2.5 million people have stroke and more than 1 million die from stroke-related causes every year. The total cost of hospitalization for patients with stroke was twice as much as per capita annual income of China and still growing [4]. Conventional cardiovascular risk factors, such as abnormal lipid metabolism, smoking, diabetes, and hypertension, account for a considerable portion of stroke events [5]. However, most subjects exhibiting these risk factors do not develop stroke during their lifetime, suggesting that additional factors are involved.

The tissue kallikrein- (TK-) kinin/bradykinin system is recognized as an important modulator of the cardiovascular, renal, and central nervous systems [6]. TK, a major member of the ubiquitously expressed kallikrein family, releases vasoactive bradykinin and kinin peptides from low molecular weight kininogen [7]. Kinins exert their action through two G-protein-coupled receptors, kinin B1 and kinin B2 receptors in the endothelium [8], which mediate regulation of blood pressure, smooth muscle contraction and relaxation, vascular cell growth, vascular permeability, inflammatory cascades, electrolyte balance, and pain induction [9, 10]. The role of TK was studied in numerous experimental studies focusing on this disease using strategies like kallikrein gene transfer, tissue kallikrein infusion, and/or human kallikrein over expressing animals [11]. These basic studies have demonstrated that TK can reduce elevated blood pressure and inhibit remodeling in the heart and arteries [12, 13]; attenuate ischemic stroke in an animal model [14]; reduce the rate of smooth muscle cell proliferation [15], atherosclerosis, and apoptosis [16]; protect against ischemia/reperfusion damage [17]; and enhance angiogenesis [18].

Early clinical studies have indicated an inverse relationship between urinary TK activity and blood pressure in patients with hypertension [19, 20]. Our previous study investigated the association of TK protein content in plasma with stroke and coronary artery disease (CAD) [21, 22]. In a multicenter case-control study conducted in China, we found that the plasma TK level was negatively associated with incident and recurrence of stroke. However, the relationship between plasma TK level and stroke recurrence disappeared when the plasma TK level exceeded 0.200 mg/L. We also found that the elevated TK levels are positively associated with the presence of CAD and negatively associated with the severity of CAD and that the TK level might be a strong and independent biomarker for stroke. However, no study to date has investigated the relationship between TK activity and stroke. We therefore developed a novel method for determining TK activity in urine and assessed its association with stroke and the long-term recurrence of cerebrovascular and cardiovascular events in a 5-year follow-up study of Chinese patients with first-ever stroke.

## 2. Methods

*2.1. Study Population and Data Collection.* The study population has been described in detail in a previous publication [21]. Experiments were conducted in accordance with the principles of Declaration of Helsinki. The study protocol was approved by the Ethics Committee of Tongji Hospital, and informed written consent was obtained from all participants. We recruited participants from November 2000 to November 2001 from 5 hospitals in Wuhan, China. Stroke patients, described previously, included cerebral infarction (atherothrombosis and lacunar infarction) and cerebral hemorrhage. Other types of stroke (transient ischemic attack, subarachnoid hemorrhage, embolic brain infarction, brain tumors, cerebrovascular malformation, cardioembolic stroke, and documented atrial fibrillation); severe systemic disease; inflammatory and autoimmune diseases; and serious chronic diseases were excluded from the study. Confirmation of stroke was based on strict neurological examination, computed tomography (CT), or magnetic resonance imaging (MRI) according to the International Classification of Diseases, Ninth Revision as described previously [21]. Ethnically matched controls were randomly selected from inpatients with minor illness who were free of neurological diseases. In total, 321 patients (174: ischemic stroke, 147: hemorrhagic stroke) and 323 control subjects were recruited. All participants underwent a standardized interview, and data on traditional stroke risk factors were recorded for all subjects. These included gender, age, body mass index (BMI), systolic blood pressure (SBP), diastolic blood pressure (DBP), triglyceride (TG), total cholesterol (TC), high-density lipoprotein (HDL), cholesterol, history of diabetes mellitus, hypertension, hyperlipidemia, and smoking habits. These criteria were described in a previous study [21].

To evaluate the association of TK activity with long-term clinical outcomes in stroke patients, follow-up visits of patients for a median of 5 years (range: 4–5.5 years) were performed by telephone or household contact after the initial stroke. The primary endpoint was recurrence of stroke. The onset of coronary heart disease or death was secondary endpoints.

*2.2. TK Activity Assays.* Plasma and urinary samples were collected after an overnight fast and stored at −80°C. Specimens collected from stroke patients were taken after the acute phase of the initial stroke (between 1 month and 1 year after the onset). TK activity was measured using a novel assay utilizing TK immunological characteristics and the catalysis of benzoyl arginine ethyl ester hydrochloride (BAEE). To generate a polyclonal antibody specific for TK, a synthetic TK peptide consisting of 11 amino acids (AC-Glu-Asn-His-Thr-Arg-Gln-Ala-Asp-Glu-Asp-Thr-COOH) was fused to keyhole limpet hemocyanin (KLH) and used to immunize rabbits. The antibody was purified by affinity column chromatography. SDS-PAGE (12%) and Western blot were used to visualize the specificity of the purified antibody. The polyclonal antibody was pure (Figure 1) and had a high titer (1 : 25600 dilution). The antibody specific for TK was precoated onto microplates and incubated for 24 hours at 4°C. After aspirating each well and washing, 1% BSA-PBS was used as a blocking buffer for 1 hour at 37°C. All samples consisted of 10 $\mu$L of urine added to 90 $\mu$L of PBS. Samples were then added to the appropriate microplate wells and incubated for 1 hour at 37°C. After aspirating each well and washing, TK-catalyzed BAEE and the remaining BAEE were reacted with hydroxylamine and ferric chloride. TK activity was then detected by its esterolytic activity on synthetic ester substrates [23–26].

*2.3. Statistical Analysis.* Statistical and association analyses were performed using SPSS 18.0 software (SPSS Inc., Chicago, IL, USA). Continuous variables were expressed as mean ± standard deviation and statistical significance was tested using the independent samples $t$-test or a 1-way analysis of variance. Categorical variables were analyzed using the chi-square statistic test. Bivariate analyses were conducted to assess the relationship between plasma TK level and urinary TK activity. Pearson's and Spearman's correlation coefficient $r$ was calculated to test for associations between both continuous and categorical variables. The relationships of TK activity with traditional cardiovascular risk factors of stroke patients were tested in multivariable forward stepwise linear regression analysis. The distribution of continuous variables was tested based on skewedness and kurtosis. Because TK activity had a skewed distribution, for further analysis the TK activity levels in stroke patients and controls were categorized by 4 quartiles. TK activity was then used as a continuous, categorical variable in the subsequent analysis. Correlations between TK activity and other risk factors were also calculated. Unconditional logistic regression analysis was run for stroke and separately for ischemic and hemorrhagic stroke to estimate odds ratio (OR), together with 95% confidence intervals (CIs). Multivariate Cox proportional hazard

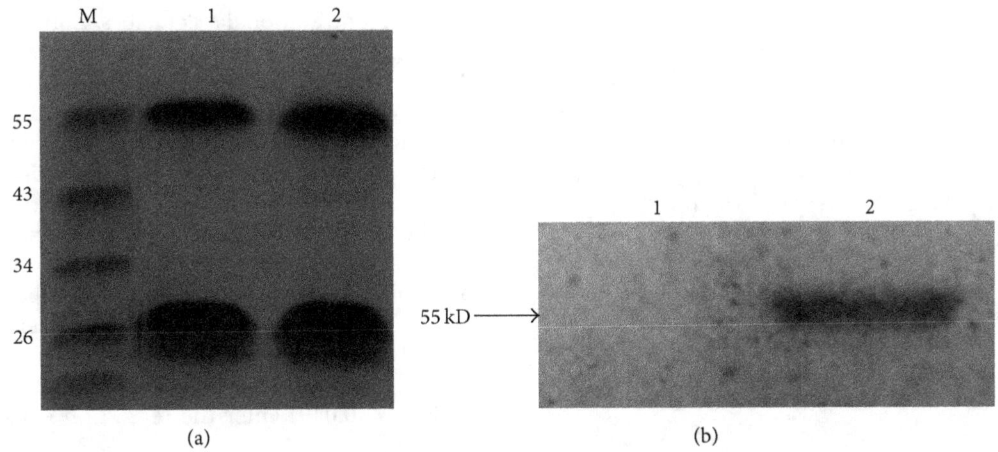


FIGURE 1: SDS-PAGE and Western blotting with polyclonal and monoclonal antibodies. (a) the purified polyclonal antibody (lanes 1 and 2) was separated using SDS-PAGE with the molecular mass markers indicated in lane M. (b) PEGX-4T1 control protein (lane 1) and GST-TK fusion protein (lane 2) were transferred onto nitrocellulose membranes for Western blotting using a polyclonal antibody.

models were then performed to estimate relative risks (RRs) and 95% CIs for the effect of TK activity on independent risk of recurrent stroke. Unadjusted models and models adjusted for traditional cardiovascular risk factors (described above) were calculated. Kaplan-Meier survival estimates were used to examine the association between TK activity, stroke recurrence, and event-free survival time. A $P$ value of less than 0.05 was considered as statistically significant and all probabilities were two-tailed.

## 3. Results

*3.1. Descriptive Statistics of TK Activity in Urine.* Results generated using TK activity assays indicated that TK activity is linear ($r = 0.995$, Figure 2). The range of detection of the assay was 1.27 Eu–0.040 Eu. Of the 20 people for whom 3 TK activity measurements during a 6-month period were obtained, the intraindividual coefficient of variation was 6.9%, reflecting the long-term stability of TK activity. The assay remained stable, as indicated by an intraindividual coefficient of variation of 4.7% for 15 samples over 5 freeze-thaw cycles.

The distribution of TK activity was positively skewed (skewedness = −0.602, standard error = 0.096; kurtosis = 1.879, standard error = 0.192). There was a significant correlation between plasma TK levels and urinary TK activity when the plasma TK level was below 0.200 mg/L ($r = -0.100$; $P = 0.016$). This result is similar to our other study, in which we found that plasma TK levels below 0.200 mg/L were negatively associated with recurrent stroke [21]. However, this association disappeared when the plasma TK level was over 0.200 mg/L ($r = 0.150$; $P = 0.244$).

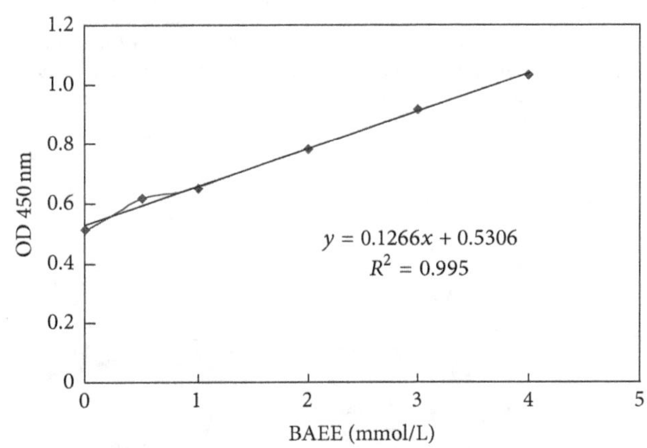


FIGURE 2: Standard curve of TK activity measurement.

*3.2. Study Population Characteristics.* A total of 321 stroke patients (174: ischemic stroke, 147: hemorrhagic stroke) and 323 local control subjects were enrolled in the study. The clinical and laboratory characteristics of the participants at baseline are presented in Table 1. Stoke patients had a significantly higher proportion of hypertension ($P = 0.034$), diabetes ($P = 0.016$), cigarette smoking habits ($P < 0.001$), increased body weight ($P = 0.022$), higher levels of triglycerides ($P < 0.001$), lower levels of HDL cholesterol ($P < 0.001$), and total cholesterol ($P < 0.001$). There were no statistically significant group differences in terms of gender, age, SBP, and BMI. In particular, TK activity was significantly lower in total stroke patients than in controls (1.583 ± 0.673 versus 1.934 ± 0.284 Eu/mL, $P < 0.001$).

Significant differences in TK activity were not observed between ischemic stroke patients and hemorrhagic stroke patients ($P = 0.962$). Further study by the type of stroke showed that both ischemic stroke (1.582 ± 0.601 versus 1.934 ± 0.284 Eu/mL, $P < 0.001$) and hemorrhagic stroke patients (1.585 ± 0.751 versus 1.934 ± 0.284 Eu/mL, $P < 0.001$; Figure 3) had lower TK activity levels than controls.

*3.3. Association of TK Activity with Stroke.* The TK activity values were divided into 4 levels by quartiles as follows: quartile 1 (<1.600 Eu/mL), quartile 2 (1.600 to 1.936 Eu/mL), quartile 3 (1.936 to 2.052 Eu/mL), and quartile

TABLE 1: General characteristics of stroke patients and controls.

| Variable | Stroke patients | Controls | $P$ value |
|---|---|---|---|
| $N$ (male %) | 321 (65) | 323 (34) | 0.121 |
| Age, y | 62.0 ± 10 | 62.6 ± 8 | 0.703 |
| Hypertension, number (%) | 203 (63) | 136 (42) | 0.034 |
| Diabetes, number (%) | 37 (12) | 14 (4) | 0.016 |
| Hyperlipidemia, number (%) | 60 (19) | 91 (28) | 0.003 |
| Current smoker, number (%) | 135 (42) | 49 (15) | <0.001 |
| DBP, mmHg | 90 ± 15 | 81 ± 11 | 0.002 |
| SBP, mmHg | 147 ± 25 | 137 ± 21 | 0.887 |
| Weight, kg | 66 ± 12 | 62 ± 9 | 0.022 |
| BMI, kg/m$^2$ | 24 ± 4 | 24 ± 3 | 0.23 |
| Total cholesterol, mmol/L | 4.49 ± 1.01 | 5.23 ± 1.09 | <0.001 |
| Triglyceride, mmol/L | 1.95 ± 1.0 | 1.65 ± 1.1 | <0.001 |
| HDL cholesterol, mmol/L | 0.88 ± 0.3 | 1.29 ± 0.4 | <0.001 |
| TK activity, Eu/mL | 1.583 ± 0.673 | 1.934 ± 0.284 | <0.001 |

SBP: systolic blood pressure; DBP: diastolic blood pressure; BMI: body mass index; HDL: high-density lipoprotein cholesterol; TK: tissue kallikrein.
$P$ values for the difference between stroke patients and controls, tested with independent samples $t$-test.

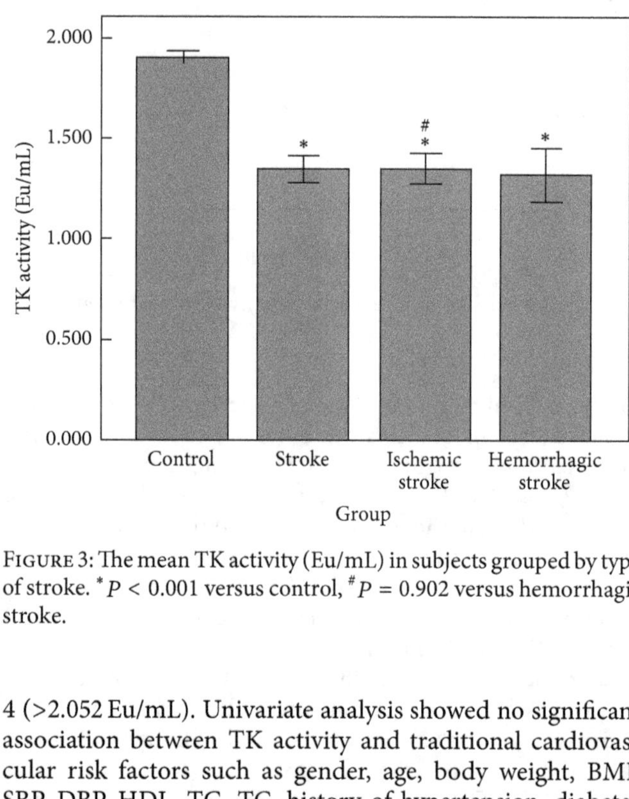


FIGURE 3: The mean TK activity (Eu/mL) in subjects grouped by type of stroke. $^*P < 0.001$ versus control, $^\#P = 0.902$ versus hemorrhagic stroke.

4 (>2.052 Eu/mL). Univariate analysis showed no significant association between TK activity and traditional cardiovascular risk factors such as gender, age, body weight, BMI, SBP, DBP, HDL, TG, TC, history of hypertension, diabetes mellitus, hyperlipidemia, and smoking habits in controls grouped by quartiles, except for a univariate correlation with hyperlipidemia ($P = 0.027$) (Table 2).

TK activity level showed a strong negative association with risk of first-ever stroke in unconditional logistic regression analysis (OR, 0.47; 95% CI, 0.38–0.58; $P < 0.001$), when TK activity was used as a continuous variable after adjusting for traditional risk factors. Compared with quartile 1 of TK activity, the adjusted ORs of total stroke were 0.14 (95% CI, 0.07–0.29), 0.02 (95% CI, 0.01–0.04), and 0.10 (95% CI, 0.05–0.20) in quartiles 2, 3, and 4, respectively. These outcomes indicate that higher TK activity is independently associated with a significantly decreased risk of ischemic and hemorrhagic stroke (Table 3).

There were nonsignificant differences in TK activity among stroke patients with and without traditional cardiovascular risk factors, with the exception of SBP ($r = 0.164$, $P = 0.003$) and DBP ($r = 0.206$, $P < 0.001$). Further analysis by multivariable forward stepwise linear regression analysis showed that TG (Bata = −0.115; $P = 0.040$) and SBP (Bata = 0.110; $P = 0.049$) enter the regression equation in patients with stroke.

*3.4. TK Activity Predicted Follow-Up Outcomes.* Among the 321 patients of first-ever stroke, a total of 105 patients (including 47 ischemic stroke patients and 58 hemorrhagic stroke patients) experienced stroke recurrence during a median follow-up of 5 years (range, 4–5.5 years). We used multivariate Cox proportional hazard models to estimate the association of TK activity in both ischemic and hemorrhagic stroke patients with the recurrence of stroke after adjusting for traditional risk factors. The result of this analysis showed a dose-response relationship between higher TK activity and a markedly lower risk of recurrent stroke (adjusted RR, 0.69; 95% CI, 0.57–0.84; $P < 0.001$). In an unadjusted model using the lowest quartile as a reference group, the second, third, and fourth quartiles were associated with decreased risk of total recurrent stroke ($P < 0.05$). After adjusting for traditional risk factors, those in the higher quartiles of TK activity continued to have decreased risk of recurrent stroke. The adjusted RRs of total recurrent stroke were 0.59 (95% CI, 0.35–0.99), 0.44 (95% CI, 0.25–0.78), and 0.33 (95% CI, 0.18–0.61) in quartiles 2, 3, and 4, respectively (Table 4).

Kaplan-Meier survival analysis was used to examine the association between TK activity, stroke recurrence, and event-free survival time. At 5-year follow-up, the rates of total stroke recurrence were 52.5%, 31.3%, 26.3%, and 21% for stroke patients in quartiles 1, 2, 3, and 4, respectively. The event-free survival time of patients in quartile 1 was 44.4 ± 2.3 months. Compared with patients in quartile 1, the event-free survival times of patients in quartiles 2, 3, and 4 were 48.1 ± 2.3 months (Log Rank test, $P = 0.018$), 52.1 ± 1.7 months (Log Rank test, $P = 0.001$), and 56 ± 1.3 months (Log Rank test, $P < 0.001$) (Figure 4). These data suggested that higher TK activity is predictive of fewer stroke recurrences and a longer event-free survival time.

## 4. Discussion

We examined TK activity in urine and evaluated the relationship between urinary TK activity and plasma TK levels for the first time. The results showed that urinary TK activity was correlated with plasma TK levels when the plasma TK level was below 0.200 mg/L. Patients with ischemic and hemorrhagic stroke exhibit markedly reduced TK activity,

TABLE 2: The relationship between TK activity and cardiovascular disease risk factors in controls.

| Variable | Quartile 1 | Quartile 2 | Quartile 3 | Quartile 4 | *P* value |
|---|---|---|---|---|---|
| TK activity, Eu/mL | <1.600 | 1.600–1.936 | 1.936–2.052 | >2.052 | |
| Number of participants | 16 | 79 | 131 | 97 | |
| Male sex, number (%) | 10 (63) | 25 (32) | 44 (34) | 30 (31) | 0.091 |
| Age, y | 60 ± 7 | 63 ± 8 | 63 ± 8 | 62 ± 7 | 0.236 |
| Hypertension, number (%) | 4 (25) | 34 (43) | 52 (40) | 45 (46) | 0.390 |
| Diabetes, number (%) | 0 (0) | 6 (1) | 4 (0) | 4 (0) | 0.300 |
| Hyperlipidemia, number (%) | 0 (0) | 19 (24) | 38 (29) | 34 (35) | 0.027 |
| Current smoker, number (%) | 4 (25) | 9 (11) | 23 (18) | 13 (13) | 0.407 |
| Weight, kg | 63 ± 9 | 62 ± 10 | 61 ± 9 | 62 ± 9 | 0.392 |
| BMI, kg/m$^2$ | 24 ± 2 | 24 ± 3 | 23 ± 3 | 24 ± 3 | 0.555 |
| SBP, mmHg | 136 ± 6 | 138 ± 20 | 137 ± 21 | 136 ± 21 | 0.883 |
| DBP, mmHg | 85 ± 6 | 82 ± 11 | 81 ± 11 | 81 ± 11 | 0.481 |
| Total cholesterol, mmol/L | 4.89 ± 1.04 | 5.41 ± 0.91 | 5.13 ± 1.16 | 5.26 ± 1.13 | 0.192 |
| Triglyceride, mmol/L | 2.05 ± 1.28 | 1.62 ± 0.99 | 1.59 ± 1.25 | 1.69 ± 1.07 | 0.462 |
| HDL, mmol/L | 1.21 ± 0.33 | 1.30 ± 0.38 | 1.33 ± 0.44 | 1.24 ± 0.32 | 0.286 |

TK: tissue kallikrein; BMI: body mass index; SBP: systolic blood pressure; DBP: diastolic blood pressure; HDL: high-density lipoprotein cholesterol.

TABLE 3: Unconditional logistic regression analysis for stroke and TK activity.

| Group measure | Quartile 1 | Quartile 2 | Quartile 3 | Quartile 4 |
|---|---|---|---|---|
| TK activity, Eu/mL | <1.600 | 1.600–1.936 | 1.936–2.052 | >2.052 |
| Total stroke | 145 | 82 | 30 | 64 |
| Unadjusted (OR)$^{\dagger}$ | 1 | 0.11 (0.06–0.21) | 0.03 (0.013–0.05) | 0.07 (0.04–0.12) |
| Adjusted (OR)$^{\dagger}$ | 1 | 0.14 (0.07–0.29) | 0.02 (0.01–0.04) | 0.10 (0.05–0.20) |
| Ischemic stroke | 66 | 58 | 20 | 30 |
| Unadjusted (OR)$^{\dagger}$ | 1 | 0.81 (0.52–1.27) | 0.20 (0.11–0.37) | 0.32 (0.19–0.52) |
| Adjusted (OR)$^{\dagger}$ | 1 | 1.12 (0.66–1.88) | 0.30 (0.16–0.59) | 0.55 (0.32–0.97) |
| Hemorrhagic stroke | 79 | 24 | 10 | 34 |
| Unadjusted (OR)$^{\dagger}$ | 1 | 0.18 (0.11–0.31) | 0.07 (0.03–0.14) | 0.26 (0.16–0.41) |
| Adjusted (OR)$^{\dagger}$ | 1 | 0.20 (0.10–0.38) | 0.07 (0.03–0.16) | 0.37 (0.21–0.68) |

TK: tissue kallikrein; ORs: odds ratios.
$^{\dagger}$ORs (95% confidence interval). Adjusted ORs have been adjusted for age, sex, presence or absence of hypertension, diabetes, hyperlipidemia, smoking, weight, BMI, SBP, DBP, total cholesterol, triglyceride, and HDL.

independent of other factors related to the risk of arterial disease. These results are consistent with our previous study, which showed that lower plasma TK levels were independently associated with the first occurrence of stroke [21]. These results further suggest that TK may be an independent endogenous protective factor against stroke in the Chinese population.

Previous studies have typically measured TK activity in urine using radioimmunoassay [27, 28]. Immunological and chemical technologies result in less radiocontamination and are comparatively safer. We therefore developed a novel assay to measure TK activity by utilizing its immunological characteristics [29] and the chemical characteristics of BAEE [23]. The results of this assay indicated that the TK activity is correlated with plasma TK levels. However, this association disappeared when the plasma TK level exceeded 0.200 mg/L.

TK has been demonstrated to elicit a broad spectrum of biological effects, such as reducing hypertension, cardiovascular and renal damage, restenosis, ischemic stroke, and skin wound injury. TK attenuates cardiovascular, renal, and brain damage by inhibiting oxidative stress, cell proliferation, apoptosis, inflammation, hypertrophy, atherosclerosis, and fibrosis and promoting angiogenesis and neurogenesis [14–18]. Transgenic and somatic gene transfer approaches have been used to achieve a continuous supply of TK and have shown that TK significantly reduces aortic thickening and the stroke-induced death rate in Dahl salt-sensitive rats [30]. TK provides neuroprotection against cerebral ischemia injury by enhancing glial cell survival and migration and inhibiting apoptosis through the suppression of oxidative stress and activation of the Akt-Bcl-2 signaling pathway [31].

In our previous study, higher plasma TK levels (below 0.200 mg/L) predicted a lower risk of stroke recurrence and a longer stroke-free interval over the course of a 5-year follow-up study. However, this association did not exist when the plasma TK level was over 0.200 mg/L [21]. In this report, subjects experiencing a subsequent stroke had significantly lower TK activity than first-ever stroke patients who had not

Table 4: The association between TK activity and stroke recurrence.

| Stroke recurrence | Quartile 1 | Quartile 2 | Quartile 3 | Quartile 4 |
|---|---|---|---|---|
| Total stroke, *n* | 80 | 80 | 80 | 81 |
| Events, number (%) | 42 (52.5) | 25 (31.3) | 21 (26.3) | 17 (21) |
| Unadjusted (RR)[†] | 1 | 0.55 (0.34–0.91) | 0.43 (0.25–0.72) | 0.32 (0.18–0.54) |
| *P* value | | 0.019 | 0.001 | <0.001 |
| Adjusted (RR)[†] | 1 | 0.59 (0.35–0.99) | 0.44 (0.25–0.78) | 0.33 (0.18–0.61) |
| *P* value | | 0.048 | 0.005 | <0.001 |
| Ischemic stroke | 40 | 37 | 55 | 42 |
| Events, number (%) | 22 (55) | 14 (37.8) | 15 (27.3) | 7 (16.7) |
| Unadjusted (RR)[†] | 1 | 0.71 (0.36–1.39) | 0.45 (0.23–0.87) | 0.25 (0.11–0.58) |
| *P* value | | 0.321 | 0.018 | 0.001 |
| Adjusted (RR)[†] | 1 | 0.90 (0.43–1.89) | 0.59 (0.28–1.22) | 0.30 (0.12–0.75) |
| *P* value | | 0.779 | 0.155 | 0.01 |
| Hemorrhagic stroke | 40 | 43 | 25 | 39 |
| Events, number (%) | 20 (50) | 11 (25.6) | 6 (24) | 10 (25.6) |
| Unadjusted (RR)[†] | 1 | 0.44 (0.21–0.92) | 0.39 (0.16–0.98) | 0.39 (0.18–0.84) |
| *P* value | | 0.028 | 0.046 | 0.016 |
| Adjusted (RR)[†] | 1 | 0.27 (0.12–0.63) | 0.16 (0.06–0.46) | 0.17 (0.07–0.46) |
| *P* value | | 0.002 | 0.001 | <0.001 |

TK activity in quartile 1 (<1.063 Eu/mL), quartile 2 (1.063–1.667 Eu/mL), quartile 3 (1.667–1.988 Eu/mL), and quartile 4 (>1.988 Eu/mL).

TK: tissue kallikrein; RRs: relative risks. [†]RRs (95% confidence interval). Adjusted RRs have been adjusted for age, sex, presence or absence of hypertension, diabetes, hyperlipidemia, smoking, weight, BMI, SBP, DBP, total cholesterol, triglyceride, and HDL.

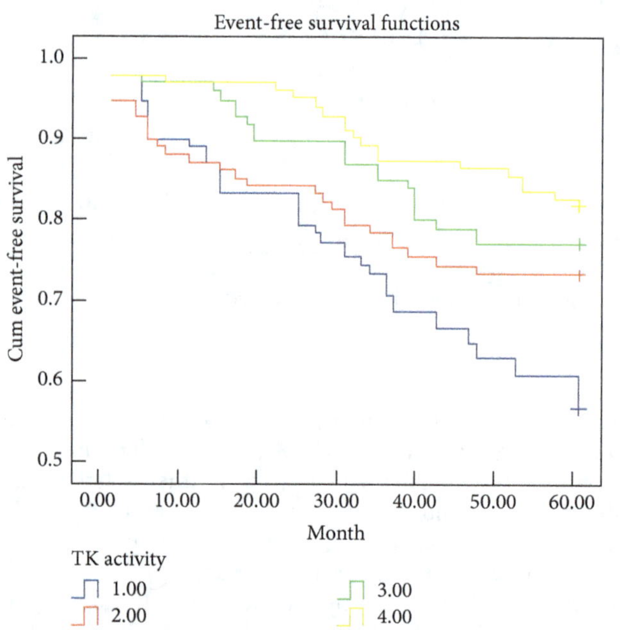


Figure 4: Kaplan-Meier survival curves based on TK activity. 1 = quartile 1; 2 = quartile 2; 3 = quartile 3; 4 = quartile 4.

experienced a recurrence. Our data showed that TK activity is negatively associated in a dose-dependent manner with overall stroke recurrence. These results might have several explanations. First, TK may both directly and indirectly activate the kinin B2 receptor and trigger an array of biological effects by increasing nitric oxide (NO)/cyclic 3′, 5′-guanosine monophosphate and cyclic adenosine monophosphate (cAMP) levels, thus reducing nicotinamide adenine dinucleotide phosphate oxidase activity and proinflammatory cytokine levels and activating the intracellular PI3 kinase/Akt and MAP kinase pathways, thereby protecting against atherosclerosis and cerebral injuries and preventing initial or recurrent stroke [32]. Second, traditional risk factors for stroke might impact plasma TK levels or TK activity. However, our previous study evaluated the association between TK level and activity in control subjects and found no significant statistical correlations by multivariate stepwise linear regression analysis, except for those with lipid metabolism. Cox proportional hazard models showed that plasma TK levels below 0.200 mg/L were independently and negatively associated with event and recurrent total stroke in a dose-dependent manner, regardless of whether adjustments were made for traditional stroke risk factors [21]. Therefore, these risk factors did not significantly impact plasma TK levels. In addition, an effect of these risk factors on TK activity was not observed. Third, TK protected humans from initial or recurrent stroke by activating endothelial NO synthase and increasing NO production, which triggers a broad spectrum of biological effects, including vasodilatation; smooth muscle contraction and relaxation; inhibition of apoptosis, atherosclerosis, inflammation, hypertrophy, and fibrosis; protection against ischemia/reperfusion damage; and promotion of angiogenesis and neurogenesis [14, 15]. Fourth, when plasma TK levels were above 0.200 mg/L, there was no association between plasma TK level and urinary TK activity, and there was no relationship between plasma TK level and the risk of stroke recurrence and stroke-free interval. Therefore, we suspected that plasma TK levels above 0.200 mg/L might inactivate the kinin B2 receptor and then suppress TK activity in urine. Further prospective and basic studies are needed to determine why plasma TK levels above 0.200 mg/L were not associated with urinary TK activity or the risk of stroke recurrence. Therefore, urinary TK activity may act as a protective factor against initial and recurrent stroke, and urinary TK activity may be a stronger predictor than plasma TK level of the recurrence of both ischemic and hemorrhagic strokes. Fifth, elevated TK may directly inhibit the proliferation, migration, and phenotype transformation of vascular smooth muscle cells by Rho/ROCK signaling pathway and protect human from stroke [33, 34]. In addition, DNA methylation, a powerful epigenetic regulator of endothelial transcription, plays an important role in the process of atherosclerosis [35, 36]. We, therefore, suspect that the methylation of KLK1 promoter region may affect TK activity and the occurrence of stroke. Therefore, studies on DNA methylation of the kallikrein-kinin genes will enhance the understanding of their role in stroke protection and provide insights into the predictor of stroke recurrent.

There are several limitations in the current study that should be addressed. First, both plasma TK levels and urinary TK activity were measured after stroke; therefore, we could not create a causal connection between stroke and reduced plasma TK level or urinary TK activity, nor could we determine whether changes in TK level and TK activity are predictors or consequences of first-ever stroke. Second, even though we adjusted for traditional risk factors in the multivariate stepwise linear regression analysis, the possibility of residual confounding elements remains. Third, the influence of diet on TK activity cannot be ruled out. Fourth, a causal link between reduced TK activity and recurrent stroke is biologically plausible and is supported by temporal and long-term associations and a dose-dependent correlation between urinary TK activity and long-term prognosis for stroke patients. Compared with plasma TK levels, urinary TK activities may be a stronger predictor of recurrent stroke. These issues can only be addressed through additional prospective studies of the association between TK activity and first-ever stroke. Additional studies could elucidate why stroke patients exhibit lower urinary TK activity.

## 5. Conclusions

This work, combined with our previous study, suggests that both the plasma TK level and urinary TK activity have a significant inverse relationship with first-ever stroke and stroke recurrence in the Chinese population. Furthermore, urinary TK activity may be a stronger predictor of recurrent stroke than plasma TK level. Large prospective human studies, as well as cellular and animal research, are needed to establish causality between stroke and TK activity.

## Conflict of Interests

The authors declare that they have no conflict of interests regarding the publication of this paper.

## Authors' Contribution

Qin Zhang and Dao Wen Wang conceived and designed the experiments; Xiao Ran and Qin Zhang performed the experiments; Xiao Ran and Qin Zhang analyzed the data and wrote the paper.

## Acknowledgments

The authors would like to thank all the participants in this study. This work was supported by Grants from the National Natural Science Foundation of China (no. 81100864).

## References

[1] S. C. Johnston, S. Mendis, and C. D. Mathers, "Global variation in stroke burden and mortality: estimates from monitoring, surveillance, and modelling," *The Lancet Neurology*, vol. 8, no. 4, pp. 345–354, 2009.

[2] S. Sidney, W. D. Rosamond, V. J. Howard, and R. V. Luepker, "The 'heart disease and stroke statistics—2013 update' and the need for a national cardiovascular surveillance system," *Circulation*, vol. 127, no. 1, pp. 21–23, 2013.

[3] G. Xu, X. Liu, W. Wu, R. Zhang, and Q. Yin, "Recurrence after ischemic stroke in chinese patients: impact of uncontrolled modifiable risk factors," *Cerebrovascular Diseases*, vol. 23, no. 2-3, pp. 117–120, 2007.

[4] L. Liu, D. Wang, K. S. L. Wong, and Y. Wang, "Stroke and stroke care in China: huge burden, significant workload, and a national priority," *Stroke*, vol. 42, no. 12, pp. 3651–3654, 2011.

[5] J. S. Kim, H.-W. Nah, S. M. Park et al., "Risk factors and stroke mechanisms in atherosclerotic stroke: intracranial compared with extracranial and anterior compared with posterior circulation disease," *Stroke*, vol. 43, no. 12, pp. 3313–3318, 2012.

[6] C. Golias, A. Charalabopoulos, D. Stagikas, K. A. Charalabopoulos, and A. Batistatou, "The kinin system—bradykinin: biological effects and clinical implications. Multiple role of the kinin system—bradykinin," *Hippokratia*, vol. 11, no. 3, pp. 124–128, 2007.

[7] N. Emami and E. P. Diamandis, "Human tissue kallikreins: a road under construction," *Clinica Chimica Acta*, vol. 381, no. 1, pp. 78–84, 2007.

[8] R. Mahabeer and K. D. Bhoola, "Kallikrein and kinin receptor genes," *Pharmacology & Therapeutics*, vol. 88, no. 1, pp. 77–89, 2000.

[9] J. Chao, B. Shen, L. Gao, C.-F. Xia, G. Bledsoe, and L. Chao, "Tissue kallikrein in cardiovascular, cerebrovascular and renal diseases and skin wound healing," *Biological Chemistry*, vol. 391, no. 4, pp. 345–355, 2010.

[10] P. Li, T. Kondo, Y. Numaguchi et al., "Role of bradykinin, nitric oxide, and angiotensin II type 2 receptor in imidapril-induced angiogenesis," *Hypertension*, vol. 51, no. 2, pp. 252–258, 2008.

[11] D. Westermann, H.-P. Schultheiss, and C. Tschöpe, "New perspective on the tissue kallikrein-kinin system in myocardial infarction: role of angiogenesis and cardiac regeneration," *International Immunopharmacology*, vol. 8, no. 2, pp. 148–154, 2008.

[12] L. Potier, L. Waeckel, C. Richer, R. Roussel, N. Bouby, and F. Alhenc-Gelas, "Tissue kallikrein, blood pressure regulation, and hypertension: insight from genetic kallikrein deficiency," *Biological Chemistry*, vol. 394, no. 3, pp. 329–333, 2013.

[13] Y.-Y. Yao, H. Yin, B. Shen, L. Chao, and J. Chao, "Tissue kallikrein and kinin infusion rescues failing myocardium after myocardial infarction," *Journal of Cardiac Failure*, vol. 13, no. 7, pp. 588–596, 2007.

[14] R.-Y. Lu, D.-F. Luo, S.-H. Xiao et al., "Kallikrein gene transfer induces angiogenesis and further improves regional cerebral blood flow in the early period after cerebral ischemia/reperfusion in rats," *CNS Neuroscience & Therapeutics*, vol. 18, no. 5, pp. 395–399, 2012.

[15] H.-Z. Yu, L.-D. Xie, P.-L. Zhu, C.-S. Xu, and H.-J. Wang, "Human tissue kallikrein 1 gene delivery inhibits PDGF-BB-induced vascular smooth muscle cells proliferation and upregulates the expressions of $p27^{Kip1}$ and $p21^{Cip1}$," *Molecular and Cellular Biochemistry*, vol. 360, no. 1-2, pp. 363–371, 2012.

[16] H. Yin, L. Chao, and J. Chao, "Kallikrein/kinin protects against myocardial apoptosis after ischemia/reperfusion via Akt-glycogen synthase kinase-3 and Akt-Bad.14-3-3 signaling pathways," *The Journal of Biological Chemistry*, vol. 280, no. 9, pp. 8022–8030, 2005.

[17] Z. Wang, X. Han, M. Cui, K. Fang, Z. Lu, and Q. Dong, "Tissue kallikrein protects rat hippocampal CA1 neurons against cerebral ischemia/reperfusion-induced injury through the B2R-Raf-MEK1/2-ERK1/2 pathway," *Journal of Neuroscience Research*, vol. 92, no. 5, pp. 651–657, 2014.

[18] Y. Yao, Z. Sheng, Y. Li et al., "Tissue kallikrein-modified human endothelial progenitor cell implantation improves cardiac function via enhanced activation of akt and increased angiogenesis," *Laboratory Investigation*, vol. 93, no. 5, pp. 577–591, 2013.

[19] N. Ura, K. Shimamoto, T. Nakao et al., "The excretion of human urinary kallikrein quantity and activity in normal and low renin subgroups of essential hypertension," *Clinical and Experimental Hypertension A*, vol. 5, no. 3, pp. 329–337, 1983.

[20] W. J. Lawton and A. E. Fitz, "Urinary kallikrein in normal renin essential hypertension," *Circulation*, vol. 56, no. 5, pp. 856–859, 1977.

[21] Q. Zhang, H. Ding, J. Yan et al., "Plasma tissue kallikrein level is negatively associated with incident and recurrent stroke: a multicenter case-control study in China," *Annals of Neurology*, vol. 70, no. 2, pp. 265–273, 2011.

[22] Q. Zhang, X. Ran, and D. W. Wang, "Relation of plasma tissue kallikrein levels to presence and severity of coronary artery disease in a Chinese population," *PLoS ONE*, vol. 9, no. 3, Article ID e91780, 2014.

[23] T. Nikai, Y. Komori, S. Kato, and H. Sugihara, "Biological properties of kinin-releasing enzyme from *Trimeresurus okinavensis* (himehabu) venom," *Journal of Natural Toxins*, vol. 7, no. 1, pp. 23–35, 1998.

[24] A. O. Aasen, W. Frolich, O. D. Saugstad, and E. Amundsen, "Plasma kallikrein activity and prekallikrein levels during endotoxin shock in dogs," *European Surgical Research*, vol. 10, no. 1, pp. 50–62, 1978.

[25] P. S. Roberts, "Measurement of the rate of plasmin action on synthetic substrates," *The Journal of Biological Chemistry*, vol. 232, no. 1, pp. 285–291, 1958.

[26] J. M. Da Costa Castro, F. Deschamps, M. Benbachir, J. Henrichsen, P. J. Volle, and R. M. F. Guinet, "Highly sensitive biotin-avidin sandwich ELISA for the rapid detection of pneumococcal capsular polysaccharide antigens," *Journal of Immunological Methods*, vol. 104, no. 1-2, pp. 265–270, 1987.

[27] O. A. Carretero, N. B. Oza, A. Piwonska, T. Ocholik, and A. G. Scicli, "Measurement of urinary kallikrein activity by kinin radioimmunoassay," *Biochemical Pharmacology*, vol. 25, no. 20, pp. 2265–2270, 1976.

[28] S. H. Zinner, H. S. Margolius, B. Rosner, and E. H. Kass, "Stability of blood pressure rank and urinary kallikrein concentration in childhood: an eight-year follow-up," *Circulation*, vol. 58, no. 5, pp. 908–915, 1978.

[29] J. Chao, L. Chao, D. M. Tillman, C. M. Woodley, and H. S. Margolius, "Characterization of monoclonal and polyclonal antibodies to human tissue kallikrein," *Hypertension*, vol. 7, no. 6, part 1, pp. 931–937, 1985.

[30] J. Chao and L. Chao, "Experimental therapy with tissue kallikrein against cerebral ischemia," *Frontiers in Bioscience*, vol. 11, no. 2, pp. 1323–1327, 2006.

[31] C.-F. Xia, H. Yin, C. V. Borlongan, L. Chao, and J. Chao, "Kallikrein gene transfer protects against ischemic stroke by promoting glial cell migration and inhibiting apoptosis," *Hypertension*, vol. 43, no. 2, pp. 452–459, 2004.

[32] G. Yuan, J. Deng, T. Wang et al., "Tissue kallikrein reverses insulin resistance and attenuates nephropathy in diabetic rats by activation of phosphatidylinositol 3-kinase/protein kinase B and adenosine 5′-monophosphate-activated protein kinase signaling pathways," *Endocrinology*, vol. 148, no. 5, pp. 2016–2026, 2007.

[33] G. S. Ceravolo, A. C. Montezano, M. T. Jordão et al., "An interaction of renin-angiotensin and kallikrein-kinin systems contributes to vascular hypertrophy in angiotensin II-induced hypertension: in vivo and in vitro studies," *PLoS ONE*, vol. 9, no. 11, Article ID e111117, 2014.

[34] A. Martinsen, N. Baeyens, X. Yerna, and N. Morel, "Rho kinase regulation of vasopressin-induced calcium entry in vascular smooth muscle cell: comparison between rat isolated aorta and cultured aortic cells," *Cell Calcium*, vol. 52, no. 6, pp. 413–421, 2012.

[35] A. Baccarelli, R. Wright, V. Bollati et al., "Ischemic heart disease and stroke in relation to blood DNA methylation," *Epidemiology*, vol. 21, no. 6, pp. 819–828, 2010.

[36] I. A. Qureshi and M. F. Mehler, "Emerging role of epigenetics in stroke—part 1: DNA methylation and chromatin modifications," *Archives of Neurology*, vol. 67, no. 11, pp. 1316–1322, 2010.

# 30

# Modelling the Role of Dietary Habits and Eating Behaviours on the Development of Acute Coronary Syndrome or Stroke: Aims, Design, and Validation Properties of a Case-Control Study

**Christina-Maria Kastorini,[1,2] Haralampos J. Milionis,[1] John A. Goudevenos,[1] and Demosthenes B. Panagiotakos[2]**

[1] *School of Medicine, University of Ioannina, 45110 Ioannina, Greece*
[2] *Department of Nutrition Science and Dietetics, Harokopio University, 17671 Athens, Greece*

Correspondence should be addressed to Demosthenes B. Panagiotakos, d.b.panagiotakos@usa.net

Academic Editor: Christina Chrysohoou

In this paper the methodology and procedures of a case-control study that will be developed for assessing the role of dietary habits and eating behaviours on the development of acute coronary syndrome and stroke is presented. Based on statistical power calculations, 1000 participants will be enrolled; of them, 250 will be consecutive patients with a first acute coronary event, 250 consecutive patients with a first ischaemic stroke, and 500 population-based healthy subjects (controls), age and sex matched to the cases. Socio-demographic, clinical, dietary, psychological, and other lifestyle characteristics will be measured. Dietary habits and eating behaviours will be evaluated with a special questionnaire that has been developed for the study.

## 1. Introduction

Cardiovascular disease (CVD) is the leading cause of morbidity and mortality at a global level, with a significant impact on quality of life as well as an important economic burden [1]. In fact, in 2002, it is estimated that 7.2 million people died from coronary heart disease and 5.5 million from stroke, while according to the WHO estimates and due to the demographic changes, the number of CVD events is expected to increase further [2]. Therefore, prevention of CVD is now considered of major public health importance. Means for reducing the burden of the disease at population level include lifestyle interventions, and particularly dietary modifications.

During the last decades, studies from all over the world have evaluated the relationship between specific foods and dietary patterns with the development of CVD, and particularly coronary heart disease [3–8]. Healthy dietary patterns, like the Mediterranean, characterized by high consumption of foods of plant origin, fruits, vegetables, whole grain cereals, legumes, as well as poultry and fish, have been associated with decreased risk of the disease. On the contrary, more western dietary patterns, characterized by increased consumption of red and processed meat, sweets and desserts, potatoes, and refined cereal are associated with increased risk. However, the role of diet on the development of ischaemic stroke is not that well established [9, 10]. Moreover, although significant scientific evidence exists regarding the role of specific foods and dietary patterns on the development of CVD, the influence of certain dietary behaviours and practices has not been extensively studied and understood. For example, apart from the type of foods that are actually consumed, meal frequency, breakfast consumption, food consumption in parallel with other activities (such as working or television viewing), systematic consumption of heavy meals or eating alone, as well as sleeping patterns may also play an important direct or indirect role, regarding the development of coronary heart disease and stroke [11–15] (Figure 1).

Thus, the aim of the present study is to evaluate the role of dietary habits and eating behaviours on the likelihood

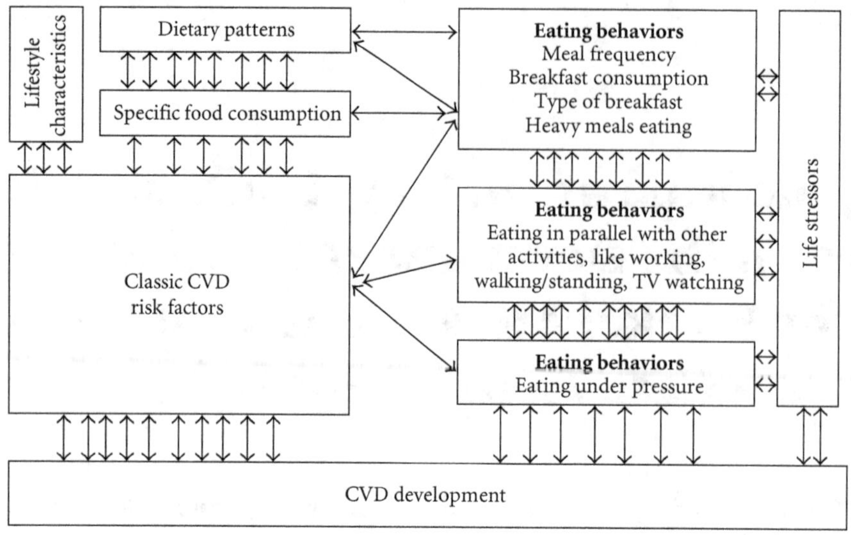


FIGURE 1: A conceptual model about dietary patterns, eating and lifestyle behaviours, and practices that will be tested in this study regarding the development of CVD.

of developing a first CVD event (acute coronary syndrome or stroke), after taking into account other lifestyle and environmental factors as well as socio-demographic and clinical characteristics.

## 2. Materials and Methods

*2.1. Design.* Multicentre, case-control with individual, age (within ±3 years) and sex matching (Figure 2).

*2.2. Sampling Procedure.* According to the sampling procedure all consecutive patients with a first acute coronary syndrome (ACS) event (acute myocardial infarction (AMI) or unstable angina (UA)) or ischaemic stroke, and without any suspicion of previous CVD, that will enter in the cardiology, pathology clinics, or the emergency units of three major General Hospitals in Greece (i.e., University General Hospital of Ioannina, Korgialeneio-Benakeio Red Cross Hospital, and Alexandra General Hospital, Athens) between October 1, 2009 and December 31, 2010 will be contacted to enrol in the study. Patients with a history of neoplasia or chronic inflammatory disease, as well as individuals with recent changes in their dietary habits, will not be included. Control subjects will be selected on a random, volunteer basis, and they will be without any clinical symptoms or suspicions of CVD in their medical history, as this will be assessed by a cardiologist. The control subjects will be allocated at population basis, and from the same region of the patients. Based on a priori statistical power analysis, a sample size of 500 patients (250 ACS, 250 stroke) and 500 age- and sex-matched healthy subjects, is adequate to evaluate two-sided odds ratios equal to 1.20, achieving statistical power greater than .80 at .05 probability level ($P$ value).

*2.3. Diagnosis of ACS or Stroke.* At hospital entry clinical symptoms will be evaluated and a 12-lead electrocardiogram will be performed, by a cardiologist. Evidence of myocardial cell death will be assessed with blood tests and measurement of the levels of troponin I and the MB fraction of total creatinine phosphokinase (CPK). According to the Universal Definition of Myocardial Infarction (Joint ESC/ACCF/AHA/WHF Task Force) [16], blood samples will be obtained on hospital admission, at 6 to 9 h, and again at 12 to 24 h if earlier samples will be negative and the clinical index of suspicion is high. Acute coronary syndromes, and particularly myocardial infarction (AMI) will be defined by detection of rise and/or fall of troponin I or CPK with at least one value above the 99th percentile of the upper reference limit as well as with at least one of the following features: (a) compatible clinical symptoms, (b) ECG changes indicative of new ischaemia (new ST-T changes or new left bundle branch block LBBB), (c) development of pathological Q waves in the ECG, (d) imaging evidence of new loss of viable myocardium or new regional wall motion abnormality [16]; unstable angina (UA) will be defined by the occurrence of one or more angina episodes, at rest, within the preceding 48 h, corresponding to class III of the Braunwald classification [17]. Ischaemic strokes will be defined through symptoms of neurologic dysfunction of acute onset of any severity, consistent with focal brain ischaemia and imaging/laboratory confirmation of an acute vascular ischaemic pathology [18].

*2.4. Anthropometric Characteristics.* Body weight (in kilograms) and height (in meters) will be measured following standard procedures (i.e., height will be measured to the nearest 0.5 cm, without shoes, back square against the wall tape, eyes looking straight ahead, while weight will be measured with a lever balance, to the nearest 100 g, without shoes, in light undergarments). Due to possible difficulties

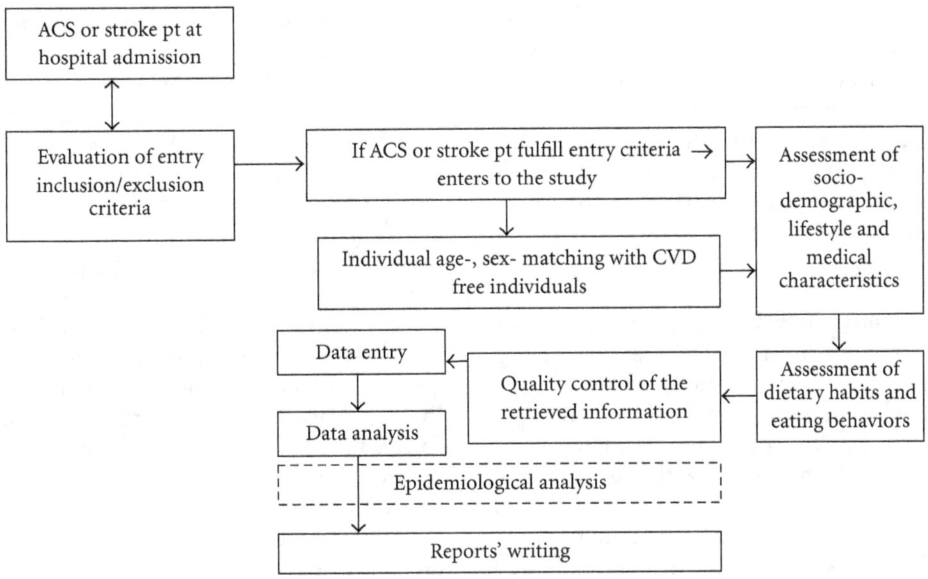


FIGURE 2: Flowchart of the study.

in the assessment of these anthropometric characteristics for the patients, it will be recorded whether the above values are self-reported or measured. Body mass index will then be calculated as weight (in kilograms) divided by standing height (in meters squared) and overweight and obesity will be defined as body mass index 25.0–29.9 kg/m$^2$ and >29.9 kg/m$^2$, respectively. Additionally participants will be asked what their lower and higher body weight was after the age of 20 years (in kilograms). Moreover, the participants will be asked if they have gained or lost weight during the last three months. In case they did, the kilograms gained or lost, and if the gain or the loss were voluntary or not will be recorded.

*2.5. Socio-Demographic Characteristics.* Socio-demographic variables that will be recorded are age and sex (for the matching procedure), educational level measured by years of school, type of occupation (in the following categories: civil servant, private employee, part-time employee, freelancer, rentier, retired, unemployed, housewife) and occupational skills that will be evaluated through a nine-point scale (values 1–3 refer to manual labour, while values from 7 to 9 refer to intellectual labour). Marital status categorised as single, married, divorced, or widowed and number of children will also be recorded. Financial status will be indirectly evaluated using (a) an index measuring how satisfied the participant is from his/her income (i.e., value 1 means not at all satisfied, to value 9 which means very satisfied), (b) the number of cars in the family, (c) the number of rooms in the house (including kitchen and bathroom), and (d) whether the residence is owned or not.

*2.6. Lifestyle Characteristics.* Physical activity will be assessed using the International Physical Activity Questionnaire (IPAQ) index [19] that has been validated for the Greek population, too [20]. Subjects will be asked to recall the number of days and hours or minutes they engaged in physical activity of different intensities for at least ten minutes, vigorous intensity and moderate intensity, walking and time spent sitting. According to their physical activity levels, participants will be classified as inactive, minimally active, or health enhancing physical activity (HEPA) active.

Furthermore, sleeping patterns will be assessed and participants will be asked about the hours they sleep at night, if they nap during the day (almost never, only on holidays, sometimes per week, almost every day), and in case they do, for how long (in minutes). They will also be asked about the frequency of night shifts at work (less than once in three months, 1–3 times per month, 2–4 times per week, almost every day). Television viewing will also be assessed by the hours of television viewed daily (less than 1 h, 1-2 h, 3–5 h, more than 5 h) and frequency of food consumption in front of the TV will be recorded (less than once in three months, 1–3 times per month, 2–4 times per week, almost every day).

Current or former smoking habits will be recorded and participants will be classified as (a) current smokers, (b) former smokers, or (c) non-smokers. Particularly, current smokers will be defined as those who smoke at least one cigarette per day, former smokers as those who had stopped smoking more than one year previously, and the rest of the participants will be defined as non-current smokers. Additionally, current and former smokers will be asked about the age they started smoking, the total number of years they smoke, and the number of cigarettes they smoke/smoked daily. Former smokers will be also asked about the number of years they have stopped smoking. Moreover, current and former smokers will be asked about the type of smoke they prefer/preferred (i.e., regular cigarettes, light cigarettes, tobacco), whether they smoke/smoked pipe or cigars, and if they smoke/smoked in their workplace, at home, or in front of their children. For the evaluation of passive smoking, participants will be asked if other colleagues smoke in front of them in the workplace for more than 30 min daily and if other people in their environment smoke in front of them for more than 30 min per day (partner, parents, children, roommates). If they are not currently exposed to passive smoking, participants will be asked if they were exposed in passive smoking in the past and the years of exposure to passive smoking will be recorded.

*2.7. Assessment of Dietary Habits.* Dietary habits of the past year will be assessed through a 90-item, validated semi-quantitative food-frequency questionnaire (FFQ). Its validation properties will be briefly presented below. Regarding the dietary assessment, the participant will be asked how often (i.e., less than 3 months, 1-2 times/3 months, 1-2 times/month, 2–4 times/month, 1-2 times/week, 3–5 times/week, almost every day, more than one time per day) he/she consumes the following foods and beverages: red meat, processed meat, poultry, fish (and more specifically baked/boiled fish, fried fish, fresh tuna, or swordfish), legumes, cooked vegetables, pasta and rice (and in particular white pasta, whole wheat pasta, white rice, brown rice), potatoes, salads and fresh vegetables (and more specifically green leafy, cruciferous, coloured or starchy vegetables), eggs, sweets (and in particular baked sweets, honey, marmalade, cakes, white or milk chocolate, dark chocolate), consumption of non-homemade food and type of food (fast-food, sandwich, restaurant), salted nuts, unsalted nuts, canned food, milk and yogurt (and in particular full fat, low fat or skim), the number of milk and yogurt servings consumed in one week, feta-cheese, low fat white cheese, yellow cheese, low fat yellow cheese, and the number of servings of cheese consumed in one week. Fruit consumption will be recorded in fruits per day. The frequency of consumption (rarely, monthly, weekly, daily) of the following sources of fat will also be evaluated: olive oil for cooking or salad dressing, olive oil for frying, seed oil for cooking or salad dressing, seed oil for frying, mayonnaise or other sauce, butter, margarine, milk cream, olives. Additionally, the type of olive oil (packed extra-virgin olive oil, packed virgin olive oil, packed refined olive oil, unpacked olive oil—production by the participant, unpacked olive oil bought from friends) and the weekly amount (in litters) consumed will be assessed. Furthermore, bread as well as rusk consumption will be evaluated according to slices of bread consumed daily (less than half a slice, 0-1, 1-2, 3-4, 5-6, over 7 slices) and according to rusks consumed daily (less than one, 1-2, 3-4, 5-6, 7-8, over 9). The type (white or whole wheat) of bread and rusk consumption will be also recorded (frequency: rarely, monthly, weekly, and daily). Salt consumption in cooking, and the use of table salt or salt substitute will also be assessed. In addition, water, beverages, and juice consumption will be assessed in glasses per day. The type of beverage (cola drink, soda, light) and juice (carbonated, non-carbonated, from fresh fruits) will be evaluated. Frequency of alcohol consumption will be assessed in four categories: rarely, monthly, weekly, and daily. The participant will be also asked if he/she consumed more alcohol in the past as compared with the present consumption. Furthermore, the type of drink consumed will be recorded (i.e., beer, white wine, red wine, whisky, vodka, or ouzo) and the amount of alcohol consumed will be measured in wineglasses per day (i.e., <1, 1-2, 3-4, 5-6, over 7 wineglasses; each wineglass will be equivalent to 12 g of ethanol). Additionally, alcohol consumption patterns will be recorded; in particular, drinking of large quantities of alcohol rarely (for example in the weekends) as well as the frequency of hangover during the last year (i.e., never, 1-2 times/year, 1-2 times/6 months, 1-2 times/month, over twice/month). Coffee consumption will be assessed regarding its frequency (i.e., rarely, monthly, weekly, and daily). The participants will be asked about the type of coffee they prefer to drink (Greek, instant coffee, filtered, espresso, decaffeinated, cappuccino) as well as about the cups of coffee consumed daily (<1, 1-2, 3-4, 5-6, over 7). Additionally, the amount of coffee added in teaspoons in each cup, the type of coffee consumed (light, medium, heavy), and whether sugar or other sweetener is added and if yes, how many teaspoons are added will be evaluated. Frequency (i.e., rarely, monthly, weekly, daily) of tea consumption, the number of cups of tea per day (i.e., 0-1, 1-2, 3–5, over 5 cups) as well as the type of tea consumed (mountain tea, green tea, black tea, chamomile tea) will be also assessed. Additionally, participants will be asked whether they add sugar or other sweetener, and if yes how many teaspoons they add. Furthermore, the participants will be asked if they are on a diet and if they have changed their dietary patterns during the last year. Participants with important recent (i.e., within a year) changes in their dietary habits will be excluded from the study.

Overall assessment of dietary habits will be performed using the MedDietScore [21], an eleven-item composite index that evaluates adherence to the Mediterranean dietary pattern. The range of the MedDietScore is between 0–55. Higher values of this diet score indicate greater adherence to the Mediterranean diet. The validation properties of the MedDietScore have been presented elsewhere in the literature [21–23].

*2.8. Validation of the FFQ.* As mentioned above, a semi-quantitative FFQ developed for the purposes of this study will be used. For the validation properties, 59 males (40 ± 14 yrs) and 77 females (40 ± 13 yrs) were asked to complete the FFQ presented above, during 2010. Participants were also asked to complete a 3-day food record of what they have eaten. The recording period included two weekdays and one weekend day, over the same time span as the FFQ. This record was used as the reference method for validating the FFQ. Agreement of the FFQ with the 3-day food records was evaluated using the Bland-Altman method and the Kendall's tau-b coefficient. Between the 3-day food records and the FFQ, moderate agreement for coffee (tau-b = 0.56, $P < .001$), fruits (tau-b = 0.48, $P < .001$), fast-food consumption (tau-b = 0.47, $P < .001$), alcohol (tau-b = 0.47, $P < .001$), sweets (tau-b = 0.36, $P < .001$), vegetables (tau-b = 0.32, $P < .001$), and red meat (tau-b = 0.31, $P < .001$) was found, while low, but still significant agreement for greens (tau-b = 0.22, $P$ = .004), cereals (tau-b = 0.21, $P$ < .001), and dairy products (tau-b = 0.18, $P$ = .007) was observed. According to the Bland-Altman method the level of agreement varied from 90% to 99%. Sensitivity analyses by sex and age category (< or >55 yrs) and obesity status showed similar validity of the FFQ in each subgroup.

*2.9. Assessment of Eating Behaviours.* As mentioned in the aim of the study, a research hypothesis that will be also tested is whether certain eating behaviours may influence the likelihood of developing ACS or stroke. Thus, a special questionnaire that has been designed for the purposes of the present study will be used to evaluate several behaviours of the participants such as meal frequency, breakfast consumption, consumption of food in parallel with other activities. Frequency of consumption (rarely, 1-2 times/week, 3–5 times/week, and almost every day) of the following meals and snacks will be assessed: breakfast, morning snack, lunch, evening snack, dinner, and bed-time snack. Consumption of any food except water will be considered as a meal or snack. Additionally, potential reasons for skipping a meal will be evaluated. Participants will be asked about how frequently (less than once in three months, 1–3 times per month, 2–4 times per week, almost every day) they skip a meal or snack, because of hard work, because of the will to lose weight, or because they are not hungry. Detailed information will be asked regarding breakfast consumption. In particular, participants will be asked about the time they eat breakfast (earlier than 6 am, 6–8 am, 8–10 am, after 10 am) and the frequency (rarely, 1-2 times/week, 3–5 times/week, almost every day) they consume the following foods for breakfast: coffee or tea without sugar, coffee or tea with sugar, milk and yogurt, juice, fruits, cereals and rusks, sandwiches, bread, marmalade, honey, bakery products (croissants, cakes etc.), eggs, omelettes, and processed meat. Moreover, duration of lunch and dinner (i.e., 0–15 min, 15–30 min, 30–45 min, 45–60 min, and over 60 min), consumption of alcohol with meals (i.e., no alcohol consumption, red wine, white wine, beer, and other) and the time (in minutes) between dinner and night sleep will be recorded.

Additionally, frequency (rarely, 1-2 times per week, 3–5 times per week, almost every day) of food consumption under stress conditions (before the participant has time to relax), while working at the same time (without being on a break), and while walking or standing (not sitting) will be recorded. Furthermore, participants will be asked about how often they consume a more heavy meal that makes them feel full (less than once in three months, 1–3 times per month, 2–4 times per week, almost every day), if they are responsible for the preparation of meals (almost never, sometimes per week, a meal of the day, almost every meal), and how frequently they eat alone (almost never, sometimes per week, a meal of the day, almost every meal).

The last meal consumed before the ACS or the stroke event will be recorded (breakfast, morning snack, lunch, evening snack, dinner, and bed-time snack) and patients will be asked if they have consumed more food than usual the day of the event or the previous day or more heavy food than usually, and which type of food. They will also be asked if they have consumed more alcohol than usually (and how many wineglasses) and if they have consumed more coffee (and how many cups) in the day of the event or the previous day. Time between the last meal consumed and the event will be also recorded. Patients will be asked if they were feeling full or hungry at the time of the event, using a 9-item scale (1: very full, 9: very hungry). Furthermore, they will be asked if the day of the event or the previous day they were feeling: angry or scared, depressed or stressed, if they had exercised more than usual, if they had not slept at night, if they were ill, and if they were exposed to cold. Controls will be asked the same questions, but regarding the day of the interview or the previous day.

To evaluate the participants' health perspectives they will be asked to value the importance of several CVD risk factors using a scale of 1 to 9 (1 means not at all important whereas 9 means very important). The factors that will be evaluated are smoking, passive smoking, sedentary lifestyle, stress, unhealthy dietary habits, overweight and obesity, diabetes, hypercholesterolemia or hypertension, family history.

*2.10. Assessment of Medical History.* In all participants, family history of CVD as well as personal and family history of hypertension, hypercholesterolemia, hypertriglyceridemia, and diabetes will be recorded. In case of positive responses regarding personal history of the above conditions, the participant will be asked about the way of management (diet and/or drugs) and the frequency of drug use (daily, weekly, monthly, rarely) in case they do not adhere to the drug prescription. Participants will be also asked if they have renal failure (and if yes for how many years), peripheral artery disease and thyroid disease (hypothyroidism, hyperthyroidism, way of management, years of thyroid disease). Women will be asked about their menopause status (premenopausal, menopausal less than 2 years, or menopausal more than 2 years) and also about potential hormone use (oral contraceptive pills, menopause hormone replacement therapy) and for how many years. Finally, angiographic data and the following clinical and biochemical values will be recorded from the latest participants' record: blood pressure, heart rate, fasting glucose, total cholesterol, LDL-cholesterol, HDL-cholesterol, triglycerides, TSH, hematocrit, white blood cells count, platelets count, urea, creatinine, and uric acid.

*2.11. Psychological Evaluation.* A previously translated and validated version of the Zung Depression Rating Scale (ZDRS) will be used for the assessment of depressive symptoms [24, 25]. The ZDRS is a self-rating scale consisting of 20 items that cover affective, psychological, and somatic symptoms for the measurement of depression, and was originally developed in order to assess depression symptoms without the bias of an administrator affecting the results. The individual specifies the frequency a symptom is experienced (i.e., little = 1, some = 2, a good part of the time = 3, or most of the time = 4). Total theoretical range of the score is 20–80, with higher scores indicating more severe depression

[24]. Scores 20–49 are considered normal, scores of 50–59 indicate mild depression, scores of 60–69 moderate to marked depression, while scores of 70–80 severe depression [25].

Moreover, the State-Trait Anxiety Inventory form Y is a brief self-rating scale for the assessment of state and trait anxiety. In the present study anxiety will be assessed only with the also previously translated and validated version of Spielberger Trait Anxiety Inventory (STAI form Y-2), which is a 20-item self-reported questionnaire evaluating how the respondent feels generally [26, 27]. The 20 items are rated from 1 to 4 according to frequency of their feelings (i.e., almost never, sometimes, often, almost always). Total theoretical range of the score ranges from 20 to 80.

*2.12. Bioethics.* The study has been approved by the Ethics Committee of the University Hospital of Ioannina and will be carried out in accordance to the Declaration of Helsinki (1989) of the World Medical Association. Prior to the collection of any information, participants will be informed about the aims and procedures of the study and will provide their written signed consent.

*2.13. Statistical Analysis Plan.* Normally distributed continuous variables will be presented as mean values ± standard deviation, skewed variables as median and quartiles and categorical variables as frequencies. Associations between categorical variables will be tested by the calculation of chi-squared test. Comparisons between normally distributed continuous variables will be performed by the calculation of Student's $t$-test. In case of skewed continuous variables, the tested hypotheses will be evaluated using the nonparametric $U$-test suggested by Mann and Whitney. Correlations between continuous variables will be evaluated using the Pearson's $r$ or Spearman *rho* coefficients. Normality of the variables will be tested using P-P plots. Estimations of the relative probabilities of developing CVD (ACS, stroke or combined) will be performed by the calculation of the odds ratio and the corresponding 95% confidence intervals through multiple logistic regression analysis. Hosmer-Lemeshow statistic will be calculated to test goodness-of-fit. All reported $P$ values will be based on two-sided tests. SPSS 18.0 software (SPSS Inc., Chicago, Il, USA) will be used for all the statistical calculations.

## 3. Study's Expectations

The findings of this case-control study will provide novel information and valuable explanations and answers on how dietary choices, from specific food consumption to eating behaviours and practices, influence the development of ACS and ischaemic strokes. Prevention of CVD is of considerable public health importance as it constitutes a major public health problem, especially in westernised world, and less than 50% of its variation has been explained by the up-to-date known risk factors. Lifestyle characteristics, like diet, smoking, and physical activity are considered to play a crucial role for the prevention of the disease, because they can be modified. However, in spite of the nutritional guidelines and recommendations for a healthy diet and lifestyle, dietary habits in the developed world, in developing countries at "nutrition transition", and even around the Mediterranean basin are changing towards the opposite direction [28, 29]. Thus, understanding of the role of dietary habits and eating behaviours on the development of CVD could offer other means to focus on prevention through emphasis on these factors. The results of the present study may suggest other possible ways to emphasize when targeting on the prevention of CVD, giving attention not only on types of food consumed and dietary guidelines, but also on eating behaviours, like meal frequency, breakfast consumption, heavy meal consumption, eating alone, activities to be followed or not while consuming a meal, like working, walking, or television viewing. Finally, attention might be needed regarding other lifestyle behaviours like hours of night sleep and napping, as they could also have an effect on the development of cardiovascular disease directly or indirectly (meaning that they could influence as well food choices).

## Authors' Contribution

C. M. Kastorini is the principal investigator of the study and wrote the paper, H. Milionis, J. Goudevenos contributed to the design of the study, and reviewed the paper and D. B. Panagiotakos had the concept, designed the study, and reviewed the paper.

## Acknowledgments

The authors would like to thank the Directors from the Department of Cardiology, Athens Red Cross Hospital and Acute Stroke Unit, Department of Clinical Therapeutics, Alexandra Hospital, University of Athens, Vasileios Nikolaou and Konstantinos N. Vemmos, for their substantial support, as well as to present and thank the field investigators of the study: Aggeliki Ioannidi, Ekavi Georgousopoulou, Eva Ntziou, Markella Symeopoulou, Zoe Konidari, Kallirroi Kalantzi, Vaia Salma, Dimitrios Kantas, Eftychia Bika, Michael Kostapanos, Antonis Kramvis, Glykeria Papagiannopoulou, Alexandra Litsardopoulou, Eirini Trichia, Dimitris Potsios, Vassiliki Vlachaki, Fani Lioliou, Labros Papadimitriou, Konstantina Siganou, and Ioanna Kousoula. C. M. Kastorini received grants to perform this study from the National Scholarships Foundation and the Hellenic Atherosclerosis Society.

## References

[1] AHA. American Heart Association, *Heart and Stroke Statistical Update*, American Heart Association, Dallas, Tex, USA, 2008.

[2] World Health Organization, "The top 10 causes of death," March 2009, http://www.who.int/mediacentre/factsheets/fs310/en/index.html.

[3] T. T. Fung, K. M. Rexrode, C. S. Mantzoros, J. E. Manson, W. C. Willett, and F. B. Hu, "Mediterranean diet and incidence of and mortality from coronary heart disease and stroke in women," *Circulation*, vol. 119, no. 8, pp. 1093–1100, 2009.

[4] S. Lee, L. Harnack, D. R. Jacobs Jr., L. M. Steffen, R. V. Luepker, and D. K. Arnett, "Trends in diet quality for coronary heart disease prevention between 1980–1982 and 2000–2002: the Minnesota Heart Survey," *Journal of the American Dietetic Association*, vol. 107, no. 2, pp. 213–222, 2007.

[5] A. Keys, A. Menotti, C. Aravanis, et al., "The seven countries study: 2,289 deaths in 15 years," *Preventive Medicine*, vol. 13, no. 2, pp. 141–154, 1984.

[6] M. de Lorgeril, P. Salen, J.-L. Martin, I. Monjaud, J. Delaye, and N. Mamelle, "Mediterranean diet, traditional risk factors, and the rate of cardiovascular complications after myocardial infarction: final report of the Lyon Diet Heart Study," *Circulation*, vol. 99, no. 6, pp. 779–785, 1999.

[7] F. B. Hu and W. C. Willett, "Optimal diets for prevention of coronary heart disease," *Journal of the American Medical Association*, vol. 288, no. 20, pp. 2569–2578, 2002.

[8] J. S. Skinner, C. J. Albers, J. Goudevenos et al., "Prospective study of patients aged 55 years or less with acute myocardial infarction between 1981 and 1985: outcome 7 years and beyond," *British Heart Journal*, vol. 74, no. 6, pp. 604–610, 1995.

[9] T. O. Cheng, "Influence of dietary patterns on stroke risk in China," *Stroke*, vol. 36, no. 2, p. 228, 2005.

[10] T. T. Fung, M. J. Stampfer, J. E. Manson, K. M. Rexrode, W. C. Willett, and F. B. Hu, "Prospective study of major dietary patterns and stroke risk in women," *Stroke*, vol. 35, no. 9, pp. 2014–2019, 2004.

[11] N. Lipovetzky, H. Hod, A. Roth, Y. Kishon, S. Sclarovsky, and M. S. Green, "Heavy meals as a trigger for a first event of the acute coronary syndrome: a case-crossover study," *Israel Medical Association Journal*, vol. 6, no. 12, pp. 728–731, 2004.

[12] F. Kronenberg, M. A. Pereira, M. K. Schmitz et al., "Influence of leisure time physical activity and television watching on atherosclerosis risk factors in the NHLBI Family Heart Study," *Atherosclerosis*, vol. 153, no. 2, pp. 433–443, 2000.

[13] H. Campos and X. Siles, "Siesta and the risk of coronary heart disease: results from a population-based, case-control study in Costa Rica," *International Journal of Epidemiology*, vol. 29, no. 3, pp. 429–437, 2000.

[14] A. Naska, E. Oikonomou, A. Trichopoulou, T. Psaltopoulou, and D. Trichopoulos, "Siesta in healthy adults and coronary mortality in the general population," *Archives of Internal Medicine*, vol. 167, no. 3, pp. 296–301, 2007.

[15] A. I. Qureshi, W. H. Giles, J. B. Croft, and D. L. Bliwise, "Habitual sleep patterns and risk for stroke and coronary heart disease: a 10-year follow-up from NHANES I," *Neurology*, vol. 48, no. 4, pp. 904–911, 1997.

[16] K. Thygesen, J. S. Alpert, and H. D. White, "Universal definition of myocardial infarction," *Journal of the American College of Cardiology*, vol. 50, no. 22, pp. 2173–2195, 2007.

[17] E. Braunwald, *Heart Disease*, W.B. Saunders, London, UK, 5th edition, 1997.

[18] C. S. Kidwell and S. Warach, "Acute ischemic cerebrovascular syndrome: diagnostic criteria," *Stroke*, vol. 34, no. 12, pp. 2995–2998, 2003.

[19] C. L. Craig, A. L. Marshall, M. Sjöström et al., "International physical activity questionnaire: 12-country reliability and validity," *Medicine and Science in Sports and Exercise*, vol. 35, no. 8, pp. 1381–1395, 2003.

[20] G. Papathanasiou, G. Georgoudis, M. Papandreou et al., "Reliability measures of the short International Physical Activity Questionnaire (IPAQ) in Greek young adults," *Hellenic Journal of Cardiology*, vol. 50, no. 4, pp. 283–294, 2009.

[21] D. B. Panagiotakos, C. Pitsavos, and C. Stefanadis, "Dietary patterns: a Mediterranean diet score and its relation to clinical and biological markers of cardiovascular disease risk," *Nutrition, Metabolism and Cardiovascular Diseases*, vol. 16, no. 8, pp. 559–568, 2006.

[22] D. B. Panagiotakos, C. Pitsavos, F. Arvaniti, and C. Stefanadis, "Adherence to the Mediterranean food pattern predicts the prevalence of hypertension, hypercholesterolemia, diabetes and obesity, among healthy adults; the accuracy of the MedDietScore," *Preventive Medicine*, vol. 44, no. 4, pp. 335–340, 2007.

[23] D. Panagiotakos, N. Kalogeropoulos, C. Pitsavos, et al., "Validation of the MedDietScore via the determination of plasma fatty acids," *International Journal of Food Sciences and Nutrition*, vol. 60, supplement 5, pp. 168–180, 2009.

[24] W. W. Zung, "A self-rating depression scale," *Archives of General Psychiatry*, vol. 12, pp. 63–70, 1965.

[25] K. Fountoulakis, A. Iacovides, S. Samolis et al., "Reliability, validity and psychometric properties of the Greek translation of the Zung Depression Rating Scale," *BMC Psychiatry*, vol. 1, Article ID 6, 2001.

[26] Spielberger, *CDGRLLRE: Manual for the State-Trait Anxiety Inventory (Self-Evaluation Questionnaire)*, Consulting Psychologists Press, Palo Alto, Calif, USA, 1970.

[27] K. N. Fountoulakis, M. Papadopoulou, S. Kleanthous et al., "Reliability and psychometric properties of the Greek translation of the State-Trait Anxiety Inventory form Y: preliminary data," *Annals of General Psychiatry*, vol. 5, article 2, 2006.

[28] D. Lairon, "Intervention studies on Mediterranean diet and cardiovascular risk," *Molecular Nutrition and Food Research*, vol. 51, no. 10, pp. 1209–1214, 2007.

[29] F. Sofi, G. Innocenti, C. Dini et al., "Low adherence of a clinically healthy Italian population to nutritional recommendations for primary prevention of chronic diseases," *Nutrition, Metabolism and Cardiovascular Diseases*, vol. 16, no. 6, pp. 436–444, 2006.

# 31

# Intravenous Thrombolysis of Occlusion in the Middle Cerebral and Retinal Arteries from Presumed Ventricular Myxoma

**Cheung-Ter Ong[1, 2] and Rei-Yeuh Chang[3]**

[1] *Department of Neurology, Chia-Yi Christian Hospital, 539 Chung-Shao Road, Chia-Yi 60002, Taiwan*
[2] *Department of Physical Therapy, Shu Zen College of Medicine and Management, Kaohsiung, Taiwan*
[3] *Department of Cardiology, Chia-Yi Christian Hospital, 539 Chung-Shao Road, Chia-Yi 60002, Taiwan*

Correspondence should be addressed to Cheung-Ter Ong, ctong98@yahoo.com.tw

Academic Editor: Halvor Naess

*Background.* Although thrombolytic therapy has been shown to be beneficial to stroke patients, the effectiveness of intravenous thrombolysis in ischemic stroke patients with ventricle myxoma is unknown. *Case Description.* A 22-year-old woman with left hemiplegia was sent to the emergency department at a teaching hospital. The magnetic resonance angiography showed occlusion of the right middle cerebral artery, and the echocardiography showed a mass in the left ventricle. Intravenous recombined tissue plasminogen activator (rt-PA) was administrated, and the postthrombolysis transcranial Doppler exam showed that her right middle cerebral artery was circulative. The patient's condition improved gradually, and no complication was observed up to 16 months of follow-up. *Conclusion.* Intravenous rt-PA is a reasonable treatment for stroke patients with ventricle myxoma.

## 1. Introduction

Myxoma represents 50% of primary cardiac tumors. Embolic stroke is the most common neurological manifestation of cardiac myxoma [1, 2], but the role of thrombolytic therapy in the treatment of stroke patients with cardiac myxoma is unknown. Considering that thrombolytic therapy has a 3-hour time-window only, physicians seldom performed a complete cardiac evaluation when applying the thrombolytic therapy to stroke patients. We hereby report a patient with left ventricle myxoma who received an intravenous recombined tissue plasminogen activator (rt-PA) treatment and showed gradual symptom improvement without complications up to 16 months of followup.

## 2. Case Report

The patient was a 22-year-old, 53 Kg, right-handed woman with a history of exertional dyspnea who had suffered from three episodes of syncope. There was no family history of stroke. She had no history of headache, smoking, or drinking and no history of taking birth control pills. She suddenly developed left-side limbs weakness and was brought to the emergency department at a teaching hospital within one hour of stroke onset. At the emergency department, her blood pressure was 104/68 mmHg, and she had a regular heart rate of 72 with normal heart sounds. She was conscious and well oriented. Her eyes were deviated to the right side, and her right eye vision was lost. She had a severe left-side hemiparesis and a left central type facial palsy. Her National Institutes of Health-Stroke-Scale (NIHSS) score was 12, and her modified rankin score (mRS) was 4. Results of her hematologic and biochemistry tests were normal, and her chest roentgenogram revealed a normal heart size. The brain computerized tomography (CT) showed no abnormal density, and the electrocardiogram (ECG) revealed sinus rhythm. There was no carotid bruit. Intravenous administration of rt-PA (0.9 mg/Kg) was given between 125 to 185 min after the stroke onset.

On the next day, her blood sugar, cholesterol, triglyceride, protein C, protein S, antithrombin, antinuclear antibody, anticardiolipin, and homocystein values were normal.

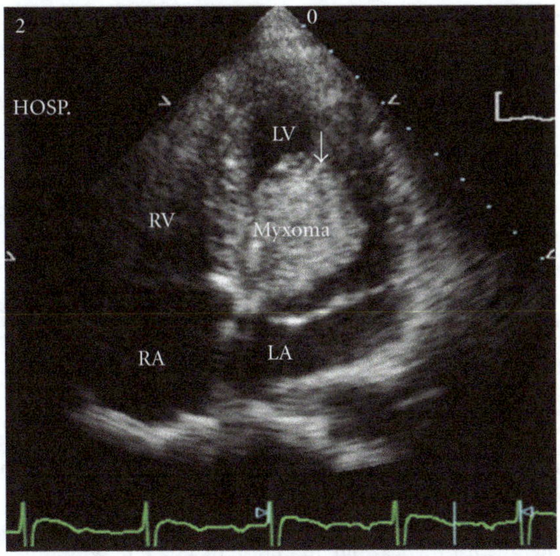


FIGURE 1: Transthoracic echocardiogram from apical 4-chamber view showed one myxoma (arrow) in the left ventricle with diameter 3 × 4 cm and stalk on middle interventricular septum.

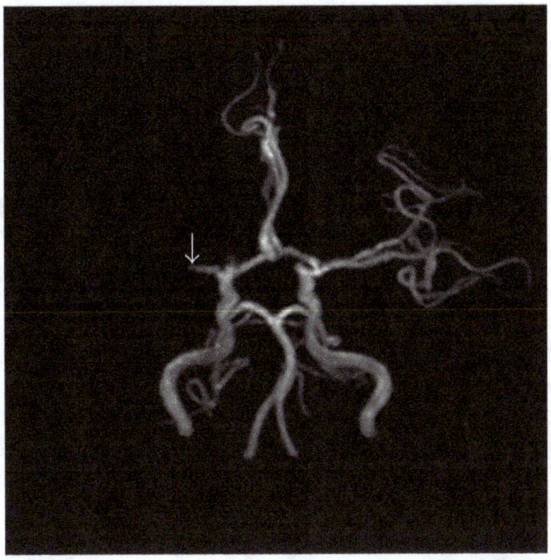

FIGURE 3: MRA shows right proximal middle cerebral artery (MCA) occlusion (arrow).

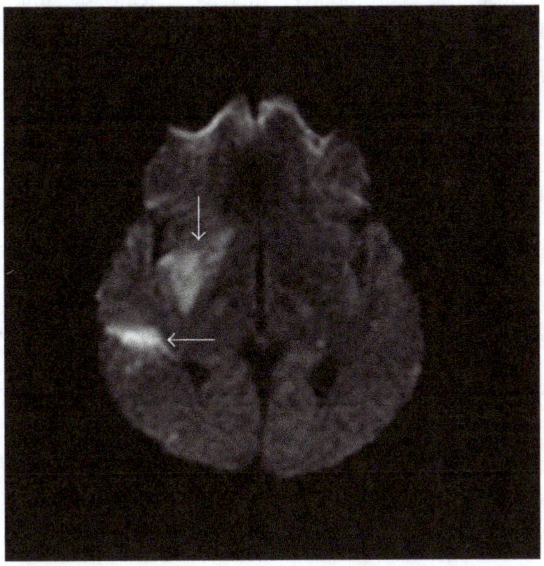

FIGURE 2: MRI of brain shows infarct in right putamen and temporal lobe (arrows).

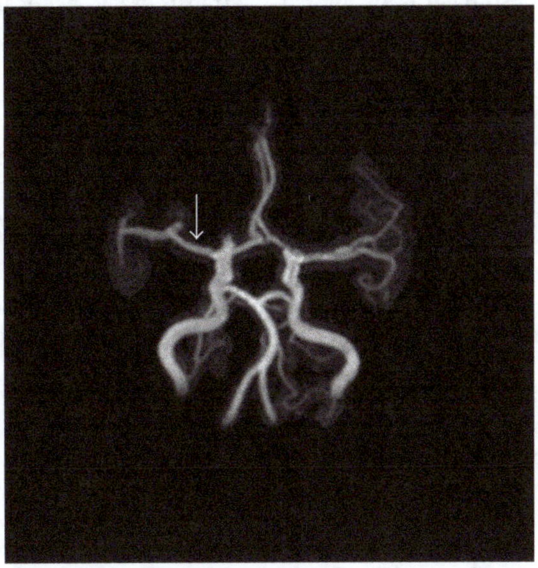

FIGURE 4: Sixteen months after thrombolytic therapy, MRA shows right middle cerebral artery recanalization (arrow).

A neurological examination showed a mild improvement, with NIHSS of 11 and mRS of 4, but no change in muscle power or facial palsy. Her transthoracic echocardiogram revealed a large (3 × 4 cm) homogenous mass with a stalk attached to the left interventricular septum (Figure 1), but her carotid duplex ultrasonography was normal. A transcranial Doppler (TCD) exam showed a decrease in blood flow in the right middle cerebral artery. From T2 and diffusion-weighted magnetic resonance image (MRI), infarcts in right basal ganglion and temporal lobe were observed (Figure 2). Magnetic resonance angiography (MRA) showed occlusion of the right middle cerebral artery in the proximal section (Figure 3). No adverse effects following the thrombolytic therapy were observed.

The patient received a tumor resection, and the pathological examination confirmed the diagnosis of left ventricle myxoma. The postoperation clinical course was uneventful without further syncope episodes. Her neurological symptoms improved gradually, but her visual acuity had no improvement. Ten months after the thrombolytic therapy, her NIHSS was 5 and mRS was 2. Sixteen months after the therapy, the MRA showed right middle cerebral artery recanalization (Figure 4).

## 3. Discussion

Approximately 75% of cardiac myxomas are located in the left atrium, and only 2.5% of them occur in the left ventricle [3, 4] Clinical manifestations of cardiac myxoma include constitutional, obstructive, and embolic symptoms. Constitutional symptoms (recurrent fever, malagia, and weight loss) occur in 34 to 90% of patients, and obstructive symptoms (fatigue, weakness, dyspnea, and syncope) occur in 54 to 95% of patients. Embolic symptoms were reported in 10 to 45% of cases [2]. Neurological symptoms present in 12 to 45% of patients, and embolic cerebral infarct is the most common event [1, 5].

Thrombolysis with intravenous rt-PA treatment within three hours of ischemic stroke is now widely applied because it has been found to be beneficial to patient's outcome. In this patient, acute occlusions of the right middle cerebral artery and retinal artery were likely to be caused by embolism from the left ventricle myxoma. This patient had received a complete dose of rt-PA before her myxoma was diagnosed by transthoracic echocardiography. After the thrombolytic therapy, the patient's neurological symptoms improved. Although MRA did not show recanalization of the right middle cerebral artery, TCD showed that the right middle cerebral artery was circulative. Approximately 41% of cardiac myxomas have surface emboli, and systemic embolization related to myxoma surface thrombus is most likely [5]. Because cases of embolic stroke following thrombolytic therapy of myocardial infarction were reported [6], cardiac myxoma was once considered as a contraindication for thrombolytic therapy, but such an argument has not been well established [7].

Successful thrombolytic therapy with rt-PA in acute ischemic stroke patients with cardiac thrombus has been reported [8, 9], and intra-arterial thrombolysis of cerebral artery occlusion with urokinase has been demonstrated to be capable of causing partial recannalization [10]. However, a previous report showed that thrombolytic therapy in patients with ventricular thrombous may cause embolic stroke [6]. The response to intravenous thrombolysis by myxomatous embolic stroke patients is unpredictable.

Using "ventricular myxoma," "thrombolytic therapy," "stroke," and "cerebrovascular disease" as key words, we did not find any reports on similar cases in the PubMed databases. Intravenous thrombolytic therapy in acute ischemic stroke patients, caused by left atrial myxoma, had been reported to be an effective treatment [11]. However, thrombolytic therapy in patients caused by ventricular myxoma has not been reported. Therefore, the case described in this paper is probably the first reported evidence of a successful thrombolytic therapy in a stroke patient with presumed left ventricular myxomatous embolism. Based on this case, thrombolytic therapy with IV rt-PA is reasonable for ischemic stroke patients with ventricular myxoma.

## References

[1] L. E. Knepper, J. Biller, H. P. Adams Jr., and A. Bruno, "Neurologic manifestions of atrial myxoma. A 12-year experience and review," *Stroke*, vol. 19, no. 11, pp. 1435–1440, 1988.

[2] F. O'Rourke, N. Dean, M. S. Mouradian, N. Akhtar, and A. Shuaib, "Atrial myxoma as a cause of stroke: case report and discussion," *Canadian Medical Association Journal*, vol. 169, no. 10, pp. 1049–1051, 2003.

[3] M. F. Bauer, H. Aebert, H. Zurbrugg, J. Ruschoff, and D. E. Birnbaum, "Torsades de pointes arrhythmia in a patient with left ventricular myxoma," *Chest*, vol. 105, no. 6, pp. 1876–1878, 1994.

[4] W. K. Nasser, "Atrial myxoma," *Chest*, vol. 60, no. 3, pp. 207–209, 1971.

[5] V. H. Lee, H. M. Connolly, and R. D. Brown Jr., "Central nervous system manifestations of cardiac myxoma," *Archives of Neurology*, vol. 64, no. 8, pp. 1115–1120, 2007.

[6] R. E. D. Bautista, "Embolic stroke following thrombolytic therapy for myocardial infarction in a patient with preexisting ventricular thrombi," *Stroke*, vol. 26, no. 2, pp. 324–325, 1995.

[7] V. M. Abascal, J. Kasznica, G. Aldea, and R. Davidoff, "Left atrial myxoma and acute myocardial infarction: a dangerous duo in the thrombolytic agent era," *Chest*, vol. 109, no. 4, pp. 1106–1108, 1996.

[8] L. Derex, N. Nighoghossian, M. Perinetti, J. Honnorat, and P. Trouillas, "Thrombolytic therapy in acute ischemic stroke patients with cardiac thrombus," *Neurology*, vol. 57, no. 11, pp. 2122–2125, 2001.

[9] C. C. Trabuco, P. A. Pereira de Jesus, A. S. Bacellar, and J. Oliveira-Filho, "Successful thrombolysis in cardioembolic stroke from Chagas disease," *Neurology*, vol. 64, no. 1, pp. 170–171, 2005.

[10] I. Bekavac, J. P. Hanna, R. C. Wallace, J. Powers, N. B. Ratliff, and A. J. Furlan, "Intra-arterial thrombolysis of embolic proximal middle cerebral artery occlusion from presumed atrial myxoma," *Neurology*, vol. 49, no. 2, pp. 618–620, 1997.

[11] C. D. Nagy, M. Levy, T. J. Mulhearn 4th et al., "Safe and effective intravenous thrombolysis for acute ischemic stroke caused by left atrial myxoma," *Journal of Stroke and Cerebrovascular Diseases*, vol. 18, no. 5, pp. 398–402, 2009.

# 32

# Haematological Indices and Antioxidant Enzyme Activity in Ghanaian Stroke Patients

**Richard Harry Asmah**,[1] **Pomah Sackey,**[2] **Patrick Adjei,**[3] **Timothy N. Archampong,**[3] **Seth Attoh,**[4] **Derek Doku,**[2] **Marjorie Quarchie,**[2] **Felix Botchway,**[5] **David Adedia**,[6] **and Eric Sampene Donkor**[7]

[1]*Department of Biomedical Sciences, School of Basic and Biomedical Sciences, University of Health and Allied Sciences, Ho, Ghana*
[2]*Department of Medical Laboratory Sciences, School of Biomedical and Allied Health Sciences, University of Ghana, Ghana*
[3]*Department of Medicine and Therapeutics, University of Ghana Medical School, Ghana*
[4]*Division of Pathology, 37 Military Hospital, Accra, Ghana*
[5]*Child Health Department, Korle-Bu Teaching Hospital, Accra, Ghana*
[6]*Department of Basic Sciences, School of Basic and Biomedical Sciences, University of Health and Allied Sciences, Ho, Ghana*
[7]*Department of Medical Microbiology, University of Ghana Medical School, Ghana*

Correspondence should be addressed to Richard Harry Asmah; rhasmah@chs.edu.gh

Academic Editor: Dorota Formanowicz

*Background.* Stroke is a cardiovascular disorder causing mortality globally and long-lasting harm worldwide. The disease occurs when the blood flow to the brain is either interrupted or blocked. This disruption leads to the increase in reactive oxygen species (ROS), especially superoxide free radicals, resulting in oxidative stress. The superoxide radicals are removed by superoxide dismutase (SOD), a key antioxidant enzyme. In this work, we investigated haematological indices and superoxide dismutase enzyme activity in Ghanaian patients with stroke and healthy control participants. *Materials and Methods.* Thirty stroke patients attending a stroke clinic and thirty apparently healthy control participants were recruited into the study. Blood samples were collected to determine haematological indices and SOD enzyme activity in red blood cells. *Results.* The stroke patients had significantly high blood parameters such as white blood cell ($p < 0.001$), neutrophil ($p < 0.001$), lymphocyte ($p = 0.003$), and eosinophil ($p < 0.001$) comparing with study participants without stroke, who were the control group in the study. Other blood parameters such as red blood cell, ($p < 0.001$), haemoglobin ($p < 0.001$), and haematocrit ($p < 0.001$) levels and mean cell haemoglobin concentration ($p = 0.030$), platelet ($p = 0.010$), and plateletcrit ($p = 0.027$) were high in stroke patients comparing with study control participants and statistically significant. Blood lymphocyte levels observed in stroke patients correlated negatively and significantly with SOD activity levels. SOD activity levels were significantly lower in stroke patients compared with the control group ($p < 0.001$). Low values of the antioxidant enzyme SOD activity levels, lymphocytes, and high values of plateletcrit were significant predictors of stroke. *Conclusion.* Haematological parameters such as WBC, lymphocyte, platelet levels, and red cell indices were significantly different in the stroke patients being studied. There was negative correlation between lymphocyte significantly with SOD activity and high oxidative stress in stroke patients compared with the control group. Lymphocytes and plateletcrit levels were also good predictors of the occurrence of stroke.

## 1. Introduction

Stroke is a cardiovascular disorder causing mortality globally and long-lasting harm worldwide [1, 2]. The disease is a leading cause of adult disability [3], the second cause of dementia [4], and the third cause of mortality in most developed countries such as sub-Saharan Africa [5]. These conditions result in about 70 percent of death and 87% of disabilities in low- and middle-level-income countries [1]. According to the World Health Organization, stroke is the second leading cause of death among people over 60 years of age and the fifth leading cause among those 15 to 59 years of age [6]. In Africa, especially sub-Saharan Africa, currently, there is an increase in stroke cases in middle-age lives [7, 8]. The reported annual incidence of stroke in Africa was reported as 316 per 100,000 individuals [1]. Stroke is classified mainly into two types: ischaemic and haemorrhagic [9]. There are reports of high-level small-vessel disease-(ischaemic-) related stroke and intracerebral lesion on the continent of Africa than elsewhere in the world [10]. Hypertension remains the most important risk factor in Africa including other such as diabetes, stress, dyslipidaemia, cardiac disease, and obesity [11]. There are gaps in the general understanding of stroke care, practice, and policy in Africa [1]. Research insights into the disease would offer useful comprehension into stroke prevention and care.

Reactive oxygen species produced during ischaemic and perfusion phases in acute ischaemic stroke can lead to brain injury [12]. Also, unstable haemostasis in the brain causes the increased production of free radicals, especially reactive oxygen species such as superoxide. Increasing evidence suggests that reactive oxygen molecules are closely linked to tissue injury during stroke [13]. Elevation in reactive oxygen species can be injurious and also lead to adverse changes to biomolecules such as lipids, proteins, DNA, RNA, and enzymes in cells [14]. These changes include cell protein denaturation, DNA breaks, and alterations of cell membrane fluidity and eventually may lead to cell death. Furthermore, an increase in reactive oxygen species also leads to adverse oxidative stress situations in the stroke patients [15]. Biological functions such as apoptosis, necrosis, and phagocytosis are mediated by reactive oxygen species. These reactive metabolites are selectively neutralized by the body's defensive mechanism. Principal defensive agents are antioxidant enzymes such as superoxide dismutase, catalase, and glutathione peroxidase [16].

The imbalance caused by oxidative stress results in red blood cell dysfunction, platelet destruction, and tissue injury. In stroke patients, such abnormalities may affect blood cell function as well as the coagulation system, leading to anaemia, infection, and hypercoagulability [17]. In the pathogenesis of acute ischaemic stroke, low-molecular weight antioxidants are involved in the reactions with free radicals generated during physiological cellular reactions resulting in oxidative stress [18]. The antioxidant enzyme superoxide dismutase and its derivatives cause vasodilation by opening potassium channels as well as deterioration of vascular reactivity [19]. Cerebrovascular thrombosis and subsequent cerebral perfusion injury in stroke necessitates constant monitoring of haemostatic parameters in stroke patients for effective management and care. In this study, we investigated haematological indices and superoxide dismutase activity in Ghanaian patients with stroke and study participants without stroke.

## 2. Materials and Methods

*2.1. Study Design and Site.* This cross-sectional study was conducted between May and July 2017 recruiting 60 study participants following informed consent by random sampling. Of these, thirty were diagnosed with stroke and were on admission at the stroke clinic of Korle-Bu Teaching Hospital (KBTH). The control group ($n = 30$) comprised of persons without clinical evidence of stroke or any history of the disease which were recruited from relatives of patients in the out-patient clinic of the healthcare facility. Structured questionnaire was used to collect data about subject demographic, life style, alcohol intake, disease condition, treatment history, and family history of stroke.

*2.2. Inclusion Criteria.* Inclusion criteria: patients (males and females) between the ages of 20 and 80 who were clinically diagnosed with stroke and who are in recovery during the first three to four months, were included in the study. Apparently, healthy subjects between the ages of 20 to 80, without any clinical evidence of stroke, served as control participants.

*2.3. Clinical Evaluation.* The clinical history of all participants including demographic data, diagnosis, treatment history, and family history of stroke was recorded.

*2.4. Blood Sample Collection.* Three millilitres of venous blood was collected from each study participant into an ethylenediaminetetraacetate (EDTA) tube for full blood count analysis. The blood samples were then centrifuged at 4000 rpm for 10 minutes at 4°C. Red blood cells obtained were stored by refrigeration for further analysis, while plasma and buffy coat were aliquoted into separate microcentrifuge tubes and stored at −20°C until use.

*2.5. Sample Analyses.* Full blood count was carried out at the central laboratory (KBTH), and SOD activity assay was carried out at the laboratories of the School of Biomedical and Allied Health Sciences, University of Ghana, Accra, Ghana.

*2.6. Full Blood Count.* The haematological parameters including white blood cell (WBC), neutrophil (NEUT), lymphocyte (LYM), eosinophil (EOS), basophil (BAS), red blood cell (RBC), count, haemoglobin concentration (HGB), haematocrit (HCT), mean cell volume (MCV), mean cell haemoglobin (MCH), mean cell haemoglobin concentration (MCHC), and platelet concentration (PLT) were determined by an automated blood analyzer (Mindray BC-5300, China).

*2.7. Superoxide Dismutase (SOD) Assay.* Superoxide dismutase activity was determined using a commercial kit, SOD Assay Kit-WST (Sigma-Aldrich, St. Louis, MO, USA), following the manufacturer's protocol. Red blood cell lysate of the study participants was used. Prepared briefly as follows, 50 $\mu l$ of RBC pellets from each participant was lysed on ice for 5 min using double-distilled ice-cold sterile water followed by centrifugation at 13000 g for 15 min at 4°C. The supernatant was diluted 100x using double-distilled ice-cold sterile water. The manufacturer's protocol required that twenty microlitres of the supernatant from each sample processed is added to the wells of a 96-microtitre plate. Three wells on the microtitre plate are designated as blanks

1, 2, and 3. Two hundred microlitres of water-soluble formazan (WST) working solution was added to each well and mixed well. Also added was 20 $\mu l$ of sample dilution buffer to blanks wells, labeled 2 and 3. Twenty microlitres of enzyme working solution was added to samples and blank 1 except blanks 2 and 3. The microtitre plate was mixed thoroughly by incubating briefly on a rocking platform. The reaction mixture was incubated at 37°C for 20 min and absorbance was read at 450 nm using a spectrophotometer (LabSystems Multiskan MS, LabSystems, Finland). SOD activity was calculated per formula described by the kit manufacturer. The SOD activity assays were done in duplicates [20, 21].

*2.8. Statistical Analysis.* The data obtained from the study was entered into Microsoft Excel 2010 and analyzed statistically using XLSTAT, R and Statistical Package for Social Sciences (SPSS) 25.0 software for Windows to arrive at the summary statistics of mean and standard deviation for numerical variables and proportions for categorical variables. An independent $t$-test was used to determine the mean differences between quantitative variables. Pearson's correlation analysis was used to look at association between variables. A $p$ value less than 0.05 was interpreted as significant. Receiver operating characteristic (ROC) analysis was used to assess ability of SOD enzyme activity and various haematological indices (lymphocyte (LYM), mean cell haemoglobin, (MCH), mean cell haemoglobin concentration (MCHC), monocyte (MON), mean platelet volume (MPV), platelet distribution width (PDW), platelet (PLT), total white blood cell (WBC), neutrophil (NEUT), eosinophil (EOS), basophil (BAS), red blood cells (RBC), haemoglobin (HGB), haematocrit (HCT), mean cell volume (MCV), and plateletcrit (PCT)) in predicting stroke. The ROC curve, area under the curve, sensitivity, specificity, and accuracy of prediction were the criteria used. Sensitivity measures the probability that a person has stroke given that the person actually has stroke, whilst specificity measures the probability that a person does not have stroke given that the person does not have stroke [22].

*2.9. Ethics.* Ethical clearance was sought from the ethics and protocol review committee of the School of Biomedical and Allied Health Sciences (SBAHS), University of Ghana, prior to the commencement of the study and enrollment of subjects. Also, permission was sought from the head of the stroke unit of Korle-Bu Teaching Hospital before the start of the study. Written informed consent was obtained from the study participants.

## 3. Results

*3.1. Demographic and Clinical Characteristics.* Tables 1 summarizes the distribution of demographic and clinical characteristics of study participants. The numbers of males in the study were 20 (66.7%) and 18 (60%) for stroke patients and controls, respectively (Table 1). The numbers of females in the study were 10 (33.3%) and 12 (40.0%) for stroke patients and controls, respectively (Table 1). The mean age of the stroke group was significantly higher than that of the control group ($p = 0.003$). The mean period of stroke for the cases was $1.93 \pm 1.0$ weeks (Table 1). Risk factors identified were hypertension 13 (43.3%), diabetes mellitus 10 (33.3%), physical inactivity 3 (10%), and smoking 2 (6.7%). The spectra of stroke cases were haemorrhagic 10 (33.3%), 10 (33.3%), recurrent 2 (6.7%), infarctive 6 (20%), and transient ischaemic attack 2 (6.7%).

*3.2. White, Red Blood Cell and Platelet Parameters.* In Table 2, stroke participants had significantly higher numbers of white blood cell (WBC) ($p < 0.001$), neutrophil (NEU) ($p < 0.001$), lymphocyte (LYM) ($p = 0.003$), and eosinophil (EOS) ($p < 0.001$) as compared with the control group. However, for mean monocyte (MON) ($p = 0.4570$), as well as basophil (BAS) ($p = 0.226$), the difference between stroke and control groups was not significant. Table 2 also shows the mean platelet volume (MPV) ($p = 0.523$) and mean platelet distribution width (PDW) ($p = 0.235$). Differences between stroke patients and control group were not statistically significant. For the mean platelet count (PLT) ($p = 0.010$) and mean plateletcrit (PCT) ($p = 0.027$), differences between stroke patients and controls were statistically significant. In Table 3, red blood cell (RBC), ($p < 0.001$) haemoglobin (HGB) ($p < 0.001$), and haematocrit (HCT) ($p < 0.001$) levels and mean cell haemoglobin concentration (MCHC) ($p = 0.030$) were statistically significant comparing stroke patients with the control group. Mean cell volume (MCV) ($p = 0.583$) and mean cell haemoglobin (MCH) ($p = 0.207$) levels were not significantly different between stroke patients and the control group.

*3.3. Superoxide Dismutase Activity.* Figure 1 shows a box plot with mean SOD activity after analysis of blood samples. Superoxide dismutase activity among the control group ($n = 30$; $18.46 \pm 3.53$) was significantly ($p < 0.001$) compared with that among stroke patients ($n = 30$; $12.54 \pm 2.74$).

*3.4. Correlation between SOD Activity and Blood Parameters.* As seen in Table 4, neutrophil (NEU) ($r = -0.135$), lymphocyte (LYM) ($r = -0.326$), and monocyte (MON) ($r = -0.015$) correlated negatively with SOD activity. WBC ($r = 0.018$), EOS ($r = 0.005$), and BAS ($r = 0.137$) correlated positively with SOD activity. The correlation between SOD activity and lymphocyte was significant ($p = 0.014$). In Table 4, the SOD activity correlated negatively with MPV ($r = -0.011$) and PCT ($r = -0.041$) and there was positive correlation between SOD activity with PLT ($r = 0.044$) and PDW ($r = 0.070$). In Table 4, HGB ($r = 0.137$), HCT ($r = 0.137$), MCV ($r = 0.321$), MCH ($r = 0.330$), and MCHC ($r = 0.054$) positively correlated with SOD activity. There were significant correlations between SOD activity levels with MCV ($p = 0.015$) and MCH ($p = 0.013$) in stroke patients.

*3.5. Receiver Operator Characteristic Curve Analysis.* Lower values of superoxide dismutase (SOD) enzyme activity, lymphocyte (LYM), mean cell haemoglobin (MCH), mean cell haemoglobin concentration (MCHC), monocyte (MON), mean platelet volume (MPV), and platelet distribution width (PDW) were related with stroke, whilst SOD enzyme

TABLE 1: Demographic parameters of patients.

| Variable | Stroke patients ($n = 30$) | Controls ($n = 30$) | $p$ value |
|---|---|---|---|
| Mean age (SD) | 57.0 (16.2) | 41.6 (14.4) | 0.003* |
| Duration of stroke (weeks) mean (SD) | 1.93 (1.0) | | |
| Age groups | Stroke patients (%) | Controls (%) | |
| 20–29 | 0 (0.0) | 7 (23.3) | |
| 30–39 | 7 (23.3) | 10 (33.3) | |
| 40–49 | 4 (13.3) | 6 (20.0) | |
| 50–59 | 1 (3.4) | 2 (6.7) | |
| 60–69 | 11 (36.7) | 3 (10) | |
| 70–79 | 7 (23.3) | 2 (6.7) | |
| Gender (%) | | | |
| Male | 20 (66.7) | 18 (60.0) | |
| Female | 10 (33.3) | 12 (40.0) | |

SD: standard deviation; %: percentage. Values are presented as mean (standard deviation) or value (percentage or range). $p$ value was set at 0.05.

TABLE 2: White blood cell and platelet parameters.

| Variable (×10^9/L) | Mean (SD) Stroke patients ($n = 30$) | Control ($n = 30$) | $p$ value |
|---|---|---|---|
| WBC | 8.72 (4.61) | 5.05 (2.93) | <0.001* |
| NEU | 7.6 (6.7) | 2.57 (2.4) | <0.001* |
| LYM | 1.5 (0.85) | 2.16 (0.66) | 0.003 * |
| MON | 1.04 (4.34) | 0.44 (0.64) | 0.457 |
| EOS | 0.27 (0.19) | 0.12 (0.09) | <0.001* |
| BAS | 0.14 (0.54) | 0.02 (0.01) | 0.226 |
| PLT | 267.58 (103.0) | 202.97 (77.6) | 0.008* |
| MPV (fL) | 9.76 (1.04) | 9.96 (1.35) | 0.523 |
| PDW | 16.15 (0.36) | 16.31 (0.60) | 0.235 |
| PCT (mL/L) | 2.74 (.63) | 0.21 (0.09) | <0.001* |

WBC: total white blood cell; NEU: neutrophil; LYM: lymphocyte; MON: monocyte; EOS: eosinophil; BAS: basophil; PLT: platelet; MPV: mean platelet volume; PDW: platelet distribution width; PCT: plateletcrit; SD: standard deviation. Values are presented as mean (standard deviation). *Mean difference is statistically significant at $p < 0.05$.

TABLE 3: Red blood cell parameters.

| Variable | Mean (SD) Stroke patients ($n = 30$) | Control ($n = 30$) | $p$ value |
|---|---|---|---|
| RBC (×10^12/L) | 5.57 (1.79) | 4.18 (1.02) | <0.001* |
| HGB (g/dL) | 14.5 (1.9) | 11.4 (3.4) | <0.001* |
| HCT | 0.48 (0.06) | 0.37 (0.1) | <0.001* |
| MCV (fL) | 91 (6.3) | 89.73 (11.0) | 0.583 |
| MCH (pg) | 27.6 (1.93) | 28.3 (2.3) | 0.207 |
| MCHC (g/dL) | 30.37 (1.0) | 31.59 (2.76) | 0.030* |

$n$: sample size; RBC: red blood cells; HGB: haemoglobin; HCT: haematocrit; MCV: mean cell volume; MCH: mean cell haemoglobin; MCHC: mean cell haemoglobin concentration; SD: standard deviation. Values are presented as mean (standard deviation). *Mean difference is statistically significant at $p < 0.05$.

activity, LYM, and MCHC were significant predictors of stroke. SOD enzyme activity (0.9000) had the highest accuracy in predicting stroke and was followed by LYM (0.8167). They also had higher area under curve (AUC) values as well as sensitivity and specificity (Table 5; Figure 2(a)). Higher values of platelet (PLT), white blood cell (WBC), neutrophil (NEUT), eosinophil (EOS), basophil (BAS), red blood cells (RBC), haemoglobin (HGB), haematocrit, (HCT), mean cell volume (MCV), and plateletcrit (PCT) were related with stroke. MCV was not a significant predictor of stroke. Other markers were significant determinants of stroke, with PCT being the highest predictor of stroke having the highest sensitivity, specificity, accuracy, and AUC values (Table 5; Figure 2(b)).

## 4. Discussion

The economic impact of stroke causes financial cost to a country's health care system as well as loss of income and productivity on the part of those affected, either directly by the disease or indirectly as caregivers to those with stroke [23]. In this work, we investigated haematological indices and superoxide dismutase enzyme activity in Ghanaian patients with stroke and healthy control participants. White blood cells in the stroke patients and control participants were significantly different as seen in Table 2. Hu et al. [24] reported that high white cell indices were predictive of stroke severity and the results of the study was in agreement with the present one. In addition, the stroke patients with haemorrhagic stroke had elevated WBC. There are reports in a study that elevated levels of WBC and lymphocytes could be due to atherosclerosis, an inflammatory process, and could result in cerebral infarction [25]. There were

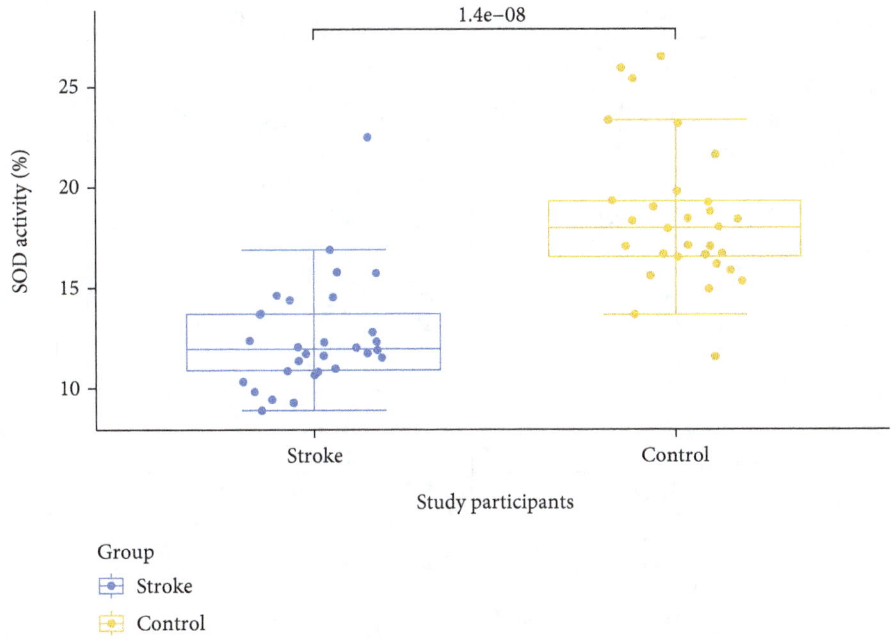


FIGURE 1: Box plot distribution of SOD activity among control and stroke study participants.

TABLE 4: Correlation between SOD activity, WBC, platelets, and RBC parameters.

| Correlation test | Pearson's $r$ value | $p$ value |
|---|---|---|
| *SOD*WBC* | 0.018 | 0.891 |
| *SOD*NEUT* | −0.135 | 0.310 |
| *SOD*LYM* | −0.326* | 0.014* |
| *SOD*MON* | −0.015 | 0.910 |
| *SOD*EOS* | 0.005 | 0.970 |
| *SOD*BAS* | 0.137 | 0.301 |
| *SOD*PLT* | 0.044 | 0.740 |
| *SOD*MPV* | −0.011 | 0.934 |
| *SOD*PDW* | 0.070 | 0.597 |
| *SOD*PCT* | −0.041 | 0.757 |
| *SOD*RBC* | −0.064 | 0.629 |
| *SOD*HGB* | 0.137 | 0.300 |
| *SOD*HCT* | 0.137 | 0.301 |
| *SOD*MCV* | 0.321* | 0.015* |
| *SOD*MCH* | 0.330* | 0.013* |
| *SOD*MCHC* | 0.054 | 0.684 |

SOD: superoxide dismutase; WBC: total white blood cell; NEU: neutrophil; LYM: lymphocyte; MON: monocyte; EOS: eosinophil; BAS: basophil; PLT: platelet; MPV: mean platelet volume; PDW: platelet distribution width; PCT: plateletcrit; RBC: red blood cells; HGB: haemoglobin; HCT: haematocrit; MCV: mean cell volume; MCH: mean cell haemoglobin; MCHC: mean cell haemoglobin concentration. *Association is statistically significant at $p < 0.05$.

TABLE 5: Receiver operator characteristics results for predicting stroke.

| Variable | Sensitivity | Specificity | Accuracy | AUC | $p$ value |
|---|---|---|---|---|---|
| *Smaller test result indicates more positive test* | | | | | |
| SOD | 0.8667 | 0.9333 | 0.9000 | 0.9267 | <0.001 |
| LYM | 0.7333 | 0.9000 | 0.8167 | 0.7744 | <0.001 |
| MCHC | 0.9000 | 0.5667 | 0.7333 | 0.7083 | 0.002 |
| MCH | 0.3667 | 0.8667 | 0.6167 | 0.6033 | 0.158 |
| PDW | 0.7667 | 0.4333 | 0.6000 | 0.5939 | 0.202 |
| MON | 0.8000 | 0.5333 | 0.6667 | 0.5711 | 0.338 |
| MPV | 0.5667 | 0.5667 | 0.5667 | 0.5361 | 0.630 |
| *Larger test result indicates more positive test* | | | | | |
| PCT | 1.0000 | 1.0000 | 1.0000 | 1.0000 | <0.001 |
| BAS | 0.9000 | 0.7667 | 0.8333 | 0.8917 | <0.001 |
| RBC | 0.8000 | 0.8333 | 0.8167 | 0.8978 | <0.001 |
| HCT | 0.8333 | 0.7000 | 0.7667 | 0.8356 | <0.001 |
| HGB | 0.7333 | 0.8667 | 0.8000 | 0.8133 | <0.001 |
| EOS | 0.6333 | 0.9000 | 0.7667 | 0.7694 | <0.001 |
| NEUT | 0.9000 | 0.5667 | 0.7333 | 0.7922 | <0.001 |
| WBC | 0.5667 | 0.8333 | 0.7000 | 0.7294 | <0.001 |
| PLT | 0.5000 | 0.9000 | 0.7000 | 0.7056 | 0.002 |
| MCV | 0.6000 | 0.7333 | 0.6667 | 0.6289 | 0.074 |

SOD: superoxide dismutase enzyme activity; LYM: lymphocyte; MCHC: mean cell haemoglobin concentration; MCH: mean cell haemoglobin; PDW: platelet distribution width; MON: monocyte; MPV: mean platelet volume; PCT: plateletcrit; BAS: basophil; RBC: red blood cells; HCT: haematocrit; HGB: haemoglobin; EOS: eosinophil; NEU: neutrophil; WBC: total white blood cell; PLT: platelet; MCV: mean cell volume.

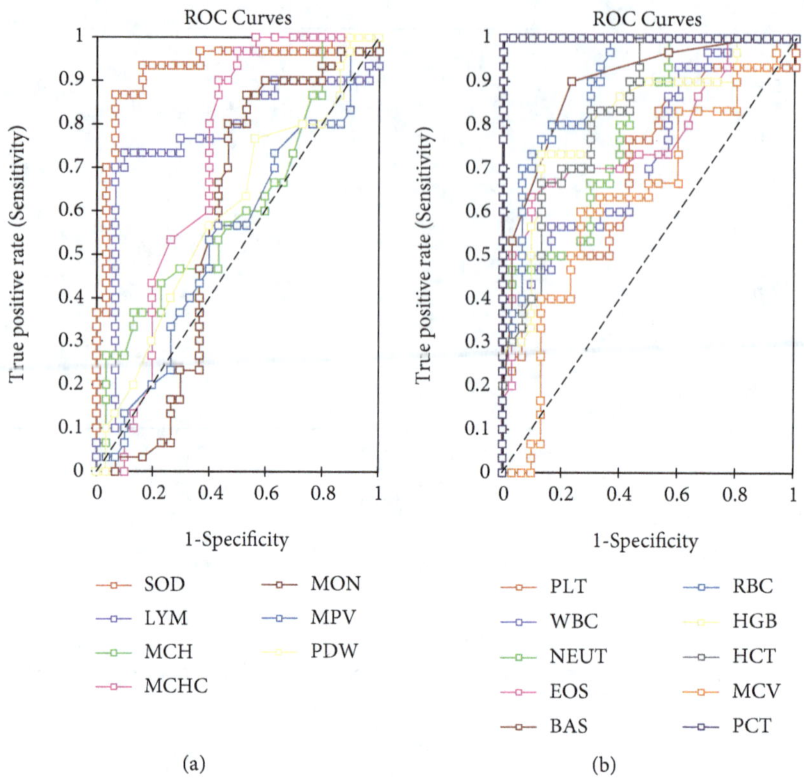


FIGURE 2: Receiver operator characteristic curve for predicting stroke.

significant differences in blood parameters such as mean cell haemoglobin concentration (MCHC) and haematocrit (HCT) levels (Table 3). There are reports that an increase in RBC above normal levels thickens blood and makes clots likely and increases the risk for stroke as this contributes to cerebrovascular blood viscosity [26]. This could possibly explain the high levels of RBC indices observed in the stroke patients in this study; increased levels of RBC indices are reported as risk factors of ischaemic stroke, cardiovascular disease, and venous thromboembolism [27]. There was significant difference in the platelet number, with stroke patients having high values (Table 2). Agreeing with reports that increase in platelet levels may imply augmented platelet aggregation and activity in early stroke, and the value of platelet counts may possibly be predictive of an event of stroke [28].

Reduced SOD activity levels in this study observed in the stroke patients (Figure 1) agree with those reported by Cherubini et al. [29]. Additionally, there was also negative correlation between SOD activity levels and lymphocyte levels that was significant (Table 4). SOD activity levels weakly correlated with neutrophil, eosinophil, and monocyte levels. This could be explained by reports that leucocytes are endogenous sources of ROS and could possible explain the low SOD activity levels in the stroke patients [12]. The sensitivity and specificity of biological markers are useful in predicting stroke if their sum is greater or equal to 1.5 using receiver operator characteristic analysis [30]. We also assessed the stroke predictive ability of haematological indices and superoxide dismutase activity using the sensitivity, specificity, accuracy, and area under the curve (Table 5, Figures 2(a) and 2(b)). For biological markers where smaller test values indicate more positive test, the area under curve (AUC) values show that SOD enzyme activity was a better predictor of stroke. Lymphocytes were also a good predictor of stroke, looking at sensitivity, specificity, and AUC values. For markers where larger test values indicate a more positive test, the AUC values showed that PCT excellently predicts stroke, with very high sensitivity and specificity values. However, the study has limitations including the small sample size used and we could not analyze other antioxidant enzymes such as catalase and glutathione peroxidase.

## 5. Conclusion

Haematological parameters such as WBC, lymphocyte levels, and red cell indices were significantly different in the stroke patients being studied. There was negative correlation of lymphocytes significantly with SOD activity and high oxidative stress in stroke patients compared with the control group. Lymphocytes and plateletcrit levels were also good predictors of the occurrence of stroke. Further investigations of these parameters would allow better clinical management and care of stroke outcome.

## Conflicts of Interest

The authors declare no conflicts of interest for this paper.

## Acknowledgments

We express our sincere appreciation to the staff of the Department of Medical Laboratory Sciences, University of Ghana, for the excellent technical assistance. We also thank the medical personnel of the stroke unit, Korle-Bu Teaching Hospital, Accra, Ghana, for all their support and help. To our study participants, for their permission and agreeing to be part of the study, we say thank you.

## References

[1] A. Waugh and G. A. Ross, *Wilson Anatomy and Physiology in Health and Illness*, Churchill Livingstone, Philadelphia, USA, 13th edition, 2018.

[2] R. O. Akinyemi, B. Ovbiagele, O. A. Adeniji et al., "Stroke in Africa: profile, progress, prospects and priorities," *Nature Reviews Neurology*, vol. 17, no. 10, pp. 634–656, 2021.

[3] C. J. Murray and A. D. Lopez, "Global mortality, disability, and the contribution of risk factors: Global Burden of Disease Study," *Lancet*, vol. 349, no. 9063, pp. 1436–1442, 1997.

[4] L. Fratiglioni, L. J. Launer, K. Anderson et al., "Incidence of dementia and major subtypes in Europe: a collaborative study of population-based cohorts. Neurologic diseases in the elderly research group," *Neurology*, vol. 54, 11 Supplement 5, pp. S10–S15, 2000.

[5] B. S. Schoenberg, E. H. Kokmen, and B. Y. Okazaki, "Alzheimer's disease and other dementing illnesses in a defined United States population: incidence rates and clinical features," *Annals of Neurology*, vol. 22, no. 6, pp. 724–729, 1987.

[6] World Health Organization, *STEPS-Stroke Manual: The WHO STEPwise Approach to Stroke Surveillance*, WHO, Geneva, Switzerland, 2006.

[7] D. Komsiiska, "Oxidative stress and stroke: a review of upstream and downstream antioxidant therapeutic options," *Comparative Clinical Pathology*, vol. 28, no. 4, pp. 915–926, 2019.

[8] J. Kim, T. Thayabaranathan, G. A. Donnan et al., "Global stroke statistics 2019," *International Journal of Stroke*, vol. 15, no. 8, pp. 819–838, 2020.

[9] F. S. Sarfo, J. Akassi, D. Awuah et al., "Trends in stroke admission and mortality rates from 1983 to 2013 in central Ghana," *Journal of the Neurological Sciences*, vol. 357, no. 1-2, pp. 240–245, 2015.

[10] M. O. Owolabi, F. Sarfo, R. Akinyemi et al., "Dominant modifiable risk factors for stroke in Ghana and Nigeria (SIREN): a case-control study," *The Lancet Global Health*, vol. 6, no. 4, pp. e436–e446, 2018.

[11] GBD 2016 Stroke Collaborators, "Global, regional, and national burden of stroke, 1990-2016: a systematic analysis for the Global Burden of Disease Study 2016," *Lancet Neurology*, vol. 18, no. 5, pp. 439–458, 2019.

[12] I. Žitňanová, P. Šiarnik, B. Kollár et al., "Oxidative Stress markers and their dynamic changes in patients after acute ischemic stroke," *Oxidative Medicine and Cellular Longevity*, vol. 2016, Article ID 9761697, 7 pages, 2016.

[13] T. Raynes, T. Shirakura, Orui et al., "A population genetic survey of stroke patients in Melanesia. Nihon Ronen Igakki Zasshi," *Japanese Journal of Geriatrics*, vol. 28, no. 4, pp. 509–514, 1991.

[14] G. Poli, G. Leonarduzzi, F. Biasi, and E. Chiarpotto, "Oxidative stress and cell signalling," *Current Medicinal Chemistry*, vol. 11, no. 9, pp. 1163–1182, 2004.

[15] M. A. Rodriguez-Martinez and A. Ruiz-Torres, "Homeostasis between lipid peroxidation and antioxidant enzyme activities in healthy human aging," *Mechanisms of Ageing and Development*, vol. 66, no. 2, pp. 213–222, 1992.

[16] O. M. Ighodaro and O. A. Akinloye, "First line defence antioxidants-superoxide dismutase (SOD), catalase (CAT) and glutathione peroxidase (GPX): their fundamental role in the entire antioxidant defence grid," *Alexandria Journal of Medicine*, vol. 54, no. 4, pp. 287–293, 2018.

[17] S. Cuzzocrea, D. Riley, A. Caputi, and D. Salvemini, "Antioxidant therapy: a new pharmalogical approach in shock, inflammation and ischemic/reperfusion injury," *Pharmacological Reviews*, vol. 53, no. 1, pp. 153–159, 2001.

[18] B. Halliwell and J. Gutteridge, *Free Radicals in Biology and Medicine*, Oxford University Press, Cary, 2015.

[19] A. Zheleva, G. Nikolova, Y. Karamalakova, E. Hristakieva, R. Lavcheva, and V. Gadjeva, "Comparative study on some oxidative stress parameters in blood of vitiligo patients before and after combined therapy," *Regulatory Toxicology and Pharmacology*, vol. 94, pp. 234–239, 2018.

[20] R. H. Asmah, B. Y. Amoah, S. Adukpo et al., "Uncomplicated malaria infection in pediatric patients in Ghana: relationship with superoxide dismutase," *Oxidants and Antioxidants in Medical Science*, vol. 4, no. 3, pp. 133–137, 2015.

[21] R. H. Asmah, G. Yeboah, H. Asare-Anane et al., "Relationship between oxidative stress and haematological indices in patients with diabetes in the Ghanaian population," *Clinical Diabetes and Endocrinology*, vol. 1, no. 1, p. 7, 2015.

[22] D. Adedia, A. A. Boakye, D. Mensah, S. Y. Lokpo, I. Afeke, and K. O. Duedu, "Comparative assessment of anthropometric and bioimpedence methods for determining adiposity," *Heliyon*, vol. 6, no. 12, article e05740, 2020.

[23] E. S. Donkor, "Stroke in the century: a snapshot of the burden, epidemiology, and quality of life," *Stroke Research and Treatment*, vol. 2018, Article ID 3238165, 10 pages, 2018.

[24] Z. Hu, Z. X. Lu, F. Zhu et al., "Higher total white blood cell and neutrophil counts are associated with an increased risk of fatal stroke occurrence: the Guangzhou Biobank Cohort Study," *BMC Neurology*, vol. 21, no. 1, p. 470, 2021.

[25] E. Zia, O. Melander, H. Björkbacka, B. Hedblad, and G. Engström, "Total and differential leucocyte counts in relation to incidence of stroke subtypes and mortality: a prospective cohort study," *Journal of Internal Medicine*, vol. 272, no. 3, pp. 298–304, 2012.

[26] C. Chen, M. Lee, Y. Yang, S. Huang, and C. Lin, "Association between clinical and laboratory markers and 5-year mortality among patients with Stroke," *Scientific Reports*, vol. 9, no. 1, article 11521, 2019.

[27] N. Cay, O. Unal, M. G. Kartal, M. Ozdemir, and M. Tola, "Increased level of red blood cell distribution width is associated with deep venous thrombosis," *Blood Coagulation & Fibrinolysis*, vol. 24, no. 7, pp. 727–731, 2013.

[28] M. M. Miller, N. Henninger, and A. Słowik, "Mean platelet volume and its genetic variants relate to stroke severity and

1-year mortality," *Neurology*, vol. 95, no. 9, pp. e1153–e1162, 2020.

[29] A. Cherubini, M. Polidori, M. Bregnocchi et al., "Antioxidant profile and early outcome in stroke patients," *Stroke*, vol. 31, no. 10, pp. 2295–2300, 2000.

[30] M. Power, G. Fell, and M. Wright, "Principles for high-quality, high-value testing," *BMJ Evidence-Based Medicine*, vol. 18, no. 1, pp. 5–10, 2013.

33

# Stroke in Patients with Schistosomiasis: Review of Cases in Literature

**Valeria Silvestri**[1], **Vivian Mushi**[1], **Billy Ngasala**[1], **Jacqueline Kihwele**[2], **Deodatus Sabas**[3] **and Lorenzo Rocchi**[4]

[1]*Department of Parasitology and Medical Entomology, Muhimbili University of Health and Applied Science, P.O. Box 65011, Dar es Salaam, Tanzania*
[2]*Department of Internal Medicine, Muhimbili University of Health and Applied Science, P.O. Box 65001, Dar es Salaam, Tanzania*
[3]*Directorate of Library Service, Muhimbili University of Health and Allied Sciences, Dar es Salaam, Tanzania*
[4]*Department of Medical Sciences and Public Health, University of Cagliari, Cagliari, Italy*

Correspondence should be addressed to Valeria Silvestri; silvestri.valeria82@gmail.com

Academic Editor: Matthew Gavino Donadu

*Introduction.* Cerebral vascular comorbidities may occur in patients with schistosomiasis, as described in case reports. *Aim and Methods.* We have summarized general clinical and neurological features in patients with stroke associated with schistosomiasis, through a review of case reports in the literature. *Investigation Outcomes.* A total of eight case reports were retrieved. The mean age of patients was $36.42 \pm 16.7$ (19 to 56 years), four females, three males, and one anonymous sex. Eosinophilia was the most frequent feature at presentation, followed by cardiac abnormalities, confusion, fever, ataxia, hemiplegia, headache, urticaria, dysphasia, and memory impairment. Patients usually present with watershed infarction or intracranial vasculitis. In one case, extracranial carotid arteries presented with inflammation and stenosis. The patient's serology was positive on admission in five cases. Full neurological recovery was reported in three cases, and partial improvement in another three. In two cases, information on neurological outcomes was incomplete. Stroke in schistosomiasis can be caused by haemodynamic impairment, direct lesion to the arterial wall, vasa vasorum obliterative endarteritis, contiguity with a focus of inflamed tissue, or inflammatory intimal damage. Schistosomiasis needs to be included in the differential diagnosis of stroke in people living or coming back from endemic areas. *Conclusions.* Further studies addressing the noncommunicable comorbidity issues related to this condition are needed.

## 1. Introduction

First described in 1851 by the German physician Theodor Bilharz, bilharziasis (or schistosomiasis) is an infestation caused by one of six species of trematode worms of the genus *Schistosoma*, which have different geographic distributions. *S. haematobium* is the most common species, occurring in sub-Saharan Africa and the Middle East [1]. Globally, 779 million people are at risk, and about 250 million are infested by Schistosoma spp., of which 201.5 million live in Africa. According to the Global Burden of Disease Study 2016, the estimated schistosomiasis global burden is 1.9 million disability-adjusted life years (DALYs) [1]. Recently, increased population movements due to climate change are directly linked to the spread of schistosomiasis [1].

Schistosome infestation in humans occurs by contact with fresh water contaminated by free-swimming cercariae, which represents the infectious stage of schistosomes, that are released by an intermediate host snail and can penetrate the intact human skin. Acute schistosomiasis, also known as Katayama fever, occurs after a primary infestation, usually between 2 weeks and 3 months after exposure to larvae, which enter small venous or lymphatic vessels, to be later transported to their maturation site in the liver. Symptoms such as fever, myalgia, and hematuria are caused by the formation of immune complexes in response to antigens released during schistosomula migration [1]. The acute stage is followed by an established phase of the invasion, which is usually asymptomatic due to the presence of somatic stem cells that regenerate the surface tegument of adult schistosome and can bind to host antigens, thus escaping the host's immune system [1]. The third stage of infestation is caused by the deposition of schistosome eggs in blood vessels, where they actively secrete antigenic glycoproteins that facilitate their passage to the lumen of the guts or urinary bladder, with the aid of the induced inflammatory response. Inflammation may also induce the formation of granulomas and consequent entrapment of eggs in surrounding tissues.

Organ-specific morbidity, according to the infecting Schistosoma spp., can develop in chronic stages. Clinical manifestations are caused by the inflammatory response of the host to the accumulation of parasite eggs in vessels and organs. For example, the involvement of mesenteric veins and small portal branches in the liver may cause liver fibrosis and portal hypertension [2]. Urogenital schistosomiasis can develop as a consequence of pelvic venous plexus involvement; hydronephrosis and kidney insufficiency may occur in severe cases, and an association with squamous cell carcinoma of the urinary bladder has also been described [1]. Schistosome worms and eggs can sometimes locate in the spleen, lungs, skin, and central nervous system, causing site-specific manifestations. For instance, in pulmonary schistosomiasis, caused by portal-caval shunting, eggs are transported to the lung capillaries, where they induce granulomas in the perialveolar area, leading to fibrosis and potentially resulting in pulmonary hypertension and cor pulmonale [1, 3].

Vascular complications of schistosomiasis are less described than the involvement of other organs or systems. Arterial damage can occur by direct lesion of arterial walls due to obliterative endarteritis involving vasa vasorum or contiguity with a focus on inflammation in surrounding tissues [4]. The vasculitic process has been described in intra- and extracranial carotid arteries [5, 6]. Therefore, the need to include the suspicion of schistosomiasis in the differential diagnosis of stroke and cerebral vasculitis has been emphasized in literature [6], especially since the prevalence of schistosomiasis is likely to increase in the near future due to climate changes and migrations [1]. Noncommunicable diseases (NCD) have been included in sustainable development goal (SDG) target 3.4, aiming to reduce premature mortality from these conditions by one-third by 2030 [7]. Still, the lack of easy-to-consult sources of data and information in many sub-Saharan settings [8] may lead to underreporting and underestimation of many conditions that could be relevant in this specific geographic-epidemiological setting, such as stroke occurring in areas with a high incidence of schistosomiasis and associated with schistosoma infestation. This highlights the need for preliminary studies that could guide further research in this specific area, in which parasitological and neurovascular interests overlap.

## 2. Aims and Methods

Our review aims to report the cerebrovascular involvement during schistosomiasis, as well as to clarify the features of cerebrovascular involvement and the possible outcome after established neurological damage.

*2.1. Search Strategy and Inclusion Criteria.* Current literature has been reviewed consulting MEDLINE, EMBASE, and Scopus for studies involving patients with a history of schistosomiasis presenting with stroke or cerebral vasculitis, using "Schistosomiasis AND stroke" OR "Schistosomiasis AND cerebral vasculitis" as keywords. All articles published between 1980 and April 2021 and written in English and French were considered.

A flow chart of the review process is provided in Figure 1.

*2.2. Quality Assessment.* Quality assessment of studies was carried out according to the checklist by Murad and colleagues [9], based on selection, ascertainment, causality, and reporting domains. More specifically, the checklist assesses for each paper availability of data from the whole investigator's experience; adequate addressing of exposure; clear report of outcome; details on differential diagnosis; description of challenges; dose-response effect description; sufficient length of follow-up; report of sufficient details to allow inference-making. Details on treatment, neurological, and general outcomes were collected, where available. Given the paucity of cases reported in the literature, the lack of details related to patients outcome was not considered an exclusion criterion.

*2.3. Data Analysis.* Due to the heterogeneity of reports, a qualitative approach was used to analyze the studies and summarize findings. Percentages and frequencies were generated for qualitative variables. Descriptive statistics (mean, standard deviation, median, and interquartile range) were used to present quantitative variables. The review of literature has been reported using a standard format [10].

## 3. Investigation Outcomes

From the literature review, we found seven papers describing eight cases (Table 1). According to Murad's checklist [9], seven out of eight case reports had a quality score between 7 and 8. The lack of follow-up was the feature of the quality checklist most frequently lacking. Incomplete differential diagnosis (or lack of diagnosis of certainty through a histology specimen) was responsible for other missing points on the checklist. The mean age of patients with schistosomiasis and stroke was $36.42 \pm 16.7$, ranging from 19 to 56 years. About 50% (four cases) were female and three (37.5%) were males, while in one case information on sex was missing.

*3.1. Summary of Cases.* Sarazin and colleagues reported the case of a 25-year-old female with a history of recent travel to

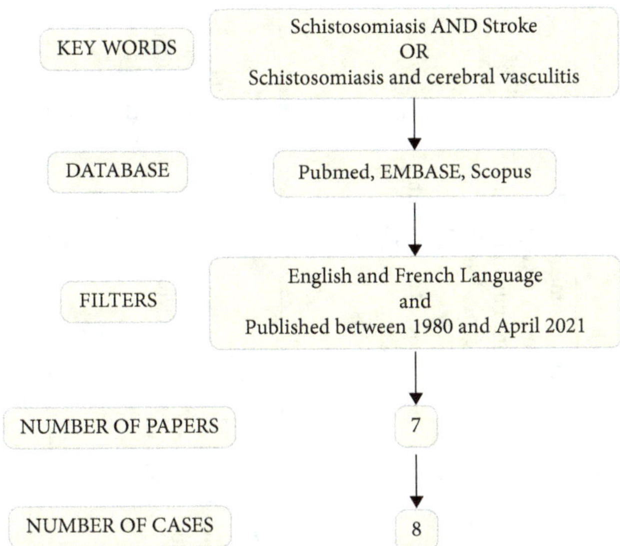


FIGURE 1: Review of literature from research strategy to number of papers included in the study.

Madagascar, presenting with fever for a week, rapidly progressive headache, limb ataxia, and memory impairment. She was diagnosed with watershed bilateral infarction. Stool positivity and seroconversion occurred only 3 weeks after neurological presentation. The case was complicated by progressive cardiomyopathy requiring surgery. No neurological recurrence occurred [11].

Sonneville and co-workers described a case of a 56-year-old woman with sudden onset of hemiplegia due to watershed infarction. Acute pericarditis and myocarditis complicated the case. The outcome was favorable with steroidal therapy, and neurological recovery was reported after 6 months [12].

Two case reports were published by Jaureguiberry. A 54-year-old man living in Mali for several years, where he had been repeatedly exposed to fresh groundwater, was medically examined due to a history of fever for 10 days, followed by acute cerebellar syndrome, hemiparesis, and confusion, with multiple cortical and subcortical infarcts caused by cerebral vasculitis. Serology and urinary positivity for the presence of schistosoma eggs was observed 4 months after the acute event when the patient still showed psychomotor slowing and insomnia [13]. The second case reported a 21-year-old male patient who bathed 1 month earlier in a lake in Mali. Four days after starting therapy with praziquantel due to a maculopapular rash and fever, he presented with confusion and anosognosia, and he was diagnosed with cerebral vasculitis. The patient had a positive serology at hospitalization, but schistosoma eggs could be detected in urine only 4 months later. The neurological features resolved after 48 hours of steroid therapy [13].

In the report by Camuset and coworkers, a 28-year-old female patient went on a mission in Burkina Faso for 1 year, where she bathed in a lake. She had a 6-month history of headaches. She was hospitalized for hemiplegia associated with an unspecified language disorder. Serology and rectal biopsy showed positivity for schistosoma. One month later, the patient presented with headache, diplopia, and VI cranial nerve palsy, with stenosis of carotid syphon. The exacerbation of vasculitis was considered due to the adverse effects of praziquantel. Minor improvement of carotid stenosis was reported at 6 months, but no details on hemiplegia were provided [6].

The case reported by Wu and colleagues lacked anagraphic details. The patient presented with acute headache and walking impairment, and multiple low densities in the alba were observed on imaging. Exposure history suggested chronic schistosomiasis [14].

Grandièr-Peréz and coworkers reported the case of a 19-year-old girl back from Kenya, where she had bathed in lake Victoria 2 weeks earlier. She presented with a 15-day history of fever and urticaria. Neurological features occurred on day 12, with the appearance of ataxia, confusion, and unilateral dysmetria. Imaging showed features of watershed infarction. Serology was positive at hospitalization, while stool and urine became positive for the presence of schistosoma eggs 4 months later. A full neurological recovery was reported 5 days after starting steroidal therapy [15].

Lastly, in the report by Nyein and colleagues, a 52-year-old patient had visited Myanmar during a schistosomiasis outbreak 1 year earlier, had swum in ponds and had eaten snails, and was hospitalized because of cognitive impairment, memory deficits, and behavioral changes, with multiple cerebral infarcts on imaging. This picture was followed, 3 weeks later, by dysarthria, hemiplegia, and facial palsy, with frontal lesions on imaging, bilateral terminal internal carotid artery narrowing, and beaded anterior cerebral artery. New frontal lesions appeared at week 9 after hospitalization. The patient had a positive serology, but no eggs were detected by optical microscopy assessment of stool. On follow-up, neurologic recovery was partial, and the patient could walk with the aid [16]. The cases are summarized in Table 1; for clarity, each case was assigned with a number, which will be used further in the text to refer to single patients. Tables 2 and 3 reports the incidence of specific neurological symptoms.

*3.2. Schistosomiasis in Differential Diagnosis for Stroke at Younger Age.* The mean age of patients was found to be $36.42 \pm 16.7$ years (min 19, max 56). It has been reported that only 10% to 15% of all strokes occur in adults aged 18 to 50 years and that the underlying pathophysiology and risk factors for stroke at younger age differ from those that occur in older patients. While the most common types of ischemic stroke in older adults are large artery atherosclerosis and small-vessel occlusions, these two subtypes accounting for only 10% to 20% of strokes in younger adults. In the latter group, other aetiologies/risk factors need to be considered, including the use of estrogens, pregnancy, migraine with aura, patent foramen ovale, inherited thrombophilia, acquired prothrombotic or hypercoagulable states, metabolic syndrome, carotid or vertebral artery dissection, and vasculitis [17]. Stroke secondary to diseases of parasitological interest, such as schistosomiasis, should be considered as a possible cause of

Table 1: Summary of case reports included in review.

| Case number | Author | Age | Sex | Schistosomiasis details | Clinical presentation | Cerebrovascular involvement | Cardiac abnormalities | Schistosomiasis diagnosis | Additional events | Outcome |
|---|---|---|---|---|---|---|---|---|---|---|
| 1 | Sarazin 2004 | 25 | F | Madagascar (3 months journey) | Day 0 = abdominal pain, diarrhea, myalgia. 1 week fever 38°C, rapidly progressive headache, limb ataxia, loss of memory | Bilateral watershed infarcts | Non-calcific endomiocardial fibrosis | Initial serology, stool and urine investigations negative. Stool positive and seroconversion after 3 weeks | Progression of cardiomyopathy in 16 months | No neurological recurrence |
| 2 | Sonneville 2006 | 56 | F | n.a. | Day 0 = hemiplegia. History of recent progressive dyspnoea | Multiple watershed infarcts | Acute pericarditis and myocarditis | Positive serology | None | Neurological recovery at 6 month |
| 3 | Jaureguiberry 2007 pt 1 | 54 | M | Lived in Mali for several years. Repeated exposure to fresh ground water | Day 0 = cerebellar syndrome and hemiparesis, confusion. 10 day history of fever 40°C | Multiple, bilateral cortical infarcts | ST tract inversion | Serology positive at 4 months | None | Psychomotor slowing and insomnia at 4 months |
| 4 | Jaureguiberry 2007 pt 2 | 21 | M | Bathed in a lake in Mali 1 month before onset (maculopapular rash) | Day 0 = myalgia, headache, fever 39°C. Day 2 = started praziquantel. Day 4 = mental confusion, anosognosia | Cerebral vasculitis | Inverted *T* waves, high troponin | Positive serology, negative stool and urine | None | Full recovery in 48 h after steroid therapy |
| 5 | Camuset 2012 | 28 | F | Burkina faso (mission-1 year), reported swimming in lake | Headache for 6 months Day 0 = transient hemiplegia, language disorders day1 = persistent hemiplegia | Watershed infarcts, carotid artery inflammation and stenosis | n.a | Positive serology, negative stool and urine, positive rectal biopsy | Development of VI cranial nerve palsy due to inflammation of carotid syphon, likely caused by praziquantel, 1 month after the first clinical observation | Minor improvement of carotid stenosis at 6 months |
| 6 | Wu 2012 | n.a. | n.a. | n.a. | Acute headache, walking impairment | Multiple frontal lobes infarcts | None | n.a | n.a. | n.a. |
| 7 | Grandiere Peréz 2013 | 19 | M | Bathed in Lake Victoria (Kenya) for 3 months | Day 0 = 15 days fever 39°C,weight loss, urticaria. Inverted T wave and positive troponin day 8 = recovery day 12 = ataxia, confusion, unilateral dysmetria | Watershed infarct | Myocarditis | Positive serology, negative stool and urine, then positive after 4 months | None | Full neurological recovery after a five-day steroid course |

Table 1: Continued.

| Case number | Author | Age | Sex | Schistosomiasis details | Clinical presentation | Cerebrovascular involvement | Cardiac abnormalities | Schistosomiasis diagnosis | Additional events | Outcome |
|---|---|---|---|---|---|---|---|---|---|---|
| 8 | Nyein 2020 | 52 | F | Visited hometown 1 year previously during schistosomiasis outbreak in Myanmar, ate snails, swam in pond | Day 0 = cognitive impairment, memory deficit, behavioral changes week 3 = dysarthria, hemiplegia, upper motor neuron facial palsy | Multiple cerebral infarcts, carotid and anterior cerebral arteries narrowing | None | Positive serology, negative stool + ova | New cerebral lesions after 3 and 9 weeks | Walked with aid at 6 months |

"Day 0" refers to the first clinical evaluation. N.a: information not available.

TABLE 2: Anagraphic data and incidence of main clinical items. Values are expressed as mean ± standard deviation of the mean.

| | |
|---|---|
| **Anagraphic data** | |
| Age | 36.42 ± 16.7 (range 19–56) |
| Sex (*N* = 7) | F: 4 (50%) M: 3 (37.5%) |
| **Clinical presentation** | |
| Disorientation/confusion | 5 (62.5%) |
| Cardiac abnormalities (myocarditis/ST or T abnormalities) | 5 (62.5%) |
| Eosinophilia | 6 (75%) |
| Fever | 4 (50%) |
| Ataxia, gait impairment | 4 (50%) |
| Hemiplegia | 4 (50%) |
| Headache | 3 (37.5%) |
| Urticaria | 2 (25%) |
| Memory impairment | 2 (25%) |
| Language impairment | 2 (25%) |
| **Cerebrovascular involvement** | |
| Cortical lesions | 3 (37.5%) |
| Cerebral vasculitis | 3 (37.5%) |
| Watershed infarcts | 5(62.5%) |
| External carotid artery involvement inflammation/stenosis | 1 (12.5%) |
| **Laboratory investigations** | |
| Exclusion of other conditions | 5 (62.5%) |
| Positive serology on admission | 5(62.5%) |
| Negative stool and urine on day 0 | 5(62.5%) |
| Late stool and urine positivity | 2(25%) |
| **Neurological and cardiac additional events** | |
| Additional events | 3 (37.5%) |
| **Neurological outcome** | |
| Partial recovery | 3 (37.5%) |
| Full recovery | 4 (50%) |
| Not specified | 1 (12.5%) |
| **Overall outcome** | |
| Alive | 5 (62.5%) |
| No follow up available | 3 (37.5%) |

TABLE 3: Clinical presentation, cerebrovascular involvement, laboratory investigation results, additional events, neurological and overall outcome details in patients with stroke and schistosomiasis.

| |
|---|
| **Clinical presentation** |
| Eosinophilia was the most frequent finding, followed by cardiac abnormalities (myocarditis/ST wave inversion), disorientation and confusion, fever, gait ataxia, hemiplegia, headache, urticaria, memory impairment, dysarthria and other non-specified speech disturbance. |
| **Cerebrovascular involvement** |
| Watershed infarction, cerebral vasculitis, vasculitis and stenosis of the extracranial portion of the carotid artery have been described in different patients affected by schistosomiasis reported. |
| **Laboratory investigations** |
| On admission patient have presented with positive serology or seroconversion occurred during hospitalization. In some cases were stool and urinary samples were negative on admission, a late stool and urine positivity has be observed. |
| **Additional events** |
| Case 5: VI nerve palsy deemed to be caused by worsening of the vasculitis at the right carotid syphon level, with consequent compression of the nerve trunk [6]. |
| Case 8: new cerebral infarcts, detected at MRI, 9 weeks after the first event [16]. |
| **Neurological outcome** |
| Case 1: no recurrence of neurological symptoms was reported, but details of outcome were not provided. |
| Cases 2, 4, 7: A full neurological recovery was reported respectively after 6 months, 48 h and 5 days after steroid therapy. |
| Case 3: psychomotor impairment and insomnia persisted at 4 months. |
| Case 5: no information on clinical improvement was reported. Diplopia due to VI nerve palsy regressed 24 hours after steroid therapy, with no relapse. Minor improvement of carotid stenosis was reported at 6 month follow-up [6]. |
| Case 6: no specified outcome |
| Case 8: partial recovery of gait occurred, which became possible without aid. |
| **Overall outcome** |
| No deaths have been reported among cases |

stroke in the young living in endemic areas or for patients coming from these regions.

*3.3. Pathophysiology of Stroke in Schistosomiasis.* Vascular complications in schistosomiasis can be caused by several pathophysiological mechanisms, including haemodynamic impairment, direct lesion to the arterial wall (obliterative endarteritis involving vasa vasorum), inflammatory intimal damage, or direct damage due to contiguity with a focus on inflammation in surrounding tissues [4]. It is interesting to note that, apart from primary schistosoma infestation [11, 13, 15], watershed infarction and cerebral vasculitis may occur during or be a delayed manifestation of chronic infestation (as in cases 5 and 8 of the present review).

*3.4. Egg-Induced Cerebral Vascular Damage.* Egg deposition usually occurs 3–4 weeks after infestation. While 20% to 55% of excreted eggs successfully reach the urinary bladder (*S. haematobium*) or the intestine (*Schistosoma mansoni* and *Schistosoma japonicum*) to be finally excreted in the environment, the remainder can embolize at various other locations, including the nervous system, where inflammation can develop [18, 19]. In the case of neuro-Schistosomiasis, the inflammatory environment established by eggs may also exacerbate established pathology or create an environment that favors other pathogen survival, suppressing the immune responses toward viral and bacterial antigens; ineffective pathogen clearance and chronicity may occur [18].

*3.5. Carotid Artery Involvement and Cerebral Vasculitis.* Two forms of vascular changes have been described in the literature in cerebral schistosomiasis caused by *S. mansoni* infestation. The first is represented by arteritis with fibrinoid necrosis involving the arterial wall, with or without ova or granulomatous lesions. The second involves arterial wall thinning, interruption of the internal elastic membrane, aneurysmal dilatation, intimal thickening, and vascular wall destruction with perivascular lymphohistiocytic infiltrate [5]. Vascular involvement in the form of cerebral [5] or carotid artery vasculitis with stenosis [6] has been also described in stroke in a patient with schistosomiasis (cases 5 and 8).

*3.6. Watershed Infarction.* Watershed infarction has been described in four of the cases reviewed here [6, 11, 12, 15]. Watershed infarcts involve the junction of the distal fields of two non-anastomosing arterial systems; in autopsy studies, they represent 10% of all brain infarcts. Being seldom fatal, the incidence is probably underestimated [20]. It is well established that severe systemic hypotension can cause bilateral watershed infarction in patients with carotid artery pathology, and watershed infarcts distal to internal carotid artery disease are more likely with a noncompetent circle of Willis [20], as in case 5. It is of interest that many of the reported cases suffered from additional cardiac complications that could have led to hypotension, including myocardial fibrosis, endocarditis, or arrhythmias (cases 1, 2, and 7).

*3.7. Laboratory Investigations.* Laboratory investigations used to diagnose schistosomiasis include optical microscopy, serological investigations, and PCR test. False-negative results at microscopy can occur in the first stages of investigations until the mature parasites start releasing eggs in the stool. Serological testing is a sensitive diagnostic method and also has high specificity (>95%), suitable for detecting low-grade infection but still not 100% sensitive: some cases of schistosomiasis may be detected by microscopy or PCR despite negative serology. This is also true for optical microscopy assessment: analysis of urine or stool samples will give negative results until the parasites are sexually mature and have started egg production: a definitive diagnosis therefore cannot be made until at least 12 weeks after the last exposure [21].

*3.8. Relation between Cerebrovascular Events and Laboratory Findings.* A positive optical microscopy investigation for Schistosoma spp. ova in the stool or urinary samples was reported in four patients. It is of interest that positivity occurred during follow-up, while the first assessment at hospitalization was reported to be negative. In case 1, optical Kato-Katz assessment of stool showed the presence of Schistosoma ova only after 3 weeks from hospitalization, when seroconversion occurred [11]. This also occurred in case 3, with a positive urinary sample 4 months after the neurological event [13], and in case 7, with watershed infarction occurring after a 2-week history of fever [15]. These findings can be explained by the fact that analysis of urine or stool samples may give negative results for the presence of ova until the parasites are sexually mature, as explained earlier [21].

*3.9. Pharmacological Management and Side Effects.* Steroids, heparin, and praziquantel have been used to treat neurological events in patients. Corticosteroids have been reported to be rapidly effective in the treatment of patients with stroke [6, 12, 13, 15, 16], intracranial vasculitis [6, 13], and in those patients with inflammatory complications occurred after the start of praziquantel therapy (see below) [13]. In this context, steroids might prevent endothelial cell damage by eosinophils [15]. Steroidal therapy has been used with success in patients with concomitant neurological and cardiological manifestations, as in the case of watershed infarction complicated by myocarditis [12].

Praziquantel can cause worsening neurological symptoms a few days after starting the treatment. This manifestation is possibly caused by schistosoma lysis and consequent immunological reaction. Clinical worsening after praziquantel treatment during acute schistosomiasis has been described in 40% of patients [15]. In case 5 of the present review, Praziquantel administration led to the exacerbation of carotid vasculitis, which was then effectively treated with intravenous methylprednisolone.

Camuset et al. report a rapid improvement in 28 years old patients with watershed infarct and carotid vasculitis with immediate treatment with anticoagulant and steroid therapy (prednisone 1 mg/kg/day). Praziquantel, added 1 week later, was tolerated in the first cycle, but induced worsening of vasculitis on the second cycle, 1 month later [6], successfully treated with methylprednisolone (500 mg/day) and switched to oral cortico-therapy (1 mg/kg/day) for 6 weeks.

Albendazole was initially started because of its wide spectrum in the 54 years old patient from Mali with cerebral vasculitis, with slow neurological improvement. In this case, seroconversion for schistosomiasis was only detected 4 months after the onset of symptoms, when praziquantel therapy was started. The patient was lost on follow-up [13].

Steroids treatment with prednisone 1 mg/kg was effective for the treatment of the 21 years old patient returning from Mali with acute schistosomiasis, which developed cerebral vasculitis 2 days after starting praziquantel therapy [13].

Prednisolone (2 mg/kg/day) tapered within 1 month also led to full clinical recovery within 5 days in the 19 years old patient who returned from Kenya, which manifested watershed infarction after acute schistosomiasis. This patient was additionally treated with praziquantel 4.8 mg on day 1, repeated after 7 days after schistosoma egg detection, which occurred 4 months after acute schistosomiasis first manifestations [22].

Praziquantel and aspirin therapy, but no steroids, was prescribed to the 25 years old patient who, after returning from Mali, presented with acute schistosomiasis followed by bilateral border-zone infarction after 1 week of fever. Concomitant progressive cardiomyopathy required surgery 16 months from onset [11].

*3.10. Pharmacological Treatment: The Role of Steroidal Therapy.* Corticosteroids have been reported to be rapidly effective in the treatment of patients with stroke and a history of schistosomiasis [6, 12, 13, 15, 16]. Steroidal therapy has been used with success in patients with associated neurological and cardiological involvement, such as those presenting myocarditis [12]. As reported by Grandière-Peréz and Caumes in their case report and discussed in the previous section of this paper, eosinophils are toxic to endothelial cells, and this toxicity may be impaired by methylprednisolone [15].

Interestingly, in the case reported by Sarazin et al., the 25 years old female patient with watershed infarction associated with progressive myocardial fibrosis finally requiring surgery, no steroidal treatment had been given [11]. Even though no conclusion can be drawn from analyzing the small number of cases, it can be speculated that steroidal therapy may have a role in arresting the progression of neurological and cardiac lesions secondary to the inflammatory burden of this specific condition.

*3.11. Neurological Complications of Anti-Parasitic Drug: Praziquantel.* Encephalopathy signs can occur a few days after a praziquantel treatment; schistosoma lysis with consequent immunological reaction can have a role in the occurrence of neurological manifestations of this anti-parasitic drug. Clinical worsening just after praziquantel treatment during acute schistosomiasis has been described in 40% of patients [15]. This was described by Camuset et al. in the 28 years old female patient returning from Burkina Faso with hemiplegia and language disorders, a junctional infarction, carotid stenosis, and contralateral carotid inflammation. Steroidal treatment was immediately started, and with the improvement of symptoms praziquantel therapy was started for schistosoma seropositivity and was initially well-tolerated, but 1 month later, the second course of praziquantel led to headache and diplopia, and sixth right cranial nerve paralysis, with new stenosis of the right carotid siphon diagnosed on magnetic resonance imaging. Exacerbation of carotid vasculitis was considered an adverse effect of praziquantel therapy, and resolution of the clinical picture, in this case, was acquired with intravenous methylprednisolone therapy [6].

## 4. Conclusions and Recommendations

Stroke might occur in patients with a history of schistosoma infestation, both acutely and in a chronic setting. The most frequent lesions are watershed infarctions. Carotid artery involvement in the form of narrowed lumen due to vasculitis may occur and have been reported in patients who were exposed up to 1 year earlier to the event, suggesting a role of chronic infestation. Clinicians should include schistosomiasis-related stroke in differential diagnosis, when assessing patients in endemic areas or travelers from those regions, given the importance of specific pharmacological management on patients' outcomes. Unfortunately, data available in the literature are limited to a small number of case reports, and are likely to be biased by understudying/underreporting of cases in endemic areas; therefore, definitive conclusions on various aspects of cerebral involvement in schistosomiasis are difficult to draw. More studies are needed to shed light on the cerebrovascular complications of schistosomiasis, following the newly-launched revised WHO 2021–2030 NTD Roadmap, which aims at the elimination of morbidity related to neglected tropical diseases in all endemic countries by 2030 [23].

## Conflicts of Interest

The authors declare that they have no conflicts of interest.

## References

[1] D. P. McManus, D. W. Dunne, M. Sacko, J. Utzinger, B. J. Vennervald, and X. N. Zhou, "Schistosomiasis," *Nature Reviews Disease Primers*, vol. 4, no. 1, pp. 13–19, 2018.

[2] J. Richter, J. G. Bode, D. Blondin et al., "Severe liver fibrosis caused by Schistosoma mansoni: management and treatment

with a transjugular intrahepatic portosystemic shunt," *Lancet Infectious Diseases*, vol. 15, no. 6, pp. 731-737, 2015.

[3] M. Abdelnaby, A. Almaghraby, Y. Saleh, and K. Ziada, "A bilharzial pulmonary artery aneurysm with a large calcified mural thrombus," *International Journal of Cardiovascular Imaging*, vol. 35, no. 3, pp. 549-550, 2019.

[4] M. M. Ramadan and M. M. Ramadan, "A huge thrombosed pulmonary artery aneurysm without pulmonary hypertension in a patient with hepatosplenic schistosomiasis," *American Journal of Case Reports*, vol. 16, pp. 140–145, 2015.

[5] A. L. Berkowitz, P. Raibagkar, B. S. Pritt, and F. J. Mateen, "Neurologic manifestations of the neglected tropical diseases," *Journal of the Neurological Sciences*, vol. 349, no. 1–2, pp. 20–32, 2015.

[6] G. Camuset, V. Wolff, C. Marescaux et al., "Cerebral vasculitis associated with Schistosoma mansoni infection," *BMC Infectious Diseases*, vol. 12, no. 1, pp. 220–225, 2012.

[7] P. M. Ezzati, "Health policy NCD countdown 2030: worldwide trends in non-communicable disease mortality and progress towards sustainable development goal target," *Lancet*, vol. 3, p. 392, 2018.

[8] A. Adindu, "The need for effective management in african health systems," *Journal of Health Management*, vol. 15, 2014.

[9] M. H. Murad, S. Sultan, S. Haffar, and F. Bazerbachi, "Methodological quality and synthesis of case series and case reports," *BMJ Evidence-Based Medicine*, vol. 23, no. 2, pp. 60–63, 2018.

[10] P. G. M. Behzadi and M. Gajdacs, "Writing a strong scientific paper in medicine and the biomedical sciences: a checklist and recommendations for early career researchers," *Biologia Futura*, vol. 72, no. 4, pp. 395–407, 2021.

[11] M. Sarazin, E. Caumes, A. Cohen, and P. Amarenco, "Multiple microembolic borderzone brain infarctions and endomyocardial fibrosis in idiopathic hypereosinophilic syndrome and in Schistosoma mansoni infestation," *Journal of Neurology Neurosurgery and Psychiatry*, vol. 75, no. 2, pp. 305–307, 2004.

[12] R. Sonneville, M. Lagrange, C. Guidoux et al., "[The association of cardiac involvement and ischemic stroke in churg strauss syndrome]," *Revue Neurologique*, vol. 162, no. 2, pp. 229–232, 2006.

[13] S. Jauréguiberry, S. Ansart, L. Perez, M. Danis, F. Bricaire, and E. Caumes, "Acute neuroschistosomiasis: two cases associated with cerebral vasculitis," *American Journal of Tropical Medicine and Hygiene*, vol. 76, no. 5, pp. 964–966, 2007.

[14] L. Wu, M. Wu, D. Tian et al., "Clinical and imaging characteristics of cerebral schistosomiasis," *Cell Biochemistry and Biophysics*, vol. 62, no. 2, pp. 289–295, 2012.

[15] L. Grandière-Pérez and E. Caumes, "Corticosteroids for watershed infarction in acute schistosomiasis," *Clinical Infectious Diseases*, vol. 57, no. 6, pp. 918-919, 2013.

[16] A. M. Nyein, A. A. Sann, N. N. Aye, and C. T. Tan, "Delayed onset cerebral vasculitis from chronic schistosoma mansoni infection in Myanmar: a case report," *Neurology Asia*, vol. 25, no. 2, pp. 203–206, 2020.

[17] M. G. George, "Risk factors for ischemic stroke in younger adults a focused update," *Stroke*, vol. 51, no. 3, pp. 729–735, 2020.

[18] A. H. Costain, A. S. Macdonald, and H. H. Smits, "Schistosome egg migration: mechanisms, pathogenesis and host immune responses," *Frontiers in Immunology*, vol. 9, 2018.

[19] C. S. Nation, A. A. Da'dara, J. K. Marchant, and P. J. Skelly, "Schistosome migration in the definitive host," *PLoS Neglected Tropical Diseases*, vol. 14, no. 4, Article ID e0007951, 2020.

[20] I. Momjian-Mayor and J. C. Baron, "The pathophysiology of watershed infarction in internal carotid artery disease: review of cerebral perfusion studies," *Stroke*, vol. 36, no. 3, pp. 567–577, 2005.

[21] T. Kristiansen, F. O. Pettersen, T. Lier, S. G. Hinderaker, and G. M. K. Greve, "Schistosomiasis in norwegian students after travel to Africa," *Tidsskr Nor Laegeforen*, vol. 15, no. 141, p. 3, 2021.

[22] E. Caumes and M. Vidailhet, "Acute neuroschistosomiasis: a cerebral vasculitis to treat with corticosteroids not praziquantel," *Journal of Travel Medicine*, vol. 17, no. 5, p. 359, 2010.

[23] P. A. Mawa, J. Kincaid-smith, E. M. Tukahebwa, J. P. Webster, and S. Wilson, "Schistosomiasis morbidity hotspots: roles of the human host , the parasite and their interface in the development of severe morbidity," *Frontiers in Immunology*, vol. 12, no. 12, Article ID 635869, 2021.

# 34

# Systematic Review of Existing Stroke Guidelines: Case for a Change

**Tissa Wijeratne,[1,2,3] Carmela Sales,[1,3] Chanith Wijeratne,[4] Leila Karimi,[1,3,5] and Mihajlo Jakovljevic[6,7,8]**

[1]*School of Applied Health, Department of Psychology, RMIT University, Melbourne, Australia*
[2]*Department of Medicine, Faculty of Medicine, University of Rajarata, Saliyapura, Anuradhapura, Sri Lanka*
[3]*Department of Neurology, Western Health & University of Melbourne, AIMSS, Level Three, WHCRE, Sunshine Hospital, St Albans, 3021, Australia*
[4]*Monash Medical School, Clayton, Victoria, Australia*
[5]*Faculty of Social and Political Sciences, Tbilisi State University, Georgia*
[6]*Institute of Advanced Manufacturing Technologies, Peter the Great St. Petersburg Polytechnic University, St. Petersburg, Russia*
[7]*Institute of Comparative Economic Studies, Hosei University Chiyoda, Japan*
[8]*Department of Global Health Economics and Policy, University of Kragujevac, Serbia*

Correspondence should be addressed to Tissa Wijeratne; twi@unimelb.edu.au

Academic Editor: Abdel Rahman Al-Tawaha

*Background and Purpose.* Stroke represents one of the most important causes of morbidity (Just over hundred million patients with disabling of ongoing effects of stroke at a given time, globally) and mortality (the second leading cause of death) worldwide. Innovative system biology-based approach is likely to increase the understanding of the underpinning of acute stroke promise to enhance stroke prevention, acute treatment, and neurorehabilitation. Recent growing body of evidence with shared pathobiology with COVID-19 and the critically important role of inflammation in the context of stroke points to far-reaching consequences of acute stroke, just as in the case of COVID-19 (postacute event issues as well as long term issues). So far, stroke is typically defined by late-appearing disease manifestation by the range of stroke subtypes as defined by the WHO or American Stroke Association. This definition neglects the underlying pathobiological mechanisms such as low-grade chronic inflammation and already compromised vascular system. Diseases such as stroke are hardly a simple result of a single problem but rather a complex cascade of pathobiological processes and interactions in a complex biochemical environment. The evidence of changes in innate immunity and adaptive immunity during the index event of acute stroke and recovery over next 3-12 months can be easily elicited with simple bedside blood tests such as neutrophil-lymphocyte ratio (NLR) with well over 300 published papers including several systematic reviews and meta-analyses confirming this. Global standard operating procedures (SOP) of stroke care are dictated by the national and international stroke guidelines at present. It is imperative to explore the evidence of system biology approach in current stroke guidelines. This is likely to be a key turning point in managing stroke across the continuum (prevention, management of acute event, and rehabilitation). *Methods.* We systematically searched for guideline recommendation on the day-to-day use of peripheral inflammatory markers such as NLR published in the English language between January 1, 2005, and October 2020. Any other evidence of system biology-based approach or recommendation was explored within the selected guidelines for this scoping review. Only the latest guideline per writing group was selected. Each guideline was analyzed independently by 2 to 4 authors to determine clinical scenarios explained/given, scientific evidence used, and recommendations presented in the context of system biology. *Results.* The scoping review found 2,911 titles at the beginning of the search. Final review included with 15 guidelines. Stroke-related organizations wrote sixty-five percent of the guidelines while national ministries wrote a fewer number of guidelines. We were primarily interested in recommendations for acute management in AIS published in the English language. Fifteen eligible guidelines were identified from 15 different countries/regions. None of the guidelines recommended the routine use of peripheral markers of inflammation, such as NLR, among their acute assessment and management recommendations. None of the existing guidelines explored the system biology approach to one of the most complex diseases affecting the human brain, stroke. *Conclusions.* This systematic review has identified a significant evidence-practice gap in all existing national stroke guidelines published in English medium as of October 2020. These guidelines included the only current "living stroke guidelines," stroke guidelines from Australia with a real opportunity to modernize the living stroke guidelines with systems biology approach, and provide 2020 vision towards better stroke care globally. Investigation of complex disease such as stroke is best served through a systems biology approach. One of the easiest places to start is simple blood tests such as total white cell count and NLR. Systems biology approach point us towards simple tools such immune-inflammatory index (SII) and serial systemic immune inflammatory indices (SSIIi) which should pave the way for the stroke physician community address the challenges in systems biology approach in stroke care. These challenges include translating bench research to the bedside, managing big data (continuous pulse, blood pressure, sleep, oxygen saturation, progressive changes in NLR, SII, SSIIi, etc.). Working with an interdisciplinary team also provides a distinct advantage. Recent adoption of historic WHO-IGAP calls for immediate action. The 2022 World Brain Day campaign on Brain Health for All is the perfect opportunity to raise awareness and start the process.

## 1. Introduction

Evidence-based medicine calls for the utilization of widely available clinical guidelines especially for the management of common conditions which have an impact on mortality and morbidity such as acute ischemic stroke (AIS). The first of this kind was published in 1974 which was entitled "Prologue to Guidelines for Stroke Care," a compendium of articles compiled by neurologists on the management of cerebrovascular disease [1] It was not until more than 20 years later that the Cochrane Collaboration Stroke Review Group convened and initiated the task of constructing a systematic guideline for the management of acute stroke [2].

Clinical guidelines are essential tools to improve the quality of healthcare systems. Factors which are crucial for a clinical guideline to be successfully crafted are team collaboration and multidisciplinary engagement [3, 4]. Furthermore, these should be tailor-fitted to individual country needs, hence, the nonexistence of a universally implemented guideline [4]. The use of tools to assess the quality of evidence also aids clinicians to interpret the recommendations according to the weight of evidence [5]. Potential barriers to nonadherence include unfamiliarity, lack of agreement, and outcome expectancy, as well as the significant impact of the precedent guideline [6].

Perhaps one of the game changers in the history of medicine is the development of clinical guidelines for the management of AIS. The wealth of data from clinical trials on reperfusion therapies paved the way for the American Heart Association (AHA) and the Canadian Stroke Consortium to publish their respective recommendations on the acute intervention of cerebrovascular ischemia [7, 8]. Through time, various versions of clinical guidelines have also been published in different languages with the primary objective of implement ability according to the resources available in each country. While constructs behind these standard procedures are anchored on the same theory, some degree of variability still occurs [9]. To date, there are no studies which specifically look at the differences in the clinical guidelines on acute ischemic stroke globally. It is in this light that this study was conceived.

## 2. Methodology

The authors of this review used the Arksey and O'Malley methodology to identify and extract useful literature. The steps undertaken include (1) research question identification; (2) relevant literature identification; (3) screening and selection of relevant literature; (4) data charting; and (5) analyzing, summarizing, and reporting results.

MEDLINE, Cochrane, and CINHAL databases were searched to identify useful keywords. Subsequently, the identified keywords were used to search the same databases for relevant studies. Literature were first screened at the title and the abstract level and then the full text articles.

Following search terms were employed based on the PICO strategy. Topic = "country name" AND TOPIC = "guideline" OR" clinical protocols" OR "recommendations" OR" standards" AND TOPIC = stroke OR cerebrovascular disorder OR cerebrovascular accident.

Guideline repositories such as the National Guideline Clearinghouse, the Scottish Intercollegiate Guidelines Network (SIGN), and Professional stroke societies were also searched. Individual bibliographies were also manually searched. Studies were included if they met the following criteria: (a) published after year 2000, (b) guidelines on stroke and/or poststroke rehabilitation, (c) graded recommendations, and (d) written in English. Titles and abstracts were initially screened (TW), and any full-text articles were further appraised (TW, CS). Any disagreement was adjudicated by an independent reviewer (LK). Guidelines which were updated in a modular format and published over separate papers were treated as one guideline.

## 3. Results

*3.1. Guideline Characteristics.* Figure 1 shows the diagram on available stroke guidelines worldwide. Figure 2 shows the PRISMA diagram of the process. Majority of the countries have no available published national guidelines while a number have guidelines but no graded recommendations. A significant majority also have guidelines published in their own language while 14 countries have their own published, graded, English clinical guidelines, with the one from the European Stroke Organization as a separate entity.

A total of 2897 titles were identified in the electronic search. Fourteen additional records were identified through other sources. After removal of duplicates and screening at the title level, 255 articles were further reviewed at the abstract level. Hundred and eighty-one papers were

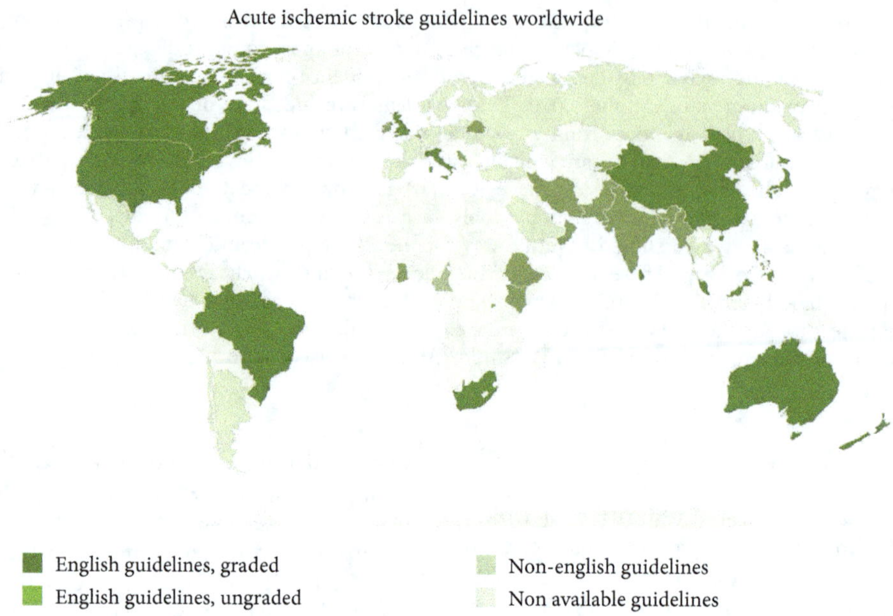


Figure 1: Acute ischemic stroke guidelines worldwide.

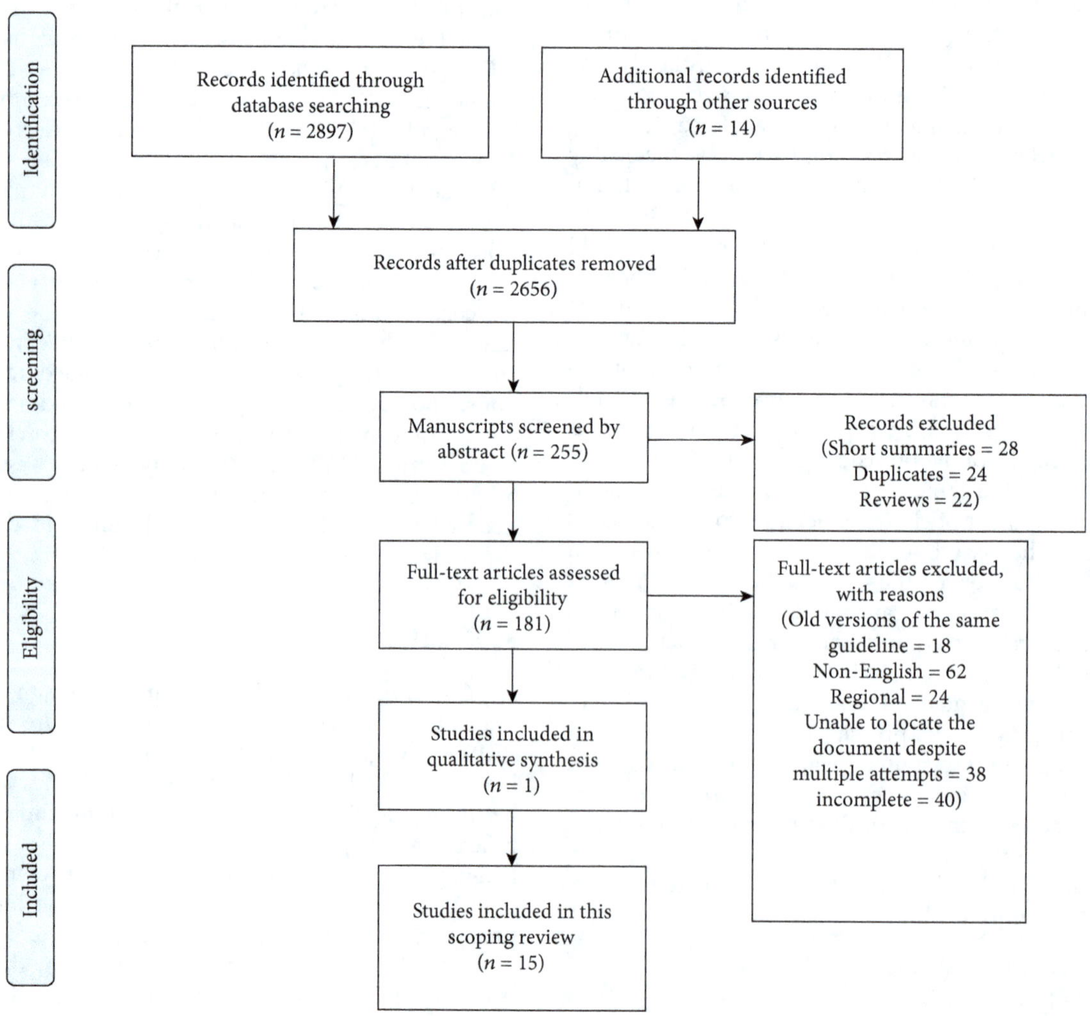


Figure 2: PRISMA diagram.

Table 1: Summary of acute ischemic stroke clinical guidelines.

| Country | Name of guideline | Year of first published version | Subsequent revisions |
|---|---|---|---|
| Australia/New Zealand [10] | Clinical Guidelines for Stroke Management | 2007 | 2010, 2019 |
| Brazil [11] | Guidelines for Acute Ischemic Stroke Treatment | 2001 | 2012 |
| Canada [12] | Canadian Best Practice Recommendations for Acute Stroke Management | 1998 | 2006, 2008, 2010, 2015, 2018 |
| China [13] | The Chinese Stroke Association scientific statement: intravenous thrombolysis in acute ischemic stroke | 2012 | 2014, 2017 |
| ESO [14] | European Stroke Organisation–Karolinska Stroke Update | 2003 | 2015, 2017, 2019 |
| Italy [15] | The Italian guidelines for stroke prevention | 2000 | |
| Japan [16] | Japanese Guidelines for the Management of Stroke | 2004 | 2009 |
| Malaysia [17] | Clinical practice guidelines, management of ischemic stroke | 2003 | 2006 |
| Qatar [18] | Clinical Guidelines for the State of Qatar, the Diagnosis and Management of Stroke and TIA | 2016 | |
| Scotland [19] | Management of patients with stroke and TIA: assessment, investigation, immediate management, and secondary prevention | 2008 | |
| Singapore [20] | Stroke and TIA: assessment, investigation, immediate management, and secondary prevention | 2009 | 2011 |
| South Africa [21] | South African guideline for management of ischemic stroke and transientischemic attack 2010: a guideline from the South African Stroke Society (SASS) and the SASS Writing Committee | 2000 | 2010 |
| Sri Lanka [22] | Clinical practice guidelines, management of stroke | 2017 | |
| UK [23] | National clinical guideline for stroke | 2000 | 2016, 2017 |
| USA [24] | Guidelines for the early Management of Patients with Acute Ischemic stroke: 2019 update to the 2018 guidelines for the early management of acute ischemic stroke | 1994 | 1996, 2003, 2005, 2007, 2013, 2015, 2018/2019 |

thoroughly assessed by the two authors (TW and CS) for eligibility. A total of 15 guidelines were included in this scoping review.

Table 1 outlines the characteristics of the 15 clinical guidelines included in this study.

*3.2. Regionalization and Adaptation from Other Clinical Guidelines.* Most countries worldwide have no available published national guidelines. However, this does not translate to lack of systematic processes and workflows in the management of acute ischemic stroke. The European Stroke Organization has successfully implemented the ESO Stroke Guidelines which is being operationalized by countries in the European region [14]. A unified approach is also being implemented in Australia and New Zealand as they both adapt the Australian Clinical Guideline for Stroke Management published in 2017 [25]. More recently, the Middle East and North Africa Stroke and Interventional Neurotherapies Organization has also created a consolidated plan to manage stroke in the midst of the pandemic [26].

Most of the conceptualized guidelines have been adapted from existing ones, usually from high-income countries [27]. A systematic review comparing stroke clinical practice guidelines (CPGs) from low- and high-income countries revealed a degree of compromise in terms of the quality on the former [27]. It is in this reason that in 2014, the World Stroke Organization conceived the *WSO Global Stroke Services Guideline and Action Plan* [28]. This initiative aims to aid country-level health authorities to set up or improve existing stroke frameworks to achieve high-quality, evidence-based recommendations and ensure that outcomes are measured to foster a milieu for continuous improvement [27].

*3.3. The Need for Grading Recommendations.* While countries have their own specific treatment recommendations, grading of evidence with the use of standardized systems is lacking. It is essential for guidelines to incorporate these as it ensures transparency and some level of confidence as these recommendations are translated into clinical practice [29]. Various country-specific guidelines make use of their own grading systems in assessing the weight and level of evidence of the recommended guidelines [12, 14, 24]. It is also essential for grading systems to be customized accordingly for low-income countries. Epidemiologists suggest the adaptation of internationally recognized approaches with efforts to integrate local evidence and weigh in appropriate resources [30].

*3.4. Clinical Trials That Changed the Guidelines.* In 1994, the AHA published the first clinical guideline on the management of acute ischemic stroke [31]. While the efficacy of thrombolytic therapy was already being recognized then, it remained to be in the sidelines for safety concerns [31, 32]. With the encouraging results of the NINDs trial and the subsequent approval of alteplase by the US-FDA for systemic reperfusion, the AHA guidelines were updated, and it was also within this period that the Canadian Stroke Guidelines were conceived [7, 8, 33]. Other major clinical guidelines from different parts of the world were also published subsequently.

With the aim of further improving stroke care, further modifications of then existing guidelines have been made. With the promising results of the ECASS3 trial, the time period for thrombolysis has been extended from three to 4.5 hours [34, 35]. The results of the J-ACT trial in 2006 has also resulted in the approval for use of the 0.6 mg/kg dose of alteplase as mandated by the revised 2009 Japanese guidelines for stroke [16, 36].

The results of five clinical trials on endovascular therapy from 2012 to 2014 have also revolutionized the landscape of stroke management in the year 2015. The MR CLEAN, ESCAPE, EXTEND-IA, SWIFT-PRIME, and the REVASCAT trials showed statistically significant improvement in clinical and radiologic outcomes after endovascular therapy (EVT) for large vessel occlusion [37–41]. Clinical guidelines were revised so that patients within six hours from onset of symptoms were deemed eligible for EVT [10, 12, 24]. A few years later, this time period was extended to 16-24 hours based on perfusion imaging parameters, as demonstrated by the DAWN and the DEFUSE 3 trials [42, 43]. Various clinical trials are still in the pipeline and are expected to make significant changes in existing guidelines worldwide in the future.

*3.5. Initial Assessment.* Guidelines included in the study are represented from all parts of the world including Asia, Australia, Europe, Africa, and America (Table 1). Sections of clinical guidelines are subdivided into initial assessment, supportive treatment, reperfusion therapy, management of complications, and rehabilitation. In most guidelines, prehospital and preventive strategies are usually included, but these are not discussed in this study. It is noted that some degree of variability in grading exists with the appraisal of different clinical guidelines.

In terms of initial assessment, there is unanimity in the clinical strategies that all patients suspected to have stroke should have neuroimaging urgently. This received the strongest recommendation among most of the countries with only ones from USA and Qatar, putting significant weight on aiming less than 20 minutes for it to be accomplished. High-income countries who have established facilities for endovascular thrombectomy also put the priority on neurovascular imaging. On the other hand, only a number of countries emphasize the use of scales for stroke severity assessment.

The importance of neuroimaging cannot be overemphasized in the management of acute stroke. While seamless processes to ensure efficiency in initial brain scanning have already been established in high-income countries, limitations in resources and logistics are still problematic most especially in rural areas of low to middle-income countries [44]. For example, a tertiary center in India identified that the lack of neuroimaging facilities posed as one of the most important barriers for thrombolysis, with even the out of pocket cost for CT scan contributing to this limitation [45]. It is also practical for other countries such as Sri Lanka, South Africa, and Malaysia not to put too much weight on neurovascular imaging as inaccessibility to neurointerventionists and comprehensive stroke centers, as well as the high cost of treatment for this sophisticated procedure, is still one of the identified problems in most developing countries [46]. On the other hand, among countries in which reputable standard operating procedures for neuroimaging are already existent, aiming to shorter door to imaging times are being optimized, as trends to improved clinical outcomes have been observed [47].

There is also homogeneity among different countries in terms of what ancillary tests are to be performed during the hyperacute management of stroke. Serum blood glucose is being specified as an absolute test to be done prior to thrombolysis in some countries while in some, this is not explicitly identified. There is also unanimity among different countries that troponin, immune cell counts, and ECG should not be deterrents to timely thrombolysis. While obtaining baseline temperature is deemed significant in almost all clinical guidelines, less degree of weight is put in this parameter as opposed to blood glucose.

It has long been recognized that hypo and hyperglycemia are known stroke masquerades [48]. A study in 2015 among 80 consecutively recruited hypoglycemic patients revealed that 11% had stroke-like presentation with symptoms reversing within one hour of administration of intravenous dextrose [49]. Furthermore, it is also essential that this parameter be recognized and corrected at an early stage as glycemic aberrations in the perithrombolysis period may significantly impact on clinical outcomes [50]. While deemed equally important, cardiac investigations should not preclude nor delay thrombolysis. It has been demonstrated in various studies that the presence of strain pattern, *t*-wave alterations, and QT dispersion may be predictors of poor outcomes among stroke patients [51–53]. Troponin is also essential to exclude the co-occurrence of AIS and acute myocardial infarction. A national registry including more than 800,000 patients with AIS identified that simultaneous occurrence of both only happens in 1.6% of the patients [54]. While the incidence is significantly low, substantial increase in hospital mortality has been observed [54].

*3.6. General Supportive Care.* There is heterogeneity in terms of supportive care among acute stroke patients with most clinical guidelines stressing moderate to strong recommendations on airway protection, correction of fluid imbalances, and treatment of sources of hyperthermia and hypoglycemia. Consensus for blood pressure targets is not uniform, with Caucasian guidelines emphasizing a threshold of 180/105 prior to thrombolysis while some Asian guidelines follow a higher target [17, 20].

It is essential that acute stroke units be organized in a manner that caters to the efficient provision of abovementioned parameters as this has been positively associated with good outcomes such as reduction of mortality, length, and cost of hospitalization as well as institutionalization [55, 56]. This is particularly problematic in low- to middle-income countries because of concerns for costs, facilities, and hospital staffing. Contrary to this, a recent prospective observational study in a tertiary hospital in South Africa demonstrated that despite the resource limitations, adaptation of the acute stroke response network which integrates organization of an acute stroke unit yields favorable thrombolysis outcomes at par to those observed in developed countries [57, 58].

Evidence proves that blood pressure optimization during thrombolysis results in good functional outcomes [59]. Prospective and retrospective studies as well as clinical trials reveal that blood pressure during thrombolysis ranging from 140 to 160 reduced the odds of poor outcomes [60–62]. To date, no studies have identified the most optimal blood pressure to achieve best outcomes post reperfusion therapy; however, clinical trial targets are set at 180/105; hence, the parameters are set in clinical guidelines [24].

*3.7. Thrombolysis and the Management of Medical and Surgical Complications.* There is also agreement between different guidelines that thrombolytic therapy (tissue plasminogen activator, alteplase) at a dose of 0.9 mg/kg be instituted among eligible patients who arrive between three and 4.5 hours from the onset of symptoms. It is only the Japanese guideline which has approved of the use of the lower dose (0.6 mg/kg). Also, only a few guidelines explicitly emphasize recommendations on the management of bleeding and angioedema after treatment. Neurosurgical recommendations for the management of malignant infarcts and obstructive hydrocephalous are also clearly defined in medium and high-income countries.

Majority of the clinical trials which looked at the safety and efficacy of the low-dose alteplase were employed among Asians, specifically Japanese. The favorable results of the J-ACT, ENCHANTED, and THAWS trial support the Japanese recommendations [36, 62–64]). Aside from practical reasons of the lower cost from the reduced dose of alteplase (which usually just consumes 1 vial per dose), physiologic advantages such as lower levels of fibrinogen and plasminogen activator inhibitor-1(PAI-1) along with less marked genetic polymorphisms that induces a higher state of coagulation compared to Caucasians have also cited by Ueshima and colleagues [65]. On the other hand, thrombolysis of patients with unclear onset of symptoms but with eligibility according the neuroimaging parameters of the WAKE-UP trial has also made the Australian and the AHA stroke guidelines recommend in favor of the later [66].

It is also interesting to note that of the guidelines reviewed, only three had explicitly stated recommendations on the management of thrombolysis-related complications such as bleeding and angioedema. More so, of the Asian countries included, only Japan had clear statements with this regard. It is equally important to address these limitations especially in resource-limited regions such as Asia and South America, where there is also a scarcity of stroke intensive care units [67, 68].

Encouraging results of various clinical trials for the management of malignant supra and infratentorial infarctions have been instrumental for the increase in confidence for guidelines to recommend these procedures especially for highly eligible patients. While this is of no question for countries with sufficient infrastructure and manpower, it has always been challenging for low- and middle-income countries. In sub-Saharan Africa, it has been previously identified that the ratio of neurosurgeon to population is as low as 1 : 64,000,000 [69]. Furthermore, a study in 2015 on the economic losses attributed to neurosurgical diseases revealed that stroke was a major contributor to the three trillion macroeconomic deficits particularly in low-income countries [70]. It is therefore critical that guidelines be crafted according to individually available resources to ensure optimal implementability.

*3.8. Poststroke Rehabilitation.* Stroke rehabilitation is another key component of stroke clinical guidelines. Majority put significant weight on early rehabilitation while moderate to weak strengths have been tagged for professional dysphagia assessment. The American, Australian, and UK guidelines likewise put high premium on functional assessment while heterogeneity exists on integrating rehabilitation on comprehensive stroke care center as well as the use of intermittent pneumatic compression for deep vein thrombosis. Majority of the guidelines have weak or no recommendations for depression screening and treatment, as well as regular skin assessment.

One of the aspects of stroke care that most clinicians fail to put attention into is postacute rehabilitation. It is important for healthcare systems to adhere to poststroke rehabilitation guidelines as various studies have shown that compliance is positively correlated with good clinical outcomes [71–73]. It has also been shown that low-cost rehabilitation with focus on exercise-based and brain training interventions, in resource-deprived settings, still translated to good clinical outcomes [74]. Commensurate rehabilitation initiated within the first seven days of stroke has been shown to initiate complex neurobiological processes which is instrumental in early neurologic recovery as evidenced in various clinical trials [75, 76]. Various clinical settings have also confirmed that poststroke dysphagia results in aspiration pneumonia which further complicates hospital outcomes [77, 78]. Additionally, evidence-based practices for the prevention of deep vein thrombosis such as the use of IPC should likewise be integrated as it may likewise impact on survival [79]. Likewise, there should be increased vigilance for poststroke depression among clinicians as it may occur in more than one third of stroke cases [80]. The need to integrate this in clinical guidelines could not be overemphasized especially in low-income to middle-income countries due to its increasing prevalence [81, 82]. Moreover, its impact on the disability-adjusted life-years lost is significantly greater in than in high-income countries [82].

*3.9. Ignored Aspects of Stroke Care.* The abundance of sophisticated techniques for stroke care has led clinicians to forget about the basic yet practical aspects of stroke management. It is noted that none of the stroke guidelines incorporate the use of basic immune biomarkers such as the neutrophil to lymphocyte ratio. In the advent of precision medicine nowadays, clinical practice is shifting towards accurate and specific disease characterization, as well as quantifying disease progression and response to therapy, for which biomarkers play critically important role [83]. The neutrophil to lymphocyte ratio is a cheap, readily available, and easy to interpret immune marker which may provide a diagnostic clue particularly for clinical outcomes poststroke [84–86].

Wijeratne and Wijeratne demonstrated the clinical utility of an easily available, universal biomarker (SSIIi) predicting the Post-Covid-19 Neurological Syndrome [87]. It is worth exploring the clinical utility of such biomarkers in the context of poststroke recovery trajectory given the shared pathobiology of these two disorders [88].

While not mentioned in any of the clinical guidelines, the importance of ocular examination in stroke care should not be discounted. Fundus photography is an emerging tool which may assist in differentiating of stroke and TIA from other causes of neurologic deficits, particularly in the emergency setting [89]. Retinal imaging otherwise known as the "window to the brain" may supplement neuroimaging particularly in providing insights for cerebrovascular neurodegenerative conditions [90]. Lastly, it may also provide additional information for identifying stroke etiology, especially that of complicated ones [91]. We have shawn the added value ot low-cost bed side functional vision testing at the bedside in the real world that should be considered in the national and international stroke guidlines [92, 93].

## 4. Discussion

Stroke and poststroke complications culminate in massive health and economic impacts globally. Stroke occurs in a compromised vascular system. The risk factors associated with stroke (both nonmodifiable risk factors such as genetic, age, and gender and modifiable risk factors such as hypertension, diabetes, high cholesterol, sedentary lifestyle, reduced fruits and vegetable intake, obesity, atrial fibrillation, poor air quality, and smoking) are linked with the build-up of low-grade chronic inflammation that perturbs the homeostasis of the vascular bed prior to the index vascular event such as acute stroke. The newly adopted WHO Intersectoral Global Action Plan calls for immediate action by national international gudiline committees in this regard (https://wfneurology.org/world-brain-day-2022) [94].

The index vascular event leads to a cascade of events that involve bioenergetic failure, disrupted cellular homeostasis, excitotoxicity, acidosis, damaged blood-brain barrier, and cell death very much akin to COVID-19 and brain involvement (Wijeratne and Crewther; https://http://www1.racgp.org.au/ajgp/coronavirus/covid-19-and-long-term-neurological-problems).

Contrary to the traditional belief that the brain and immune systems are physically separate systems, the neural and immune systems are intimately linked through sympathetic nervous system (SNS), hypothalamic pituitary adrenal (HPA) axis, and also through glymphatic systems where bidirectional communication does occur regularly [14, 27, 95, 96].

There were 80.2 million (74.1 to 86.3) prevalent strokes globally in 2016 [41, 97]. Poststroke cognitive impairment has been reported over 50% (which is still a gross underestimation) of stroke survivors with worsened disability and quality of life [42, 98]. Frequency of anxiety after stroke is very high at 24.2% (21.5%-26.9%) by rating scales [43, 99] with likely increased risk of further stroke and downward spiral from the psycho-neuroimmunological PNI point of view. Poststroke depression (PSD) is reported at 18%-33% [44, 100](gross under estimation again, see the comprehensive review on pathobiology of PSD Wijeratne and Sales [19]). Poststroke fatigue (PSF) is reported as one of the worst symptoms by 40% of the stroke survivors with prevalence of PSF that varies from 25% to 85% [45, 46, 101, 102]. Poststroke apathy (PSA) with a prevalence of 34.6% and central poststroke pain (CPSP) with a prevalence that varies from 8% to 55%,can be added to long list of poststroke neurological complications with a similar psycho-neuroimmunological pathobiology to the PCNS as we elaborated in the experimental chapters.

We suggest the desperate need of systems biology approach to all these complications and conder the complete picture with a view to optimize the best immune response after the index event of acute stroke and revisit the current guidelines as a matter of high priority. Such an approach will help the world to address one of the most disabling brain disorders affecting well over 80 million people with excellent value for money with current management approach and also the potential for individualized therapeutic and management avenues (please note that the first submission of this manuscript was published in a preprint server) [103, 104].

## 5. Conclusion

Stroke management is a dynamic process which has evolved at a very fast pace over the past two decades. With the abundance of clinical trials in this field, it is possible that trends of management now may not be applicable in the future. It is disappointing to see the lack of incorporation of easily accessible, low-cost prognostic markers such as NLR or functional vision assessment at the bed side in any of the published stroke guidelines anywhere in the world. This is despite the fact that large number of publications and metanalyses support the role of NLR in acute stroke as well as in the context of poststroke trajectory. It is therefore imperative for country-specific standard operating procedures to be updated constantly to fit to emerging needs with a systems biology-based approach. Implementability of clinical guidelines is anchored on evidence-based and well-appraised clinical guidelines which are customized according to available resources and to the beliefs of its end-users.

## Conflicts of Interest

The authors declare that they have no conflicts of interest.

## References


[1] O. M. Reinmuth, "Editorial," *Stroke*, vol. 5, no. 1, pp. 109–114, 1974.

[2] C. Counsell, C. Warlow, P. Sandercock, H. Fraser, and J. van Gijn, "The Cochrane Collaboration Stroke Review Group," *Stroke*, vol. 26, no. 3, pp. 498–502, 1995.

[3] J. Mayer, C. Kipps, and H. R. Cock, "Implementing clinical guidelines," *Practical Neurology*, vol. 19, no. 6, pp. 529–535, 2019.

[4] C. Muche-Borowski, M. Nothacker, and I. Kopp, "Leitlinienimplementierung," *Bundesgesundheitsblatt, Gesundheitsforschung, Gesundheitsschutz*, vol. 58, no. 1, pp. 32–37, 2015.

[5] G. Guyatt, A. D. Oxman, E. A. Akl et al., "GRADE guidelines: 1. Introduction-GRADE evidence profiles and summary of findings tables," *Journal of Clinical Epidemiology*, vol. 64, no. 4, pp. 383–394, 2011.

[6] M. D. Cabana, C. S. Rand, N. R. Powe et al., "Why don't physicians follow clinical practice guidelines? A framework for improvement," *JAMA*, vol. 282, no. 15, pp. 1458–1465, 1999.

[7] H. P. Adams Jr., T. G. Brott, A. J. Furlan et al., "Guidelines for thrombolytic therapy for acute stroke: a supplement to the guidelines for the management of patients with acute ischemic stroke. A statement for healthcare professionals from a Special Writing Group of the Stroke Council, American Heart Association," *Circulation*, vol. 94, no. 5, pp. 1167–1174, 1996.

[8] J. W. Norris, A. Buchan, R. Cote et al., "Canadian guidelines for intravenous thrombolytic treatment in acute stroke. A consensus statement of the Canadian Stroke Consortium," *The Canadian Journal of Neurological Sciences*, vol. 25, no. 3, pp. 257–259, 1998.

[9] A. Freixa, T. Moreira, O. Bill, and N. Anani, "Implementability of stroke guidelines: a pragmatic comparison between US and European recommendations using eGLIA," *Studies in Health Technology and Informatics*, vol. 210, pp. 256–260, 2015.

[10] Clinical guidelines — stroke foundation-Australia, 2020, http://Strokefoundation.org.au; https://strokefoundation.org.au/What-we-do/For%20health%20professionals%20and%20researchers/Clinical-guidelines.

[11] J. Oliveira-Filho, S. C. Martins, O. M. Pontes-Neto et al., "Guidelines for acute ischemic stroke treatment: part I," *Arquivos de Neuro-Psiquiatria*, vol. 70, no. 8, pp. 621–629, 2012.

[12] J. M. Boulanger, M. P. Lindsay, G. Gubitz et al., "Canadian stroke best practice recommendations for acute stroke management: prehospital, emergency department, and acute inpatient stroke care, 6th Edition, Update 2018," *International Journal of Stroke*, vol. 13, no. 9, pp. 949–984, 2018.

[13] Q. Dong, Y. Dong, L. Liu et al., "The Chinese Stroke Association scientific statement: intravenous thrombolysis in acute ischaemic stroke," *Stroke and Vascular Neurology*, vol. 2, no. 3, pp. 147–159, 2017.

[14] N. Ahmed, H. Audebert, G. Turc et al., "Consensus statements and recommendations from the ESO-Karolinska Stroke Update Conference, Stockholm 11-13 November 2018," *European Stroke Journal*, vol. 4, no. 4, pp. 307–317, 2019.

[15] D. Inzitari, "The Italian guidelines for stroke prevention. The stroke prevention and educational awareness diffusion (SPREAD) collaboration," *Neurological Sciences*, vol. 21, no. 1, pp. 5–12, 2000.

[16] Y. Shinohara, "Japanese Guidelines for the Management of Stroke 2009: important revised points necessary for the neurologist," *Rinshō Shinkeigaku*, vol. 50, no. 11, pp. 808–811, 2010.

[17] (2020), http://www.neuro.org.my/MSN_GUIDELINE/MSN_GUIDELINE_061112%20CPG%20Management%20of%20Stroke%20(ISBN%20Code)%202.pdf.

[18] (2020). http://www.researchgate.net/publication/319376697_Clinical_Guidelines_for_the_State_of_Qatar_The_diagnosis_and_management_of_stroke_and_transient_ischemic_attack.

[19] https://www.sign.ac.uk/media/1056/sign118.pdf ( updated nice version at ) https://www.nice.org.uk/guidance/ng128/resources/stroke-and-transient-ischaemic-attack-in-over-16s-diagnosis-and-initial-management-pdf-66141665603269.

[20] N. Venketasubramanian, K. H. Pwee, C. P. Chen, and on behalf of the Singapore Ministry of Health Clinical Practice Guidelines Workgroup on Stroke and Transient Ischaemic Attacks, "Singapore ministry of health clinical practice guidelines on stroke and transient ischemic attacks," *International Journal of Stroke*, vol. 6, no. 3, pp. 251–258, 2011.

[21] A. Bryer, M. Connor, P. Haug et al., "South African guideline for management of ischaemic stroke and transient ischaemic attack 2010: a guideline from the South African Stroke Society (SASS) and the SASS Writing Committee," *South African Medical Journal*, vol. 100, no. 11, p. 747, 2010.

[22] "Global-uploads," (2020), http://webflow.com, https://global-uploads, http://webflow.com/5e19f85d3feecdf9ff105b40/5e5f486f7b704fbc25d66298_CCP-stroke-guidelines-1798.pdf.

[23] A. G. Rudd, A. Bowen, G. R. Young, and M. A. James, "The latest national clinical guideline for stroke," *Clinical Medicine (London, England)*, vol. 17, no. 2, pp. 154-155, 2017.

[24] W. J. Powers, A. A. Rabinstein, T. Ackerson et al., "Guidelines for the early management of patients with acute ischemic stroke: 2019 update to the 2018 guidelines for the early management of acute ischemic stroke: a guideline for healthcare professionals from the American Heart Association/American Stroke Association," *Stroke*, vol. 50, no. 12, pp. e344–e418, 2019.

[25] K. Mahawish, P. A. Barber, A. McRae, J. Slark, and A. A. Ranta, "Why the new 'living' Australian stroke guidelines matter to New Zealand," *The New Zealand Medical Journal*, vol. 131, no. 1487, pp. 12–14, 2018.

[26] H. Al-Jehani, S. John, S. I. Hussain et al., "MENA-SINO consensus statement on implementing care pathways for acute neurovascular emergencies during the COVID-19 pandemic," *Frontiers in Neurology*, vol. 11, p. 928, 2020.

[27] H. Bayona, M. Owolabi, W. Feng et al., "A systematic comparison of key features of ischemic stroke prevention guidelines in low- and middle-income vs. high-income countries," *Journal of the Neurological Sciences*, vol. 375, pp. 360–366, 2017.

[28] P. Lindsay, K. L. Furie, S. M. Davis, G. A. Donnan, and B. Norrving, "World Stroke Organization global stroke services guidelines and action plan," *International Journal of Stroke*, vol. 9, Suppl A100, pp. 4–13, 2014.

[29] G. H. Guyatt, A. D. Oxman, G. E. Vist et al., "GRADE: an emerging consensus on rating quality of evidence and strength of recommendations," *BMJ*, vol. 336, no. 7650, pp. 924–926, 2008.

[30] M. English and N. Opiyo, "Getting to grips with GRADE–perspective from a low-income setting," *Journal of Clinical Epidemiology*, vol. 64, no. 7, pp. 708–710, 2011.

[31] H. P. Adams Jr., T. G. Brott, R. M. Crowell et al., "Guidelines for the management of patients with acute ischemic stroke. a statement for healthcare professionals from a special writing group of the stroke Council, American Heart Association," *Circulation*, vol. 90, no. 3, pp. 1588–1601, 1994.

[32] S. M. Wolpert, H. Bruckmann, R. Greenlee, L. Wechsler, M. S. Pessin, and G. del Zoppo, "Neuroradiologic evaluation of patients with acute stroke treated with recombinant tissue plasminogen activator. The rt-PA Acute Stroke Study Group," *American Journal of Neuroradiology*, vol. 14, no. 1, pp. 3–13, 1993.

[33] "Tissue plasminogen activator for acute ischemic stroke," *The New England Journal of Medicine*, vol. 333, no. 24, pp. 1581–1588, 1995.

[34] W. Hacke, M. Kaste, E. Bluhmki et al., "Thrombolysis with alteplase 3 to 4.5 hours after acute ischemic stroke," *The New England Journal of Medicine*, vol. 359, no. 13, pp. 1317–1329, 2008.

[35] E. C. Jauch, J. L. Saver, H. P. Adams Jr. et al., "Guidelines for the early management of patients with acute ischemic stroke: a guideline for healthcare professionals from the American Heart Association/American Stroke Association," *Stroke*, vol. 44, no. 3, pp. 870–947, 2013.

[36] T. Yamaguchi, E. Mori, K. Minematsu et al., "Alteplase at 0.6 mg/kg for acute ischemic stroke within 3 hours of Onset," *Stroke*, vol. 37, no. 7, pp. 1810–1815, 2006.

[37] P. S. Fransen, D. Beumer, O. A. Berkhemer et al., "MR CLEAN, a multicenter randomized clinical trial of endovascular treatment for acute ischemic stroke in the Netherlands: study protocol for a randomized controlled trial," *Trials*, vol. 15, no. 1, p. 343, 2014.

[38] M. Goyal, A. M. Demchuk, B. K. Menon et al., "Randomized assessment of rapid endovascular treatment of ischemic stroke," *The New England Journal of Medicine*, vol. 372, no. 11, pp. 1019–1030, 2015.

[39] B. C. Campbell, P. J. Mitchell, T. J. Kleinig et al., "Endovascular therapy for ischemic stroke with perfusion-imaging selection," *The New England Journal of Medicine*, vol. 372, no. 11, pp. 1009–1018, 2015.

[40] J. L. Saver, R. Jahan, E. I. Levy et al., "Solitaire flow restoration device versus the merci retriever in patients with acute ischaemic stroke (SWIFT): a randomised, parallel-group, non-inferiority trial," *Lancet*, vol. 380, no. 9849, pp. 1241–1249, 2012.

[41] A. Dávalos, E. Cobo, C. A. Molina et al., "Safety and efficacy of thrombectomy in acute ischaemic stroke (REVASCAT): 1-year follow-up of a randomised open-label trial," *Lancet Neurology*, vol. 16, no. 5, pp. 369–376, 2017.

[42] R. G. Nogueira, A. P. Jadhav, D. C. Haussen et al., "Thrombectomy 6 to 24 hours after stroke with a mismatch between deficit and infarct," *The New England Journal of Medicine*, vol. 378, no. 1, pp. 11–21, 2018.

[43] G. W. Albers, M. P. Marks, S. Kemp et al., "Thrombectomy for stroke at 6 to 16 hours with selection by perfusion imaging," *The New England Journal of Medicine*, vol. 378, no. 8, pp. 708–718, 2018.

[44] G. L. Chimatiro and A. J. Rhoda, "Scoping review of acute stroke care management and rehabilitation in low and middle-income countries," *BMC Health Services Research*, vol. 19, no. 1, p. 789, 2019.

[45] S. Badachi, T. Mathew, A. Prabhu, R. Nadig, and G. R. Sarma, "Hurdles in stroke thrombolysis: experience from 100 consecutive ischemic stroke patients," *Annals of Indian Academy of Neurology*, vol. 18, no. 4, pp. 415–418, 2015.

[46] A. C. O. Tsang, I. H. Yang, E. Orru et al., "Overview of endovascular thrombectomy accessibility gap for acute ischemic stroke in Asia: a multi-national survey," *International Journal of Stroke*, vol. 15, no. 5, pp. 516–520, 2020.

[47] S. F. Zaidi, J. Shawver, A. Espinosa Morales et al., "Stroke care: initial data from a county-based bypass protocol for patients with acute stroke," *Journal of NeuroInterventional Surgery*, vol. 9, no. 7, pp. 631–635, 2017.

[48] J. S. Huff, "Stroke mimics and chameleons," *Emergency Medicine Clinics of North America*, vol. 20, no. 3, pp. 583–595, 2002.

[49] T. Ohshita, E. Imamura, E. Nomura, S. Wakabayashi, H. Kajikawa, and M. Matsumoto, "Hypoglycemia with focal neurological signs as stroke mimic: clinical and neuroradiological characteristics," *Journal of the Neurological Sciences*, vol. 353, no. 1-2, pp. 98–101, 2015.

[50] I. Miedema, G. J. Luijckx, R. Brouns, J. De Keyser, and M. Uyttenboogaart, "Admission hyperglycemia and outcome after intravenous thrombolysis: is there a difference among the stroke-subtypes?," *BMC Neurology*, vol. 16, no. 1, p. 104, 2016.

[51] G. P. Braga, R. S. Gonçalves, M. F. Minicucci, R. Bazan, and L. A. M. Zornoff, "Strain pattern and T-wave alterations are predictors of mortality and poor neurologic outcome following stroke," *Clinical Cardiology*, vol. 43, no. 6, pp. 568–573, 2020.

[52] J. Lazar, D. Busch, E. Wirkowski, L. T. Clark, and L. Salciccioli, "Changes in QT dispersion after thrombolysis for stroke," *International Journal of Cardiology*, vol. 125, no. 2, pp. 258–262, 2008.

[53] F. Wu, W. Cao, Y. Ling, L. Yang, X. Cheng, and Q. Dong, "The predictive role of electrocardiographic abnormalities in ischemic stroke patients with intravenous thrombolysis," *International Journal of Cardiology Heart Vessel.*, vol. 4, pp. 81–83, 2014.

[54] F. Alqahtani, S. Aljohani, A. Tarabishy, T. Busu, A. Adcock, and M. Alkhouli, "Incidence and outcomes of myocardial infarction in patients admitted with acute ischemic stroke," *Stroke*, vol. 48, no. 11, pp. 2931–2938, 2017.

[55] A. Chiu, Q. Shen, G. Cheuk, D. Cordato, and D. K. Chan, "Establishment of a stroke unit in a district hospital: review of experience," *Internal Medicine Journal*, vol. 37, no. 2, pp. 73–78, 2007.

[56] L. K. Chen, J. McClaran, and A. M. Buchan, "Impact of acute stroke unit on hospital length of stay," *Archives of Gerontology and Geriatrics*, vol. 49, no. 1, pp. e12–e15, 2009.

[57] A. Bryer and S. Wasserman, "Thrombolysis for acute ischemic stroke in South Africa," *International Journal of Stroke*, vol. 8, Suppl A100, pp. 112-113, 2013.

[58] S. Wasserman and A. Bryer, "Early outcomes of thrombolysis for acute ischaemic stroke in a south African tertiary care Centre," *South African Medical Journal*, vol. 102, no. 6, p. 541, 2012.

[59] T. Waltimo, E. Haapaniemi, I. L. Surakka et al., "Post-thrombolytic blood pressure and symptomatic intracerebral hemorrhage," *European Journal of Neurology*, vol. 23, no. 12, pp. 1757–1762, 2016.

[60] C. Li, Y. Wang, Y. Chen et al., "Optimal blood pressure levels in patients undergoing intravenous thrombolysis for AIS," *Minerva Medica*, vol. 106, no. 5, pp. 255–258, 2015.

[61] L. Wu, X. Huang, D. Wu et al., "Relationship between post-thrombolysis blood pressure and outcome in acute ischemic stroke patients undergoing thrombolysis therapy," *Journal of Stroke and Cerebrovascular Diseases*, vol. 26, no. 10, pp. 2279–2286, 2017.

[62] C. S. Anderson, Y. Huang, R. I. Lindley et al., "Intensive blood pressure reduction with intravenous thrombolysis therapy for acute ischaemic stroke (ENCHANTED): an international, randomised, open-label, blinded-endpoint, phase 3 trial," *Lancet*, vol. 393, no. 10174, pp. 877–888, 2019.

[63] E. Mori, K. Minematsu, J. Nakagawara et al., "Effects of 0.6 mg/kg intravenous alteplase on vascular and clinical outcomes in middle cerebral artery occlusion: Japan Alteplase Clinical Trial II (J-ACT II)," *Stroke*, vol. 41, no. 3, pp. 461–465, 2010.

[64] M. Koga, H. Yamamoto, M. Inoue et al., "Thrombolysis with alteplase at 0.6 mg/kg for stroke with unknown time of onset: a randomized controlled trial," *Stroke*, vol. 51, no. 5, pp. 1530–1538, 2020.

[65] S. Ueshima and O. Matsuo, "The differences in thrombolytic effects of administrated recombinant t-PA between Japanese and Caucasians," *Thrombosis and Haemostasis*, vol. 87, no. 3, pp. 544–546, 2002.

[66] G. Thomalla, C. Z. Simonsen, F. Boutitie et al., "MRI-guided thrombolysis for stroke with unknown time of onset," *The New England Journal of Medicine*, vol. 379, no. 7, pp. 611–622, 2018.

[67] R. Khatib, Y. A. Arevalo, M. A. Berendsen, S. Prabhakaran, and M. D. Huffman, "Presentation, evaluation, management, and outcomes of acute stroke in low- and middle-income countries: a systematic review and meta-analysis," *Neuroepidemiology*, vol. 51, no. 1-2, pp. 104–112, 2018.

[68] G. S. Shrestha, A. Goffi, and D. Aryal, "Delivering neurocritical care in resource-challenged environments," *Current Opinion in Critical Care*, vol. 22, no. 2, pp. 1–5, 2016.

[69] M. Punchak, S. Mukhopadhyay, S. Sachdev et al., "Neurosurgical care: availability and access in low-income and middle-income countries," *World Neurosurgery*, vol. 112, pp. e240–e254, 2018.

[70] N. Rudolfson, M. C. Dewan, K. B. Park, M. G. Shrime, J. G. Meara, and B. C. Alkire, "The economic consequences of neurosurgical disease in low- and middle-income countries," *Journal of Neurosurgery*, vol. 1, pp. 1–8, 2018.

[71] P. W. Duncan, R. D. Horner, D. M. Reker et al., "Adherence to postacute rehabilitation guidelines is associated with functional recovery in stroke," *Stroke*, vol. 33, no. 1, pp. 167–178, 2002.

[72] S. Miura, R. Miyata, S. Matsumoto et al., "Quality Management Program of Stroke Rehabilitation Using Adherence to Guidelines: A Nationwide Initiative in Japan," *Journal of Stroke and Cerebrovascular Diseases*, vol. 28, no. 9, pp. 2434–2441, 2019.

[73] I. J. Hubbard, D. Harris, M. F. Kilkenny, S. G. Faux, M. R. Pollack, and D. A. Cadilhac, "Adherence to clinical guidelines improves patient outcomes in Australian audit of stroke rehabilitation practice," *Archives of Physical Medicine and Rehabilitation*, vol. 93, no. 6, pp. 965–971, 2012.

[74] M. Dee, O. Lennon, and C. O'Sullivan, "A systematic review of physical rehabilitation interventions for stroke in low and lower-middle income countries," *Disability and Rehabilitation*, vol. 42, no. 4, pp. 473–501, 2020.

[75] P. Langhorne, O. Wu, H. Rodgers, A. Ashburn, and J. Bernhardt, "A very early rehabilitation Trial after stroke (AVERT): a phase III, multicentre, randomised controlled trial," *Health Technology Assessment*, vol. 21, no. 54, pp. 1–120, 2017.

[76] F. Herisson, S. Godard, C. Volteau, E. Le Blanc, B. Guillon, and M. Gaudron, "Early sitting in ischemic stroke patients (SEVEL): a randomized controlled trial," *PLoS One*, vol. 11, no. 3, article e0149466, 2016.

[77] C. Henke, C. Foerch, and S. Lapa, "Early screening parameters for dysphagia in acute ischemic stroke," *Cerebrovascular Diseases*, vol. 44, no. 5-6, pp. 285–290, 2017.

[78] S. A. Abubakar and B. Y. Jamoh, "Dysphagia following acute stroke and its effect on short-term outcome," *The Nigerian Postgraduate Medical Journal*, vol. 24, no. 3, pp. 182–186, 2017.

[79] D. Zhang, F. Li, X. Li, and G. Du, "Effect of intermittent pneumatic compression on preventing deep vein thrombosis among stroke patients: a systematic review and meta-analysis," *Worldviews on Evidence-Based Nursing*, vol. 15, no. 3, pp. 189–196, 2018.

[80] G. L. Lenzi, M. Altieri, and I. Maestrini, "Depression postaccident vasculaire cerebral," *Revista de Neurologia*, vol. 164, no. 10, pp. 837–840, 2008.

[81] A. Ojagbemi, J. Akinyemi, M. Owolabi et al., "Predictors and prognoses of new onset post-stroke anxiety at one year in black Africans," *Journal of Stroke and Cerebrovascular Diseases*, vol. 29, no. 9, p. 105082, 2020.

[82] F. S. Sarfo, M. Nichols, S. Qanungo et al., "Stroke-related stigma among West Africans: patterns and predictors," *Journal of the Neurological Sciences*, vol. 375, pp. 270–274, 2017.

[83] A. N. Simpkins, M. Janowski, H. S. Oz et al., "Biomarker application for precision medicine in stroke," *Translational Stroke Research*, vol. 11, no. 4, pp. 615–627, 2020.

[84] J. Zhang, Q. Ren, Y. Song et al., "Prognostic role of neutrophil-lymphocyte ratio in patients with acute ischemic stroke," *Medicine (Baltimore)*, vol. 96, no. 45, p. e8624, 2017.

[85] R. Zhang, X. Wu, W. Hu et al., "Neutrophil-to-lymphocyte ratio predicts hemorrhagic transformation in ischemic stroke: a meta-analysis," *Brain and Behavior: A Cognitive Neuroscience Perspective*, vol. 9, no. 9, article e01382, 2019.

[86] J. Wan, X. Wang, Y. Zhen et al., "The predictive role of the neutrophil-lymphocyte ratio in the prognosis of adult patients with stroke," *Chinese Neurosurgical Journal*, vol. 6, no. 1, p. 22, 2020.

[87] T. Wijeratne and C. Wijeratne, "Clinical utility of serial systemic immune inflammation indices (SSIIi) in the context of post covid-19 neurological syndrome (PCNS)," *Journal of the Neurological Sciences*, vol. 423, p. 117356, 2021.

[88] T. Wijeratne, S. G. Crewther, C. Sales, and L. Karimi, "COVID-19 pathophysiology predicts that ischemic stroke

occurrence is an expectation, not an exception—a systematic review," *Frontiers in Neurology*, vol. 11, 2021.

[89] L. N. Vuong, P. Thulasi, V. Biousse et al., "Ocular fundus photography of patients with focal neurologic deficits in an emergency department," *Neurology*, vol. 85, no. 3, pp. 256–262, 2015.

[90] C. Y. Cheung, M. K. Ikram, C. Chen, and T. Y. Wong, "Imaging retina to study dementia and stroke," *Progress in Retinal and Eye Research*, vol. 57, pp. 89–107, 2017.

[91] C. Y. Cheung, C. Chen, and T. Y. Wong, "Ocular fundus photography as a tool to study stroke and dementia," *Seminars in Neurology*, vol. 35, no. 5, pp. 481–490, 2015.

[92] C. WIjesundera, A. J. Vingrys, T. Wijeratne, and S. G. Crewther, "Acquired visual deficits independent of lesion site in acute stroke," *Frontiers in Neurology*, vol. 11, no. 705, 2020.

[93] C. Wijesundera, S. G. Crewther, T. Wijeratne, and A. J. Vingrys, "Vision and visuomotor performance following acute ischemic stroke," *Frontiers in Neurology*, vol. 13, article 757431, 2022.

[94] WHO, "Draft Intersectoral global action plan on epilepsy and other neurological disorders," 2022, https://www.who.int/news/item/12-01-2022-draft-intersectoral-global-action-plan-on-epilepsy-and-other-neurological-disorders-2022-2031.

[95] G. M. Slavich and R. P. Auerbach, *Stress and Its Sequelae: Depression, Suicide, Inflammation, and Physical Illness*, J. M. Hooley and J. N. Butcher, Eds., Washington DC American Psychological Association, 2018.

[96] A. Louveau, B. A. Plog, S. Antila, K. Alitalo, M. Nedergaard, and J. Kipnis, "Understanding the functions and relationships of the glymphatic system and meningeal lymphatics," *The Journal of Clinical Investigation.*, vol. 127, no. 9, pp. 3210–3219, 2017.

[97] C. O. Johnson, M. Nguyen, G. A. Roth et al., "Global, regional, and national burden of stroke, 1990–2016: a systematic analysis for the Global Burden of Disease Study 2016," *The Lancet Neurology.*, vol. 18, no. 5, pp. 439–458, 2019.

[98] L. Mellon, L. Brewer, P. Hall, F. Horgan, D. Williams, and A. Hickey, "Cognitive impairment six months after ischaemic stroke: a profile from the ASPIRE-S study," *BMC Neurology*, vol. 15, no. 1, p. 31, 2015.

[99] P. Knapp, A. Dunn-Roberts, N. Sahib et al., "Frequency of anxiety after stroke: an updated systematic review and meta-analysis of observational studies," *International Journal of Stroke*, vol. 15, no. 3, pp. 244–255, 2020.

[100] G. C. Medeiros, D. Roy, N. Kontos, and S. R. Beach, "Post-stroke depression: a 2020 updated review," *General Hospital Psychiatry*, vol. 66, pp. 70–80, 2020.

[101] M. Acciarresi, J. Bogousslavsky, and M. Paciaroni, "Post-stroke fatigue: epidemiology, clinical characteristics and treatment," *European Neurology*, vol. 72, no. 5-6, pp. 255–261, 2014.

[102] M. Paciaroni and M. Acciarresi, "Poststroke Fatigue," *Stroke*, vol. 50, no. 7, pp. 1927–1933, 2019.

[103] T. Wijeratne, C. Sales, L. Karimi, and M. Jakovljevicd, "Scoping review of existing stroke guidelines; argument for a value-added change," 2021.

[104] T. Wijeratne and C. Sales, "Understanding why post-stroke depression may be the norm rather than the exception: the anatomical and neuroinflammatory correlates of post-stroke depression," *Journal of Clinical Medicine*, vol. 10, no. 8, p. 1674, 2021.

# The Effect of Stroke Subtypes on Baroreceptor Sensitivity, a Predict for Acute Stroke Outcome

**Wan-Chen Tsai,[1] Hui-Chen Lin,[1] Yun-Ru Lai,[1,2] Che-Wei Hsu,[1,2] Chih-Cheng Huang,[1] Hung-Chen Wang,[3] Chih-Min Su,[4] Yu-Jih Su,[5] Wei-Che Lin,[6] Ben-Chung Cheng,[2,5] Wen-Neng Chang,[1] Cheng-Hsien Lu,[1,2] and Nai-Wen Tsai[1]**

[1] *Department of Neurology, Chang Gung Memorial Hospital-Kaohsiung Medical Center, Chang Gung University College of Medicine, Kaohsiung, Taiwan*
[2] *Department of Biological Science, National Sun Yat-Sen University, Kaohsiung, Taiwan*
[3] *Department of Neurosurgery, Chang Gung Memorial Hospital-Kaohsiung Medical Center, Chang Gung University College of Medicine, Kaohsiung, Taiwan*
[4] *Department of Emergency Medicine, Chang Gung Memorial Hospital-Kaohsiung Medical Center, Chang Gung University College of Medicine, Kaohsiung, Taiwan*
[5] *Department of Medicine, Chang Gung Memorial Hospital-Kaohsiung Medical Center, Chang Gung University College of Medicine, Kaohsiung, Taiwan*
[6] *Department of Radiology, Chang Gung Memorial Hospital-Kaohsiung Medical Center, Chang Gung University College of Medicine, Kaohsiung, Taiwan*

Correspondence should be addressed to Nai-Wen Tsai; tsainw@yahoo.com.tw

Wan-Chen Tsai and Hui-Chen Lin contributed equally to this work.

Academic Editor: Gelin Xu

*Background.* Reduced baroreflex sensitivity (BRS) has been reported in patients with acute cardiovascular events. We tested the hypothesis that BRS varies in different subtypes of acute ischemic stroke (AIS) and that BRS is a predictor of clinical outcomes. *Methods.* We examined autonomic parameters in 34 patients with AIS, including the small deep hemisphere infarction, the large hemisphere infarction, and the brainstem infarction groups on Day 1, Day 7, and Day 30 after AIS. Autonomic parameters were also evaluated in 18 age- and sex-matched healthy volunteers as a control group. The clinical outcomes were analyzed using the modified Rankin scale at 30 days after stroke. *Results.* The BRS, Valsalva ratio, and heart rate response to deep breathing (HR-DB) were significantly lower in patients after AIS on admission than in controls ($p<0.01$). The frequency domain of HRV (LF/HF ratio) was significantly increased in patients after AIS compared to controls ($p<0.05$). BRS was significantly reduced in patients with large hemisphere infarction or brainstem infarction compared to patients with small deep hemisphere infarction on Day 1 after AIS ($p<0.01$). Stepwise logistic regression showed that the levels of BRS and NIHSS are prognostic factors of 1-month outcomes in patients with AIS. *Conclusion.* Beside NIHSS score on admission, BRS is a potential prognostic factor of 1-month outcomes in patients with AIS. Patients with large hemisphere infarction or brainstem infarction have more blunting BRS than do those with lacunar infarction, which provides some insight into which patients may be expected to have a poor outcome.

## 1. Introduction

Autonomic dysfunction is a common complication of acute ischemic stroke (AIS) [1, 2]. Previous studies have shown that autonomic dysfunction, including increased sympathetic activity and reduced baroreflex, may increase susceptibility to sudden death and predict adverse clinical outcomes after AIS [3, 4]. The possible mechanisms associated with autonomic impairment and poor outcome in AIS include increased cardiovascular events and progression of secondary brain injury due to inflammation and altered cerebral perfusion [4, 5].

The central autonomic network (CAN) includes central areas that interconnect with the autonomic nervous system (ANS) to regulate autonomic function. The areas of the CAN include the insular cortex, anterior cingulate cortex, amygdala, hypothalamus, periaqueductal gray, parabrachial nucleus, nucleus of the solitary tract, ventrolateral reticular formation of the medulla, and medullary raphe [6]. These areas generate stimulus-specific patterns of autonomic and neuroendocrine responses [7]. Recent studies have reported evidence that supratentorial infarction, especially in the right hemisphere, shows a tendency toward increased sympathetic activity [8, 9]. Brainstem stroke correlates with a significant reduction in parasympathetic and an increase in sympathetic influence that causes cardiovascular autonomic dysregulation [10, 11]. Accordingly, we speculated that the location of infarction is an important factor affecting autonomic cardiac dysfunction and impairment of the CAN in patients with AIS [12].

In this study, we hypothesized that different stroke localizations influence the development of different autonomic responses, measured by baroreflex sensitivity (BRS) and other cardiovascular autonomic function. The aim of this study was to determine whether BRS is distinct in stroke patients with different infarction locations and whether the BRS is a predictor of clinical outcomes.

## 2. Materials and Methods

*2.1. Study Participants.* This prospective study that assessed the time course of cardiovascular function included 34 patients with AIS and 18 healthy volunteers at the Kaohsiung Chang Gung Memorial Hospital. The stroke diagnosis was based on clinical presentation, neurological examination, and results of brain magnetic resonance imaging (MRI) with diffusion-weighted images. Patients aged 18-85 years were classified into (1) large hemispheric infraction, (2) small deep hemispheric infarction, and (3) brainstem infarction group in the study [13]. The hospital's Institutional Review Committee on Human Research approved the study protocol, and all participants provided informed consent.

Patients with intracranial hemorrhage were excluded, as well as those with underlying neoplasm, vasculitis, hematological disorders, end-stage renal disease, liver cirrhosis, or congestive heart failure. Patients with cardioembolic stroke, as well as those who received intravenous thrombolytic therapy, were excluded because those patients have different therapeutic strategies and a high percentage of hemorrhagic transformation. Cardioembolism was diagnosed by clinical presentation, electrocardiography (ECG), and cardiac ultrasound.

*2.2. Clinical Assessments.* The clinical assessments followed our previous method [14]. All patients underwent complete neurological examination and detailed medical history upon enrollment and during follow-up. Brain MRI with MR angiography, extracranial carotid sonography, and transcranial color-coded sonography was performed on patients with AIS. Demographic data, history of previous vascular events (i.e., myocardial infarction, coronary artery disease, and previous stroke), and vascular risks (i.e., hypertension, diabetes mellitus (DM), dyslipidemia, and smoking) were obtained at baseline [15].

Physical disability and handicap were evaluated using the modified Rankin scale (mRS). The mRS was evaluated by investigators (Dr. Yu-Jun Lin and Yun-Ru Lai) blinded to the study group of each subject. Functional outcomes were evaluated at one month after stroke. A good outcome was defined as mRS score of 0-3 without any cardiovascular event, while a poor outcome was defined as mRS score of 4-6 [16].

*2.3. Assessment of Autonomic Function.* The methodology of autonomic functional assessment was modified from our previous publication [17]. All autonomic function studies were conducted on Days 1, 7, and 30 after stroke. The schedule was arranged between 8 and 10 AM to avoid the circadian effect. Coffee, food, alcohol, and nicotine were not permitted for 4 hours before the examination. Patients on medications known to cause orthostatic hypotension or otherwise affect autonomic testing were asked to abstain. Medication for BP control was continued, except for $\beta$-blockers, which were ceased on the day of the study and resumed after the test.

Heart rate was continuously recorded from standard three-lead ECG (Ivy Biomedical, Model 3000; Branford, CT, USA), and arterial BP was continuously measured using beat-to-beat photoplethysmographic recordings (Finameter Pro, Ohmeda; Englewood, OH, USA). The following parameters were obtained through tests computed by Testworks (WR Medical Electronics Company, Stillwater, MN, USA): HR response to deep breathing (HR_DB) and Valsalva ratio (VR) [18].

Beat-to-beat R-R interval (RRI) changes were interpolated using a third-order polynomial and were resampled with an interval of 0.5s. For spectral analysis of heart rate variability (HRV), the signals were then transformed to the frequency domain with fast Fourier transformation using 512 samples. Spectral powers were divided into three frequency domains: high frequency (HF, 0.15–0.4 Hz), low frequency (LF, 0.04–0.15 Hz), and very low frequency (VLF, 0–0.04 Hz). The unit of RRI power is $ms^2$. The normalized low and high frequency powers (LF normalized units, HF normalized units) were calculated as a percentage of overall power.

Spontaneous BRS was computed by using Nevrokard sequence BRS program [19]. The criteria in computing BRS, (1) systolic BP (SBP) changes > 1 mmHg, (2) sequences longer than 3 beats, and (3) correlation coefficient > 0.85. Both bradycardic (an increase in SBP that caused an increase in RRI) and tachycardic sequences (a decrease in SBP that caused a decrease in RRI) that fulfilled the criteria, were enrolled. The BRS was calculated using a synchronous mode and a shift mode from 1 to 6 heart beat shifts [20, 21] for each subject. The mode with the largest number of slopes was selected and the average slope of the regression lines was taken as the measure of BRS.

TABLE 1: Baseline characteristics and autonomic function of the study participants.

| | Stroke patients (n=34) | Controls (n=18) | $p$-value |
|---|---|---|---|
| Age (y) (mean ±SD) | 63.2±8.7 | 59.6±7.8 | 0.14 |
| Male/female | 26/12 | 11/7 | 0.138 |
| Mean systolic blood pressure | 169.4±28.4 | 126.70±13.1 | <0.0001* |
| Mean diastolic blood pressure | 92.5±15.5 | 68.15±6.1 | <0.0001* |
| *Underlying diseases* | | | |
| Hypertension (n,%) | 26 (76.5%) | --- | |
| Diabetes mellitus (n,%) | 19 (55.9%) | --- | |
| Dyslipidemia (n,%) | 23 (67.6%) | --- | |
| Coronary artery diseases (n, %) | 2 (5.9%) | --- | |
| Smoking | 6 (17.8%) | --- | |
| *Laboratory data* | | | |
| White blood cells($\times 10^3$/ml) | 9.4±1.7 | 5.3±1.2 | 0.08 |
| Red blood cells ($\times 10^6$/ml) | 4.7±0.6 | 4.7±0.7 | 0.68 |
| Platelet counts ($\times 10^4$/ml) | 20.4±6.6 | 24.4±7.5 | 0.06 |
| Hs-CRP (mg/L) | 6.1±2.6 | 0.8±0.2 | 0.008* |
| Total cholesterol (mg/dL) | 181.2±39.4 | 189.9±27.9 | 0.42 |
| LDL-cholesterol (mg/dL) | 106.9±31.9 | 111.9±25.8 | 0.58 |
| Triglycerol (mg/dL) | 165.2±128.9 | 92.8±48.4 | 0.03* |
| HbAlc (%) | 7.5±2.0 | 5.8±0.3 | 0.002* |
| *Autonomic function* | | | |
| Spectral analysis | | | |
| LF (n.u.) | 59.6±22.6 | 50.2±18.3 | 0.14 |
| HF (n.u.) | 40.2±22.4 | 49.7±18.3 | 0.13 |
| LF/HF ratio | 2.4±2.2 | 1.3±1.2 | 0.04* |
| Cardio-vagal autonomic function | | | |
| Valsalva ratio | 1.1±0.3 | 1.7±0.4 | 0.004* |
| HR_DB | 6.4±3.5 | 13.5±8.4 | 0.006* |
| Baroreflex function | | | |
| BRS | 4.2±1.4 | 9.6±2.3 | <0.0001* |

All values are presented as mean ± SD; $*p < 0.05$, compared to controls.
*Abbreviations.* HbAlc: glycated hemoglobin; Hs-CRP= high-sensitivity C-reactive protein; LDL: low density lipoprotein; SD: standard deviation; LF: low frequency; HF, high frequency; HR_DB: heart rate response to deep breathing; BRS: baroreflex sensitivity; n.u.: normalized unit.

*2.4. Statistical Analyses.* The quantitative data are presented as mean ± standard deviations (SD). Continuous variables between two groups (i.e., controls vs. patients, good and poor outcome group) were compared using the independent $t$-test for parametric data and the Mann-Whitney U test for nonparametric data. Chi-square or Fisher's exact test was used for the comparison of proportions between two groups. One-way ANOVA was used to compare the autonomic parameters among the three stroke subtypes. Repeated measures ANOVA was used to compare BRS and HR-DB at different time points (on Days 1, 7, and 30 post-stroke), while Scheffe's multiple comparison was performed to analyze the intraindividual course of parameters over time and compare the parameters of the good and poor outcome groups. The independent $t$-test was also used to compare the good and poor outcome groups. Multiple logistic regression analyses were used to determine the independent influence of different predictive variables on functional outcome. Statistical significance was set at $p<0.05$. All statistical calculations were performed using the SAS software package, version 9.1 (2002, SAS Statistical Institute, Cary, NC, USA).

## 3. Results

*3.1. Demographic Data of Stroke Patients and Controls.* The demographic data of the AIS patients and controls are shown in Table 1. The 34 patients with AIS (mean age: 63.2 years) included 26 males and 12 females. Age and sex were similar between the two groups. Twenty-eight subjects had one or more underlying diseases, including hypertension (26), diabetes mellitus (19), hyperlipidemia (23), coronary artery

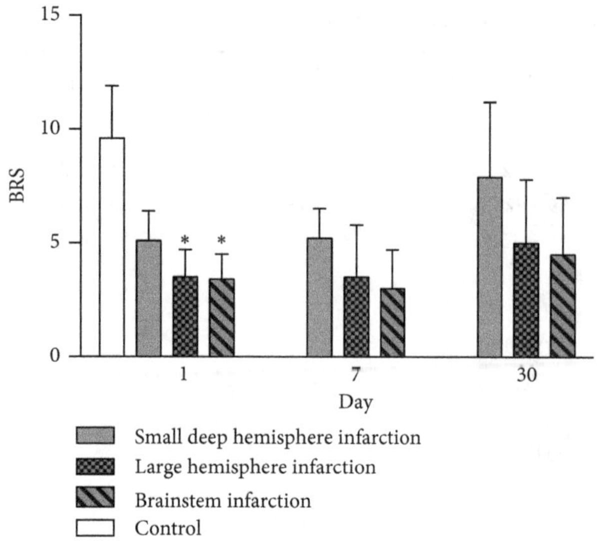


FIGURE 1: Changes in BRS level among control and the 3 stroke subtypes (small deep hemisphere infarction, large hemisphere infarction and brainstem infarction) on Day 1, Day 7, and Day 30 after acute ischemic stroke. $*p<0.05$ compared to the small deep hemisphere infarction.

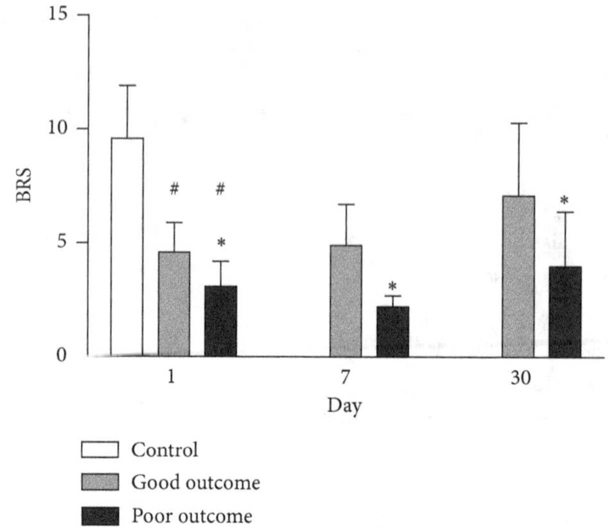


FIGURE 2: Comparison of BRS level between the good outcome group and the poor outcome group on Day 1, Day 7, and Day 30 after acute ischemic stroke. $*p<0.05$ compared to the good outcome group. $^{\#}p<0.05$ compared to the control group.

disease (2), and smoking (6). The blood pressure, serum triglycerol, HbAlc, and high-sensitivity C-reactive protein (hs-CRP) levels were significantly higher in the AIS patient group than in the control group ($p<0.05$).

*3.2. Comparison of Autonomic Function between Stroke Patients and Controls.* In terms of autonomic function testing, VR, HR_DB, and spontaneous BRS were significantly reduced in the stroke group compared to the control group ($p<0.01$). The normalized frequency power (LF/HF ratio) was significantly higher in the AIS patient group than in the control group ($p<0.05$). There were no significant differences in white blood cell counts (WBC), red blood cell counts (RBC), platelet counts, or serum total cholesterol and LDL-cholesterol levels.

*3.3. Comparison of Autonomic Function among 3 Subtypes of Acute Ischemic Stroke.* The basic demographic, stroke locations and autonomic function among 3 subtypes of stroke patients are listed in Table 2. The subtypes of AIS were small deep hemisphere infarction (14 patients), large hemisphere infarction (13 patients), and brainstem infarction (7 patients). The mall deep hemisphere infarction group had significantly higher BRS on Day 1 after stroke compared to both the large hemisphere infarction group and the brainstem infarction group. There was no statistical difference between the left and the right infarcts in each group. We had 4 patients (2 in the right hemisphere and 2 in the left hemisphere) involving insular infarction, but there was no statistical difference in autonomic parameters between the left and the right sides. Furthermore, the differences in BRS between the three subtypes were not significant on Day 7 or Day 30 after stroke (Figure 1). There were also no significant differences in the spectral analysis (LF, HF, and LF/HF ratio) parameters between the three groups.

*3.4. Prognostic Factors of Clinical Outcome.* The potential prognostic factors of the 34 acute stroke patients for one month are listed in Table 3. Among the patients, 24 had good outcomes and the remaining 10 had poor outcomes, but no patients died during the follow-up period. Statistical analysis revealed that NIHSS, BRS, and HR_DB were potential predictors of outcomes. However, age, sex, underlying disease, and laboratory data were not significantly different between the good and the poor outcome groups. Using the stepwise logistic regression model for these variables, only BRS (OR= 4.1, 95% CI 1.3-13.1) and NIHSS on admission (OR= 0.71, 95% CI 0.53-0.95) were independently associated with one-month outcome.

*3.5. Time Course of BRS Change.* The BRS values in AIS patients were initially lower and gradually increased after acute stroke compared to the control group. Furthermore, BRS values were significantly lower in patients with poor outcomes than in those with good outcomes on Day 1, Day 7 and even Day 30 (Figure 2). Similarly, the HR_DB values in patients with poor outcomes were significantly lower than those in patients with good outcomes on Day 1, Day 7 and Day 30 (Figure 3).

## 4. Discussion

The present study examined autonomic function and different subtypes of AIS and has four major findings. First, the baroreflex function (spontaneous BRS) and cardiovagal autonomic function (Valsalva ration and HR-DB) were significantly lower in patients with AIS on admission than

Table 2: The basic demographic, stroke locations, and autonomic function among 3 subtypes of stroke patients.

| | Small deep hemisphere infarction (n=14) | | | Large hemisphere infarction (n=13) | | | Brainstem infarction (n=7) | | | *p*-value |
|---|---|---|---|---|---|---|---|---|---|---|
| | Left | Right | Total | Left | Right | Total | Left | Right | Total | |
| *Age* | | | *61.7±9.9* | | | *63.5±8.7* | | | *65.6±5.8* | *0.63* |
| *Sex (female) n* | | | *6* | | | *4* | | | *2* | *0.34* |
| *NIHSS* | | | *4.3±1.5* | | | *5.3±5.3* | | | *10.4±8.3* | *0.04* |
| *SBP* | | | *172.4±24.7* | | | *163.2±29.6* | | | *175.0±34.8* | *0.60* |
| *DBP* | | | *95.8±15.9* | | | *89.5±17.5* | | | *91.4±11.0* | *0.58* |
| *Lateralization* | 6 | 8 | | 6 | 7 | | 4 | 3 | | |
| *Stroke location* | | | | | | | | | | |
| Internal capsule | 2 | 2 | *4* | | | | | | | |
| Basal ganglia | 2 | 5 | *7* | | | | | | | |
| Corona radiate | 3 | 5 | *8* | | | | | | | |
| Putamen | 0 | 1 | *1* | | | | | | | |
| Frontal lobe | | | | 5 | 3 | *8* | | | | |
| Temporal lobe | | | | 4 | 3 | *7* | | | | |
| Insula | | | | 2 | 2 | *4* | | | | |
| Parietal Lobe | | | | 2 | 5 | *7* | | | | |
| Occipital lobe | | | | 0 | 2 | *2* | | | | |
| Midbrain | | | | | | | 1 | 0 | *1* | |
| Pons | | | | | | | 3 | 3 | *6* | |
| Medulla | | | | | | | 0 | 2 | *2* | |
| *Spectral analysis* | | | | | | | | | | |
| LF (n.u) | 49.0±22.0 | 63.9±16.1 | *57.5±19.6* | 59.5±19.1 | 57.1±25.9 | *58.2±22.1* | 82.0±6.7 | 45.0±39.1 | *66.1±30.5* | *0.69* |
| HF (n.u) | 50.8±21.8 | 35.7±16.1 | *42.2±19.6* | 40.6±19.0 | 42.5±25.6 | *41.6±21.9* | 28.7±6.5 | 45.0±39 | *33.8±30.1* | *0.71* |
| LF/HF ratio | 1.2±1.1 | 2.6±2.1 | *2.0±1.9* | 2.2±2.0 | 2.3±2.2 | *2.3±2.0* | 4.2±2.5 | 2.7±1.9 | *3.7±2.8* | *0.24* |
| *Cardio-vagal function* | | | | | | | | | | |
| Valsalva ratio | 1.3±0.6 | 1.0±0.3 | *1.2±0.4* | 1.0±0.1 | 1.0±0.3 | *1.0±0.2* | 1.1±0.4 | 1.1±0.2 | *1.1±0.3* | *0.41* |
| HR_DB | 6.8±1.3 | 9.0±4.7 | *7.8±3.3* | 5.3±3.4 | 5.6±3.4 | *5.4±3.2* | 3.0±0.6 | 2.0±0.8 | *2.5±0.7* | *0.07* |
| *Baroreflex function* | | | | | | | | | | |
| BRS | 4.5±1.0 | 5.6±1.3 | *5.1±1.3* | 4.0±3.4 | 3.1±0.9 | *3.5±1.2∗* | 3.5±1.0 | 3.3±1.5 | *3.4±1.1∗* | *0.002§* |

All values are mean ± SD; § *p*-value are compared with overall mean among 3 groups; ∗$p < 0.05$, compared to small deep hemisphere infarction with post hoc analysis.
Because some patients have multiple infarction, the total number of the stroke locations is greater than the number of patients.
*Abbreviations.* SD: standard deviation; LF: low frequency; HF: high frequency; HR_DB: heart rate response to deep breathing; BRS: baroreflex sensitivity n.u.: normalized unit

TABLE 3: Prognostic factors of patients with acute ischemic stroke.

| | Good outcome (n=24) | Poor outcome (n=10) | $p$-Value | Adjusted OR (95% CI) | Adjusted $p$-Value |
|---|---|---|---|---|---|
| *Age (y)* | 62.0±9.0 | 66.1±7.2 | 0.21 | | |
| *Sex (Male/female)* | 17/7 | 9/1 | 0.23 | | |
| *Underlying diseases* | | | | | |
| Hypertension | 20 | 6 | 0.20 | | |
| Diabetes mellitus | 12 | 7 | 0.45 | | |
| Coronary artery disease | 1 | 1 | 0.51 | | |
| Hyperlipidemia | 17 | 6 | 0.54 | | |
| Smoking | 5 | 1 | 0.76 | | |
| *Clinical feature* | | | | | |
| Systolic blood pressure on admission | 171.4±27.0 | 164.7±32.3 | 0.54 | | |
| Diastolic blood pressure on admission | 94.6±15.1 | 87.4±16.2 | 0.22 | | |
| NIHSS | 4.1±2.1 | 10.3±8.2 | 0.001 | 0.71(0.53-0.95) | *0.021* |
| *Laboratory data* | | | | | |
| White blood cells($\times10^3$/ml) | 14.0±1.7 | 13.5±1.3 | 0.87 | | |
| Red blood cells ($\times10^6$/ml) | 4.7±0.6 | 4.6±0.7 | 0.77 | | |
| Platelet counts ($\times10^4$/ml) | 21.1±7.1 | 18.7±5.3 | 0.34 | | |
| Hs-CRP (mg/L) | 5.9±2.9 | 7.0±3.0 | 0.81 | | |
| Total cholesterol (mg/dL) | 186.1±42.0 | 171.5±33.5 | 0.35 | | |
| LDL-cholesterol (mg/dL) | 111.2±32.8 | 98.5±30.2 | 0.32 | | |
| Triglycerol (mg/dL) | 165.4±30.8 | 165.0±36.6 | 0.99 | | |
| HbA1c (%) | 7.4±2.1 | 7.9±1.9 | 0.74 | | |
| *Autonomic function on admission* | | | | | |
| Frequency domain | | | | | |
| LF (n.u) | 58.3±22.8 | 62.6±23.1 | 0.62 | | |
| HF (n.u) | 41.4±22.6 | 37.4±22.8 | 0.64 | | |
| LF/HF ratio | 2.2±1.9 | 3.0±2.9 | 0.32 | | |
| Cardio-vagal autonomic function | | | | | |
| Valsalva ratio | 1.1±0.3 | 1.3±0.4 | 0.52 | | |
| HR_DB | 7.0±3.5 | 3.5±1.7 | 0.02 | | |
| Baroreflex function | | | | | |
| BRS | 4.6±1.3 | 3.1±1.1 | 0.003 | 4.1(1.3-13.1) | *0.016* |

All values are mean ± SD; adjusted $p$-value was calculated by using the stepwise logistic regression model for the potential variables.
*Abbreviations.* HbA1c: glycated hemoglobin; Hs-CRP= high-sensitivity C-reactive protein; LDL: low density lipoprotein; SD: standard deviation; LF: low frequency; HF: high frequency; HR_DB: heart rate response to deep breathing; BRS: baroreflex sensitivity; n.u.: normalized unit.

in controls. Second, the frequency domain of HRV (LF/HF ratio) is significantly increased in patients with AIS compared to controls. Third, the values of BRS are significantly reduced in both large hemisphere infarction and brainstem infarction compared to small deep hemisphere infarction after AIS. Finally, the levels of BRS and NIHSS are potential prognostic factors of 1-month outcomes in patients with AIS.

BRS provides regulation of cardiovagal control and the interaction of cardiac sympathetic–parasympathetic balance. Impairment of BRS tended to have sympathetic hyperactivity, which consequently leads to an increased risk of cardiac arrhythmia, hypertensive crisis, and associated cardiac events. Furthermore, BRS impairment results in BP instability, which is likely to have a negative impact on cerebral blood perfusion, especially in patients with impaired cerebral autoregulation, such as AIS patients [22]. These mechanisms may explain the poor prognosis of the patients with impaired BRS.

A previous study has demonstrated that reduced BRS in the acute phase of stroke can predict long-term fatalities. Another study has shown that autonomic dysregulation can persist 9 months after stroke [23]. Our previous study confirmed the hypothesis that autonomic dysregulation can persist for a long time among AIS survivors and demonstrates that patients with recurrent cardiovascular events after symptomatic AIS have significantly lower HR_DB, with a trend toward reduced VR and BRS [21]. In addition to the findings in patients with AIS, our recent research shows the predictive value of BRS in patients with spontaneous intracranial hemorrhage [24]. In the current study, the BRS values in the poor outcome group were significantly lower than those in the good outcome group on Day 1, Day 7, and Day 30. Our

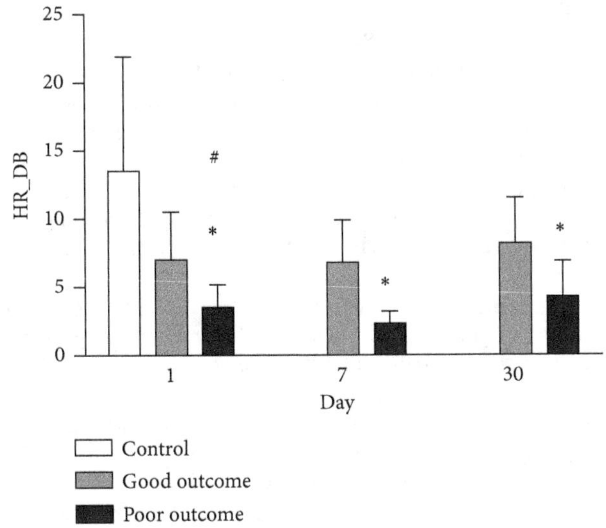


FIGURE 3: Comparison of HR_DB level between the good outcome group and the poor outcome group on Day 1, Day 7, and Day 30 after acute ischemic stroke. $*p<0.05$ compared to the good outcome group. $^{\#}p<0.05$ compared to the control group.

results are in agreement with those of previous studies that show BRS correlated to clinical outcome in patients with AIS [22, 25]. Based on this finding, it is recommended to test patients within 24 hours of symptom onset in further studies of BRS or other cardiovascular autonomic changes in stroke patients to observe the most prominent differences as these differences may diminish gradually.

The CAN, which includes the insular cortex, anterior cingulate cortex, amygdala, hypothalamus, periaqueductal gray, parabrachial nucleus, nucleus of the solitary tract, ventrolateral reticular formation of the medulla, and medullary raphe, is a group of central areas that interconnect with the peripheral ANS to regulate autonomic function [6]. Baroreceptor signaling is conducted via vagal and glossopharyngeal cranial nerves to the nucleus tractus solitarius, which in turn projects to the brainstem (e.g., ventrolateral medulla and nucleus ambiguus). The brainstem is a critical part of the baroreflex arc and participates in homeostatic tuning of the BRS. Accordingly, we speculated that the location of infarction is an important factor affecting autonomic dysfunction and CAN impairment in patients with AIS [12]. Recent evidence reported that supratentorial infarction, especially in the right hemisphere, shows a tendency toward increased sympathetic activity [8, 9]. However, our study does not show the difference of autonomic parameter between the left and the right infarcts in each group. We propose that our case number is too small to clarify this issue. Brainstem stroke correlates with a reduction in parasympathetic and an increase in sympathetic influence that caused cardiovascular autonomic dysregulation [10, 11].

The degree of autonomic dysregulation can also be influenced by stroke subtypes. One study revealed that the autonomic dysfunctions are influenced by stroke subtype, with large hemisphere arthrosclerosis showing more severe impairment of parasympathetic function [26]. Other studies have demonstrated that insults to both the brainstem and the hemispheres can result in HRV impairment [27, 28], not only in the acute phase but also on long-term follow-up. Impaired HRV is associated with severe neurological deficits and disability [29]. Low HR_DB and VR and a trend toward reduced HF in the HRV frequency domain of AIS patients are consistent with impaired cardiovagal function. This finding is corroborated by the present study that shows that patients with either large hemisphere infarction or brainstem stroke had significant reduction of BRS compared to those with small deep hemisphere infarction after AIS.

This study has several limitations. First, patients who were comatose and those who were unable to cooperate for the autonomic function test were excluded. Thus, the role of the BRS in critically ill and high-risk patients is unknown. Second, we did not enroll patients with cardioembolic stroke in this study because both BRS and other cardiovagal autonomic parameters may be influenced by the effects of cardiac arrhythmia, which would result in unreliable data. Third, some autonomic parameters may be influenced by the effects of medications (e.g., calcium channel blockers; angiotensin II receptor antagonist, $\beta$-blockers), which are commonly used by AIS patients and were not stopped during the study for ethical reasons. Furthermore, the area of each patient's cerebral infarction is not the same and the number of cases in the single stroke location is small; it is difficult to analyze the correlation between single infarct location and autonomic parameters. Finally, the number of variables considered for multiple logistic regression analysis is small and only one variable was selected as important in predicting outcome in the stepwise procedures. Thus, the maximum likelihood estimates of the coefficients are only valid in the current analysis.

In conclusion, the measurement of BRS is a potential prognostic factor of short-term outcome in patients with AIS. Patients with large hemisphere infarction or brainstem infarction have more blunting BRS than those with lacunar infarction, which may suggest that those patients are expected to have a poor outcome. The successful translation of these results may offer useful predictors of short-term outcomes after AIS.

## Abbreviations

AIS: Acute ischemic stroke
ANS: Autonomic nervous system
BP: Blood pressure
BRS: Baroreflex sensitivity
CAN: Central autonomic network
DM: Diabetes mellitus
ECG: Electrocardiography
HbA1c: Glycolate hemoglobin
HF: High frequency
HR-DB: Heart rate response to deep breathing
HRV: Heart rate variability
hs-CRP: High sensitivity C-reactive protein
LDL: Low density lipoprotein
LF: Low frequency

mRS: Modified Rankin Scale
OR: Odds ratio
RBC: Red blood cell
RRI: R-R interval
SD: Standard deviation
VLF: Very low frequency
VR: Valsalva ratio
WBC: White blood cell.

## Ethical Approval

The study was approved by Chang Gung Memorial Hospital's Institutional Review Committee on Human Research.

## Disclosure

None of the authors have any commercial association, such as consultancies, stock ownership, or other equity interests or patent-licensing arrangements.

## Conflicts of Interest

The authors declare that they have no conflicts of interest.

## Authors' Contributions

Wan-Chen Tsai and Hui-Chen Lin participated in the design of the study and drafted the manuscript. Chih-Cheng Huang and Che-Weu Hsu conducted the autonomic study. Ben-Chung Cheng and Yun-Ru Lai participated in the clinical evaluation of patients. Wei-Che Lin and Hung-Chen Wang interpreted the neuroimaging studies. Yu-Jih Su and Chih-Min Su performed the statistical analysis. Cheng-Hsien Lu and Wen-Neng Chang conceived the study. Nai-Wen Tsai participated in its design and coordination and helped draft the manuscript. All authors read and approved the final manuscript and agree on publication. Drs. Wan-Chen Tsai and Hui-Chen Lin contributed equally to this work and considered as co-first author.

## Acknowledgments

This study was supported by grants from Chang Gung Memorial Hospital Research Project CMRPG8E1051.

## References

[1] T. G. Robinson, M. James, J. Youde, R. Panerai, and J. Potter, "Cardiac baroreceptor sensitivity is impaired after acute stroke," *Stroke*, vol. 28, no. 9, pp. 1671–1676, 1997.

[2] S. M. Oppenheimer, D. F. Cechetto, and V. C. Hachinski, "Cerebrogenic cardiac arrhythmias: cerebral electrocardiographic influences and their role in sudden death," *JAMA Neurology*, vol. 47, no. 5, pp. 513–519, 1990.

[3] A. M. Mäkikallio, T. H. Mäkikallio, J. T. Korpelainen, K. A. Sotaniemi, H. V. Huikuri, and V. V. Myllylä, "Heart rate dynamics predict poststroke mortality," *Neurology*, vol. 62, no. 10, pp. 1822–1826, 2004.

[4] T. G. Robinson, S. L. Dawson, P. J. Eames, R. B. Panerai, and J. F. Potter, "Cardiac baroreceptor sensitivity predicts long-term outcome after acute ischemic stroke," *Stroke*, vol. 34, no. 3, pp. 705–711, 2003.

[5] D. Aarsland, K. Brønnick, J. P. Larsen, O. B. Tysnes, and G. Alves, "Cognitive impairment in incident, untreated parkinson disease: the Norwegian ParkWest study," *Neurology*, vol. 72, no. 13, pp. 1121–1126, 2009.

[6] E. E. Benarroch, "The central autonomic network: functional organization, dysfunction, and perspective," *Mayo Clinic Proceedings*, vol. 68, no. 10, pp. 988–1001, 1993.

[7] M. G. Cersosimo and E. E. Benarroch, "Central control of autonomic function and involvement in neurodegenerative disorders," *Handbook of Clinical Neurology*, vol. 117, pp. 45–57, 2013.

[8] M. Dütsch, M. Burger, C. Dörfler, S. Schwab, and M. J. Hilz, "Cardiovascular autonomic function in poststroke patients," *Neurology*, vol. 69, no. 24, pp. 2249–2255, 2007.

[9] S. L. Tokgözoglu, M. K. Batur, M. A. Topçuoglu, O. Saribas, S. Kes, and A. Oto, "Effects of stroke localization on cardiac autonomic balance and sudden death," *Stroke*, vol. 30, no. 7, pp. 1307–1311, 1999.

[10] C.-F. Chen, H.-F. Lin, R.-T. Lin, Y.-H. Yang, and C.-L. Lai, "Relationship between ischemic stroke location and autonomic cardiac function," *Journal of Clinical Neuroscience*, vol. 20, no. 3, pp. 406–409, 2013.

[11] J. T. Korpelainen, H. V. Huikuri, K. A. Sotaniemi, and V. V. Myllylä, "Abnormal heart rate variability reflecting autonomic dysfunction in brainstem infarction," *Acta Neurologica Scandinavica*, vol. 94, no. 5, pp. 337–342, 1996.

[12] M. Strittmatter, S. Meyer, C. Fischer, T. Georg, and B. Schmitz, "Location-dependent patterns in cardio-autonomic dysfunction in ischaemic stroke," *European Neurology*, vol. 50, no. 1, pp. 30–38, 2003.

[13] H. P. Adams Jr., B. H. Bendixen, L. J. Kappelle et al., "Classification of subtype of acute ischemic stroke: definitions for use in a multicenter clinical trial," *Stroke*, vol. 24, no. 1, pp. 35–41, 1993.

[14] N.-W. Tsai, L.-H. Lee, C.-R. Huang et al., "Statin therapy reduces oxidized low density lipoprotein level, a risk factor for stroke outcome," *Critical Care*, vol. 18, no. 1, p. R16, 2014.

[15] L. B. Goldstein, R. Adams, M. J. Alberts et al., "Primary prevention of ischemic stroke: a guideline from the american heart association/american stroke association stroke council: cosponsored by the atherosclerotic peripheral vascular disease interdisciplinary working group; cardiovascular nursing council; clinical cardiology council; nutrition, physical activity, and metabolism council; and the quality of care and outcomes research interdisciplinary working group: the american academy of neurology affirms the value of this guideline," *Stroke*, vol. 37, no. 6, pp. 1583–1633, 2006.

[16] G. Sulter, C. Steen, and J. De Keyser, "Use of the barthel index and modified rankin scale in acute stroke trials," *Stroke*, vol. 30, no. 8, pp. 1538–1541, 1999.

[17] C.-C. Huang, Y.-S. Wu, T. Chen et al., "Long-term effects of baroreflex function after stenting in patients with carotid artery

stenosis," *Autonomic Neuroscience: Basic and Clinical*, vol. 158, no. 1-2, pp. 100–104, 2010.

[18] P. A. Low, "Testing the autonomic nervous system," *Seminars in Neurology*, vol. 23, no. 4, pp. 407–421, 2003.

[19] G. Parati, M. DiRienzo, and G. Mancia, "How to measure baroreflex sensitivity: from the cardiovascular laboratory to daily life," *Journal of Hypertension*, vol. 18, no. 1, pp. 7–19, 2000.

[20] H. Malberg, N. Wessel, A. Hasart, K.-J. Osterziel, and A. Voss, "Advanced analysis of spontaneous baroreflex sensitivity, blood pressure and heart rate variability in patients with dilated cardiomyopathy," *Clinical Science*, vol. 102, no. 4, pp. 465–473, 2002.

[21] Y.-T. Chang, W.-N. Chang, N.-W. Tsai et al., "Link between cerebral blood flow and autonomic function in survivors of internal carotid artery occlusion," *Journal of the Neurological Sciences*, vol. 353, no. 1-2, pp. 143–148, 2015.

[22] P. J. Eames, M. J. Blake, S. L. Dawson, R. B. Panerai, and J. F. Potter, "Dynamic cerebral autoregulation and beat to beat blood pressure control are impaired in acute ischaemic stroke," *Journal of Neurology, Neurosurgery & Psychiatry*, vol. 72, no. 4, pp. 467–472, 2002.

[23] A. McLaren, S. Kerr, L. Allan et al., "Autonomic function is impaired in elderly stroke survivors," *Stroke*, vol. 36, no. 5, pp. 1026–1030, 2005.

[24] Y.-R. Lai, Y.-J. Lin, F.-Y. Shih et al., "Effect of baroreceptor sensitivity on outcomes in patients with acute spontaneous intracerebral hemorrhage," *World Neurosurgery*, vol. 109, pp. e754–e760, 2018.

[25] A. M. Phillips, D. L. Jardine, P. J. Parkin, T. Hughes, and H. Ikram, "Brain stem stroke ,causing baroreflex failure and paroxysmal hypertension," *Stroke*, vol. 31, no. 8, pp. 1997–2001, 2000.

[26] L. Xiong, H. W. Leung, X. Y. Chen, W. H. Leung, O. Y. Soo, and K. S. Wong, "Autonomic dysfunction in different subtypes of post-acute ischemic stroke," *Journal of the Neurological Sciences*, vol. 337, no. 1-2, pp. 141–146, 2014.

[27] V. Novak, P. Novak, M. deMarchie, and R. Schondorf, "The effect of severe brainstem injury on heart rate and blood pressure oscillations," *Clinical Autonomic Research*, vol. 5, no. 1, pp. 24–30, 1995.

[28] S. A. Barron, Z. Rogovski, and J. Hemli, "Autonomic consequences of cerebral hemisphere infarction," *Stroke*, vol. 25, no. 1, pp. 113–116, 1994.

[29] J. T. Korpelainen, K. A. Sotaniemi, H. V. Huikuri, and V. V. Myllylä, "Abnormal heart rate variability as a manifestation of autonomic dysfunction in hemispheric brain infarction," *Stroke*, vol. 27, no. 11, pp. 2059–2063, 1996.

# 36

# High Prevalence of Poststroke Depression in Ischemic Stroke Patients in Ethiopia

**Fikru Tsehayneh and Abenet Tafesse**

*Department of Neurology, Addis Ababa University School of Medicine, Addis Ababa, Ethiopia*

Correspondence should be addressed to Fikru Tsehayneh; fikru.tsehayneh@aau.edu.et

Academic Editor: Carol Milligan

*Background.* There is limited information and research carried out regarding the prevalence of poststroke depression (PSD) in the study area. Psychiatric disorders complicate a significant proportion of patients suffering from stroke. This of course have a great negative impact on our knowledge about poststroke depression in Ethiopia, and poststroke depression complicates a significant number of stroke patients and their rehabilitation. *Methods.* A cross-sectional study on all patients aged above 18 years and diagnosed with stroke in the past two years who attended the neurology follow-up clinics of Tikur Anbessa Specialized Hospital (TASH) and Zewditu Memorial Hospital (ZMH) was done by using a structured questionnaire containing Patient Health Questionnaire-9 (PHQ-9) depression screening tool. *Result.* Of 84 patients who were eligible for the study, 32.2% of patients have depressive symptoms. Women (OR 0.001, 95% CI 0.12–0.87) and aphasic patients (OR 0.034, 95% CI 0.19–1.27) were more likely to have depressive symptoms. *Conclusion.* Depressive symptoms after stroke are common in Ethiopian patients. Our study demonstrates female and aphasic patients are more likely to screen positive for PSD. Hence, screening all poststroke patients with different screening tools is practical, and further studies are needed to assess the validity of these screening tools and also to assess PSD as a predictor of stroke outcome.

## 1. Background

Stroke is becoming a leading cause of death and adult disability in the developing world. It is the second leading cause of death worldwide comprising about 10% of all the deaths which is 5.5 million people per year and with 44 million disability-adjusted life years (DALYs) lost. The global burden of disease study indicates 16.9 million stroke cases in 2010 and 70% occurred in low- and middle-income countries [1].

In Ethiopia, stroke is a common cause of mortality and morbidity. It is the most common neurological disorder seen in patients admitted to general hospitals in Ethiopia [2]. Cerebrovascular disease (CVD) was reported to account for 23.6% of all neurological admissions in Tikur Anbessa Specialized Hospital (TASH) [3].

Psychiatric disorders are known to complicate a significant proportion of patients in the poststroke period. In the acute phase of stroke, delirium and other neuropsychiatric complications become a focus of interest as they disturb the process of care and are indicators of worse outcome. Psychiatric disturbances strongly contribute to a low quality of life among stroke survivors in the long term [4].

A study showed that nonpsychiatric physicians fail to diagnose 50% to 80% of the actually existing depression. Poststroke depression has been related to physical disability and the limitations in daily activities. However, PSD is most likely not solely a psychological reflection of a physical disability. Another study showed that stroke patients were significantly more commonly depressed than orthopedic patients with equal levels of functional disability. It has been claimed that PSD is related to specific locations of ischemic brain lesions, although this has also been denied [5, 6].

Different screening tools for use in screening depression were used in previous literature studies. Evidence suggests

Table 1: Baseline sociodemographic characteristics of stroke patients at TASH and ZMH neurology clinic.

| Variables and categories | | Frequency $N = 84$ | Percentage (%) |
|---|---|---|---|
| Gender | Female | 40 | 47.6 |
| | Male | 44 | 52.4 |
| Age group | 15–24 | 2 | 2.4 |
| | 25–34 | 4 | 4.8 |
| | 35–44 | 10 | 11.9 |
| | 45–54 | 17 | 20.2 |
| | 55–64 | 24 | 28.6 |
| | >65 | 27 | 32.1 |
| Marital status | Unmarried | 24 | 28.6 |
| | Married | 60 | 71.4 |
| Education | No formal education | 30 | 35.7 |
| | Secondary school | 30 | 35.7 |
| | More than secondary | 24 | 28.6 |

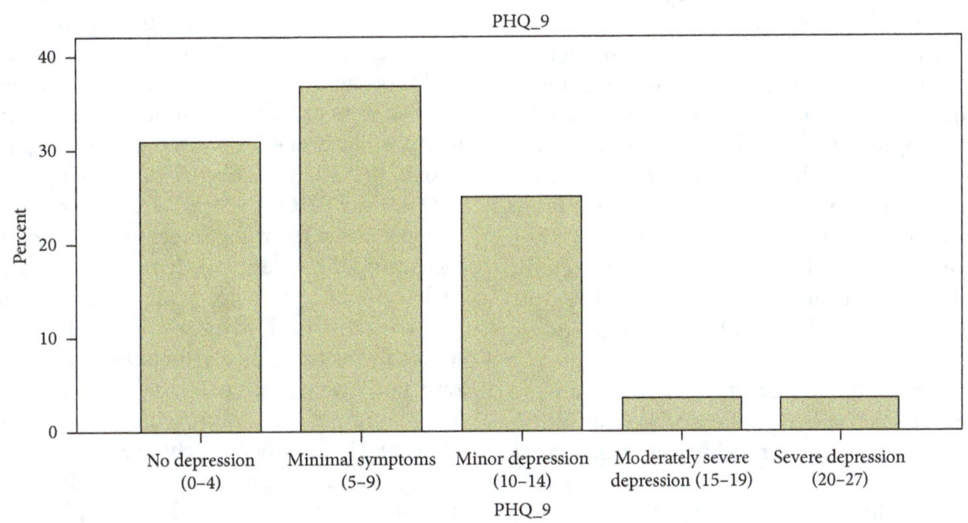


Figure 1: Frequency distribution of depression among stroke patients at TASH and ZMH neurology clinics.

Table 2: Frequency distribution of depression with age group among stroke patients at TASH and ZMH neurology clinics.

| | | Depression | | | | | Total |
|---|---|---|---|---|---|---|---|
| | | No depression (0–4) | Minimal symptoms (5–9) | Minor depression (10–14) | Moderately severe depression (15–19) | Severe depression (20–27) | |
| Age group | 15–24 | 0 | 2 | 0 | 0 | 0 | 2 |
| | 25–34 | 0 | 3 | 1 | 0 | 0 | 4 |
| | 35–44 | 4 | 2 | 4 | 0 | 0 | 10 |
| | 45–54 | 6 | 8 | 2 | 0 | 1 | 17 |
| | 55–64 | 9 | 7 | 7 | 1 | 0 | 24 |
| | >65 | 7 | 9 | 7 | 2 | 2 | 27 |
| Total | | 26 | 31 | 21 | 3 | 3 | 84 |

that the Patient Health Questionnaire-9 (PHQ-9) performs well as a brief screen for poststroke depression and has a greater sensitivity and specificity for depression [7]. The PHQ-9 is a multipurpose instrument for screening, diagnosing, monitoring, and measuring the severity of depression. It is brief and useful in clinical practice, and it can also be administered repeatedly, which can show improvement or worsening of depression in response to treatment [8].

Significant proportions of aphasic patients (62–70%) were found to have depression possibly due to loss of communication with their friends and difficulty engaging in social activities [9].

Table 3: Frequency distribution of depression with hemisphere affected on imaging among stroke patients at TASH and ZMH neurology clinics.

| | | Depression | | | | | |
|---|---|---|---|---|---|---|---|
| | | No depression (0–4) | Minimal symptoms (5–9) | Minor depression (10–14) | Moderately severe depression (15–19) | Severe depression (20–27) | Total |
| Hemisphere affected on imaging | Left | 17 | 20 | 15 | 3 | 2 | 57 |
| | Right | 8 | 7 | 5 | 0 | 0 | 20 |
| | Both | 1 | 4 | 1 | 0 | 1 | 7 |
| Total | | 26 | 31 | 21 | 3 | 3 | 84 |

Clinically significant depression is frequent after ischemic stroke. And emphasis should be given to the importance of the psychiatric examination of poststroke patients, especially those with a significant disability and with a history of prior depressive episodes [5].

It is likely that depression reduces the desire and ability to take part in rehabilitation, and depressed people are less inclined to socialize. Low social support is known to be associated with depression. Other social factors associated with depression in poststroke period are living alone or in an institution. This social isolation may be complicated by the stigma associated with mental health problems, with some people hiding symptoms so that their family and doctor are unaware of any problems. Poor adherence to medications and increased alcohol and drug intake are commonly observed in depressed and socially isolated individuals. In turn, loss of physical ability and decreased cognitive function after stroke may also lead to depression [10].

A study assessing the adequacy of SSRI treatment in PSD patients found out that those patients who responded well to the treatment has shown a better functional outcome than nonresponders to SSRI treatment. Poststroke depression remains an unfavorable factor in rehabilitating poststroke patients despite treatment with antidepressants [11]. Another study assessed the role of improvement of depression in social role functioning. Social role function is often termed as participation in the rehabilitation sciences literature. Participation is broadly defined by the World Health Organization's International Classification of Functioning, Disability and Health (ICF) 7 as a person's involvement in a life situation. It represents the societal perspective of functioning. The study found out that improvement of depression was independently associated with improvement in the social role function of patients which positively affects the rehabilitation of patients [12].

Significantly increased functional disability and poorer quality of life at 1 month poststroke was seen in patients with acute PSD after controlling for relevant confounders [13]. In another prospective study, depression detected 3 months after stroke has been independently associated with poor functional outcome [14]. These findings are not consistent, and another study showed the severity of depressive symptoms was not found to be independent predictor of length of survival in the short- and long-term follow-up of 18 years [15].

## 2. Method

A cross-sectional study on all patients aged above 18 years and diagnosed with stroke in the past two years who attended the neurology follow-up clinics of Tikur Anebessa specialized Hospital and Zewditu Memorial Hospital was done by using a structured questionnaire after obtaining informed consent.

Patients with diagnosis other than stroke, stroke patients who presented to the clinics after 2 years of sustaining stroke, and those with severe aphasia were excluded from the study.

Different variables including age, sex, marital status, ethnicity, educational level, occupation, religion, aphasia, type of stroke, hemisphere affected on imaging, previous psychiatric illness, and PHQ-9 score were assessed. PHQ-9 is a multipurpose instrument for screening, diagnosis, monitoring, and measuring the severity of depression. It assesses 9 parameters each scored 0–3 (0 = not at all, 1 = several days, 2 = more than half the days, and 4 = nearly every day). A sum of all these scores form the basis for the scale score that ranged between zero and twenty seven (score 0–4 = no depression, score of 5–9 = minimal symptoms, score of 10–14 = minor depression, score of 15–19 = moderately severe depression, and score of 20–27 = severe depression). The PHQ-9 questionnaire was translated into Amharic (the Ethiopian local language) and back translated into English to ensure quality of translation.

Descriptive statistics for all patients, as well as stratified per stroke type, are presented as frequencies for nominal and categorical data and as means ± standard deviation or median with interquartile range for continuous variables. Proportions with 95% confidence intervals have been reported for feasibility metrics. The PHQ-9 scale and extremity power were dichotomized for certain analyses (PHQ-9 > 10 as indication of depression). Univariable and multivariable logistic regression were fit to determine factors associated with PHQ-9 screening and for screening positive with the PHQ-9. Linear regression models were fit to explore association of continuous PHQ-9 score with demographic and clinical variables. In both logistic and linear models, important interactions were also assessed. All statistical tests were performed at 5% level of significance using SPSS/PC version 20.0 software packages for statistical analysis (SPSS, INC, Chicago, IL).

## 3. Results

*3.1. Characteristics of the Participants.* Eighty four patients who came for follow-up at Tikur Anbessa Specialized Hospital neurology clinic and Zewditu Memorial Hospital with stroke

TABLE 4: Factors associated with screening positive for poststroke depression imaging among stroke patients at TASH and ZMH neurology clinics.

| Variable | *p* value | Crude OR (95% CI) | *p* value | Adjusted OR (95% CI) |
|---|---|---|---|---|
| **Handedness** | | | | |
| Right | 1.00 | 1.00 | 0.99 | 0.00 (0.00–0.0) |
| Left | 0.99 | 0.00 (0.0–0.0) | | |
| **Gender** | | | | |
| Male | 1.00 | 1.00 | 0.001 | 10.21 (2.43–42.78) |
| Female | 0.26 | 0.33 (0.12–0.87) | | |
| **Age group (years)** | | | | |
| 15–24 | 0.99 | 0.00 (0.00–0.00) | 0.54 | 1.15 (0.73–1.82) |
| 25–34 | 0.55 | 0.48 (0.04–5.29) | | |
| 35–44 | 0.976 | 0.97 (0.22–4.26) | | |
| 45–54 | 0.12 | 0.31 (0.07–1.35) | | |
| 55–65 | 0.58 | 0.73 (0.23–2.28) | | |
| 65 and above | 1.00 | 1.00 | | |
| **Marital status** | | | | |
| Couples in union | 1.00 | 1.00 | 0.95 | 0.96 (0.28–3.37) |
| Not in union (separated/ divorced, widowed, and never married) | 0.84 | 0.90 (0.32–2.53) | | |
| **Duration of stroke** | | | | |
| ≤ 3 months | 1.00 | 1.00 | 0.66 | 1.17 (0.59–2.33) |
| ≤ 6 months | 0.66 | 1.33 (0.37–4.83) | | |
| ≤ 2 years | 0.97 | 1.03 (0.34–3.09) | | |
| **Employment** | | | | |
| Employed | 1.00 | 1.00 | 0.89 | 0.92 (0.28–3.02) |
| Nonemployed | 0.68 | 0.82 (0.32–2.07) | | |
| **Educational level** | | | | |
| No formal | 1.00 | 1.00 | 0.17 | 0.69 (0.42–1.16) |
| Primary | 1.0 | 1.00 (0.29–3.45) | | |
| Secondary | 0.6 | 0.67 (0.15–3.02) | | |
| More than secondary | 1.00 | 1.00 (0.32–3.12) | | |
| **Type of stroke** | | | | |
| Ischemic | 1.00 | 1.00 | 0.97 | 1.03 (0.28–3.81) |
| Hemorrhagic | 0.47 | 0.67 (0.23–1.96) | | |
| **Hemisphere affected** | | | | |
| Left | 1.00 | 1.00 | 0.56 | 0.76 (0.3–1.94) |
| Right | 0.41 | 0.62 (0.19–1.95) | | |
| Both | 0.73 | 0.74 (0.13–4.16) | | |
| **Aphasia** | | | | |
| Yes | 1.00 | 1.00 | 0.034 | 0.25 (0.07–0.90) |
| No | 0.15 | 0.50 (0.19–1.27) | | |
| **Extremity power change** | | | | |
| Improved | 1.00 | 1.00 | 0.57 | 0.71 (0.22–2.31) |
| No improvement | 0.55 | 1.33 (0.52–3.4) | | |
| **Previous psychiatric** | | | | |
| Yes | 0.99 | 0.00 (0.00) | 0.99 | 0.00 (0.0) |
| No | 1.00 | 1.00 | | |

which occurred in the past two years were enrolled consecutively into our study and analyzed. Stroke type was confirmed by head CT scan and MRI, and out of this, 61 (72.6%) had an ischemic stroke, and 23 (27.4%) had haemorrhagic stroke.

Age range was 20 to 90 years with mean age ± SD, overall was 57.1 ± 14.8 years, 52.4% were male, and 47.6% were female. Baseline sociodemographic profile of the study subjects is shown in Table 1.

Fifty seven (67.9%) of the study participants have left hemisphere affection. And 34 (40.5%) of participants have aphasia. All our patients with aphasia were able to understand the questionnaire as they were evaluated during the follow-up outpatient visit, and the language deficits were resolving.

*3.2. Factors Associated with Poststroke Depression.* Overall, almost one-third of all ischemic stroke and hemorrhagic stroke patients had depressive symptoms, as defined in our study as PHQ-9 score ≥10. Twenty seven patients out of 84 (32.2%) had depressive symptoms. Six patients' had moderate to severe depressive symptoms (Figure 1).

A majority of patients with depression are aged greater than 55 years, and two of the severely depressed patients are found in this age group as shown in Table 2. Fifteen out of twenty one patients with minor depression have left hemisphere affection on imaging (Table 3).

In both univariable and multivariable models, female sex (OR 0.97, 95% CI 0.96–0.99) and aphasia (OR 2.06, 95% CI 1.06–4.01) were associated with screening positive for PSD (Table 4). When depression score was treated as a continuous variable, none of the factor was associated with screening positive for PSD.

## 4. Discussion

The overall rate of depression in our subset of ischemic and hemorrhagic stroke patients was 32.2%, comparable to previously published data for depression in the stroke population as a whole [4, 8, 11, 16]. Fifty seven out of eighty four patients (67.8%) have unremarkable depressive symptoms.

In our study, females and aphasic patients were more likely to screen positive for depression. In accordance with our study, among United States adults, females have higher depression prevalence rates compared to males [17]. It is possible that an underlying, sex-specific predisposition to depression in females and the effect of sex hormones persists in the stroke patients as well.

In our study, 40.5% of patients screened positive for depression, and literature studies show a high prevalence of depression (62–70%) in patients with aphasia because of difficulty in communication with their friends and family members. Sixty seven (67.9%) of patients had left hemisphere affection, out of which 20 (35%) screened positive for depression, and other studies also showed that individuals with left hemisphere lesions may be particularly at a greater risk of developing depression and anxiety after stroke [18].

Out of the 84 patients enrolled in the study, 61 (72%) patients had ischemic stroke, and the rest had hemorrhagic stroke. And 21 (34.5%) of ischemic stroke patients screened positive for depression, and 6 (26%) of patients with hemorrhagic stroke also screened positive for depression. Clinically significant depression is frequent after ischemic stroke [5, 6].

Due to resource constraints, the study was limited to a small number of stroke cases on follow-up, and hence it is difficult to generalize the findings to the general stroke population. Other limitations of the study are shortage of research studies done on the topic in the study area, and comorbid psychiatric symptoms were not evaluated and may also have been common in this population.

Due to absence of a depression-control group without stroke, it is difficult to determine the degree to which the pattern of depressive symptoms discerned in this population is directly related to comorbid stroke. Other depression screening tools in aphasic patients in addition to the PHQ-9 screening tool may provide a more reliable result regarding depressive symptoms in this specific patient population.

## 5. Conclusion

In conclusion, depressive symptoms after stroke are common in Ethiopian patients as seen in the other parts of the world. Identification and treatment of PSD may positively contribute for patient recovery. Our study demonstrates female and aphasic patients are more likely to screen positive for PSD. Hence, screening all poststroke patients with different screening tools is practical, and further studies are needed to assess the validity of these screening tools and also to assess PSD as a predictor of stroke outcome.

## Ethical Approval

Ethical clearance was given from the Institutional Review Board (IRB) of the College of Health Science of Addis Ababa University and in accordance with the Helsinki Declaration of 1975.

## Consent

Study subjects provided informed written consent.

## Conflicts of Interest

The authors declare that they have no conflicts of interest.

## Authors' Contributions

The co-author has been substantially involved in the study and preparation of the manuscript. The co-authors have seen and approved the submitted version and accept responsibility for its content.

## Acknowledgments

This study was supported by the Department of Neurology, Addis Ababa University School of Medicine.

## References

[1] D. Mukherjee and C. G. Patil, "Epidemiology and the global burden of stroke," *World Neurosurgery*, vol. 76, no. 6 Suppl, pp. 85–90, 2011.

[2] T. Reda, *Neurological Disorders, Etiology of Health and Disease in Ethiopi*, pp. 483–492, West View Pres, Boulder, Colorado, 1992.

[3] A. Gebrehaymanot and A. Jamal, "CVA in Ethiopians, a review of cases," 1981.

[4] M. F. Jose, *Neuropsychiatric Symptoms of Cerebrovascular Disease*, Springer, London, UK, 2013.

[5] T. Pohjasvaara, A. Leppävuori, I. Siira, R. Vataja, M. Kaste, and T. Erkinjuntti, "Frequency and clinical determinants of poststroke depression," *Stroke*, vol. 29, no. 11, pp. 2311–2317, 1998.

[6] M. F. Folstein, R. Maiberger, and P. R. McHugh, "Mood disorder as a specific complication of stroke," *Journal of Neurology, Neurosurgery & Psychiatry*, vol. 40, no. 10, pp. 1018–1020, 1977.

[7] L. S. Williams, E. J. Brizendine, L. Plue et al., "Performance of the PHQ-9 as a screening tool for depression after stroke," *Stroke*, vol. 36, no. 3, pp. 635–638, 2005.

[8] K. Kroenke, R. L. Spitzer, and J. B. W. Williams, "The PHQ-9," *Journal of General Internal Medicine*, vol. 16, no. 9, pp. 606–613, 2001.

[9] A. Monica, A. Rolf, and A. Kjell, "Major depression in stroke patients a 3-year longitudinal study," *Stroke*, vol. 24, no. 7, pp. 976–982, 1993.

[10] K. Narushima and R. G. Robinson, "The effect of early versus late antidepressant treatment on physical impairment associated with poststroke depression," *The Journal of Nervous and Mental Disease*, vol. 191, no. 10, pp. 645–652, 2003.

[11] S. Paolucci, M. Iosa, P Coiro et al., "Post-stroke depression increases disability more than 15% in ischemic stroke survivors: a case-control study," *Frontiers in Neurology*, vol. 10, p. 926, 2019.

[12] J. P. Chau, D. R. Thompson, A. M. Chang et al., "Depression among Chinese stroke survivors six months after discharge from a rehabilitation hospital," *Clinical Nurse Specialist*, vol. 19, no. 21-22, pp. 3042–3050, 2010.

[13] T. Ellen and B. Marian, "Exclussion and inclusion criteria for people with aphasia in studies of depression after stroke: a systematic review and future recommendations," *Neuroepidemiology*, vol. 29, no. 1-2, pp. 1–17, 2007.

[14] R. R. Karamchandani, F. Vahidy, S. Bajgur et al., "Early depression screening is feasible in hospitalized stroke patients," *PLoS One*, vol. 10, no. 6, Article ID e0128246, 2015.

[15] M. . Kellermann, B. Roland, and D. . Bereczki, "Does the severity of depressive symptoms after stroke affect long-term survival? an 18-year follow-up," *PLoS One*, vol. 13, no. 12, Article ID e0209157, 2018.

[16] A. Berg, "Depression and its assessment among stroke patients and their caregivers," Doctoral Dissertation, Helsingin Yliopisto, Helsinki, Finland, 2010.

[17] NIH: National Institute of Mental Health Statistics, "Major depressive disorder among adults," 2014, http://www.nimh.nih.gov/statistics/1mdd_adult.shtm.

[18] H. Rickards, M. Way, and B. Edgbaston, "Depression in neurological disorders: Parkinson's disease, multiple sclerosis, and stroke," *Journal of Neurology, Neurosurgery & Psychiatry*, vol. 76, no. suppl_1, pp. i48–i52, 2005.

# 37

# BCI-Based Rehabilitation on the Stroke in Sequela Stage

**Yangyang Miao,[1] Shugeng Chen,[2] Xinru Zhang,[1] Jing Jin,[1] Ren Xu,[3] Ian Daly,[4] Jie Jia,[2] Xingyu Wang,[1] Andrzej Cichocki,[5,6,7] and Tzyy-Ping Jung[8]**

[1]*Key Laboratory of Advanced Control and Optimization for Chemical Processes, Ministry of Education, East China University of Science and Technology, Shanghai, China*
[2]*Department of Rehabilitation, Huashan Hospital, Fudan University, Shanghai, China*
[3]*Guger Technologies OG, Austria*
[4]*Brain-Computer Interfaces and Neural Engineering Laboratory, School of Computer Science and Electronic Engineering, University of Essex, Colchester, Essex CO4 3SQ, UK*
[5]*Skolkowo Institute of Science and Technology (SKOLTECH), 143026 Moscow, Russia*
[6]*Systems Research Institute PAS, Warsaw, Poland*
[7]*Nicolaus Copernicus University (UMK), Torun, Poland*
[8]*Institute for Neural Computation and Institute of Engineering in Medicine, University of California San Diego, La Jolla, CA, USA*

Correspondence should be addressed to Jing Jin; jinjingat@gmail.com and Jie Jia; shannonjj@126.com

Academic Editor: Jianzhong Su

*Background.* Stroke is the leading cause of serious and long-term disability worldwide. Survivors may recover some motor functions after rehabilitation therapy. However, many stroke patients missed the best time period for recovery and entered into the sequela stage of chronic stroke. *Method.* Studies have shown that motor imagery- (MI-) based brain-computer interface (BCI) has a positive effect on poststroke rehabilitation. This study used both virtual limbs and functional electrical stimulation (FES) as feedback to provide patients with a closed-loop sensorimotor integration for motor rehabilitation. An MI-based BCI system acquired, analyzed, and classified motor attempts from electroencephalogram (EEG) signals. The FES system would be activated if the BCI detected that the user was imagining wrist dorsiflexion on the instructed side of the body. Sixteen stroke patients in the sequela stage were randomly assigned to a BCI group and a control group. All of them participated in rehabilitation training for four weeks and were assessed by the Fugl-Meyer Assessment (FMA) of motor function. *Results.* The average improvement score of the BCI group was 3.5, which was higher than that of the control group (0.9). The active EEG patterns of the four patients in the BCI group whose FMA scores increased gradually became centralized and shifted to sensorimotor areas and premotor areas throughout the study. *Conclusions.* Study results showed evidence that patients in the BCI group achieved larger functional improvements than those in the control group and that the BCI-FES system is effective in restoring motor function to upper extremities in stroke patients. This study provides a more autonomous approach than traditional treatments used in stroke rehabilitation.

## 1. Introduction

Stroke is one of the most common cerebrovascular diseases worldwide. It causes numerous problems and is the leading cause of serious and long-term disability in many countries [1]. Motor disorders, including hemiplegia of the upper limbs, are a frequent consequence of stroke. Therefore, timely and effective treatments are needed for functional motor recovery to help survivors perform daily activities better. However, many stroke patients missed the best time period for recovery and entered the chronic sequela stage. Effective treatments for patients after stroke are a challenge.

Different approaches have been used for poststroke rehabilitation, including conventional therapy, robotic therapy, stem cell therapy, noninvasive brain stimulation techniques, and other novel therapies [2, 3]. However, during conventional rehabilitation, there is no objective way to determine whether the patients are performing the expected motor imagery task [4]. Although the rehabilitation may result in an improvement in upper limb mobility and function, this benefit did not persist months after stroke [2].

Brain-computer interface (BCI) can directly translate brain activity to specific commands and are reaching their technological maturity [5]. It could provide an alternative communication way to disabled patients. For instance, reference [6] proposed a peripheral-display speller based on BCI technology for amyotrophic lateral sclerosis (ALS) patients, which yielded a performance comparable to the conventional matrix-based speller. In addition, motor imagery- (MI-) based BCI, one of the widely used BCI systems, could also be used in stroke rehabilitation to translate brain signals into intended movements [7]. Different from other paradigms such as event-related potentials (ERP) [8, 9] and steady-state visual evoked potentials (SSVEP) [10], MI by the BCI user elicits an event-related (de)synchronization (ERD/S) in the electroencephalogram (EEG), which represents the result of conscious access to the content of the intention of a movement [11–13]. Therefore, the ERD/S features may be used to detect motor intention in stroke patients. Additionally, the strength and topology of the ERD/S have been shown to vary as a function of the degree of upper limb motor impairment in stroke patients [14], suggesting that it may also be used as an objective correlate of stroke recovery.

MI, the mental rehearsal of physical movement tasks, represents a new approach to access the motor system and rehabilitation at all stages of stroke recovery [15, 16]. Some groups have tested the applicability of MI-based BCI in stroke rehabilitation and demonstrated clinical improvements [17, 18]. Different from the preceding results, a magnetoencephalography- (MEG-) based BCI system was used for stroke rehabilitation and six out of eight stroke patients could control the system, but no significant motor improvements were found [19]. Moreover, to help patients modulate their brain activity proficiently, many training methods with feedback have been developed to attempt to improve the performance of MI-based BCIs [4, 20]. The feedback provided by these systems typically includes playing rewarding sounds or a real-time visual display and may not directly or accurately reflect the true intention of the patient. To provide patients with closed-loop sensorimotor integration for motor rehabilitation, functional electrical stimulation (FES) has been explored as a feedback stimulus in some studies [20, 21]. In order to induce muscle movement to improve or restore muscle function, FES uses pulses of electrical current to stimulate one or more muscle groups and can provide efficient proprioceptive feedback [21]. In reference [4], a rehabilitation system using FES as a feedback stimulus was investigated. The results show that EEG activity in the patients' motor cortex was significantly increased. In reference [20], researchers used an FES system and a bar as the feedback. After 10 training sessions, one stroke patient partially regained control of dorsiflexion in her paretic wrist.

In many studies, patients with shorter onset time were selected since it is hard to recover for patients in the sequela stage. In addition, single pathway feedback is the main form of feedback used in existing research. There is some evidence that viewing real or artificial body parts results in a stronger desynchronization than viewing nonbody part movements [22, 23]. Hence, we selected stroke patients in the sequela stage and sought to investigate the benefits of BCI for stroke rehabilitation using a multimodal feedback paradigm, in which cues were presented to patients via audio stimuli, by virtual limbs, and via FES.

## 2. Material and Methods

*2.1. BCI-FES System.* This study used the recoveriX system (g.tec medical engineering GmbH, Austria) for experiments, which is a BCI-FES system. In the BCI system, 16 channels (FC3, FCz, FC4, C5, C3, C1, Cz, C2, C4, C6, CP3, CP1, CPz, CP2, CP4, and Pz) were used for EEG signal recording, as shown in Figure 1. The ground electrode (GND) was placed over the forehead (FPz), and the reference electrode (REF) was located at the right earlobe. The signals were sampled at 256 Hz through a g.USBamp (g.tec medical engineering GmbH, Austria). The band-pass filter was set to 0.1-30 Hz. It stimulated appointed muscle groups, with the stimulation modes triggered by the BCI system.

Figure 2(a) shows the schematic of the BCI-FES system. As stroke patients suffer neurological damage, the brain regions associated with motor functions might be compromised and unable to control limb movements directly. The BCI system attempts to acquire, analyze, and recognize the EEG data of motor imagery from patients. The FES system will then be activated if the BCI system detects that the user is imagining hand movement on the instructed side of the body. The muscle contraction caused by FES is calibrated to be sufficient to cause movement in the affected hand. In this study, the FES muscle stimulators were placed in the extensor carpi radialis longus, extensor carpi radialis brevis, and extensor carpi ulnaris to improve the wrist dorsiflexion function of patients [24]. Before each run, stimulation parameters (current amplitude and pulse duration) were calibrated as follows. First, we set the pulse duration of the current to 300 $\mu$s. Then, we increased slowly the current amplitude until the stimulators could visibly cause wrist dorsiflexion. Verbal feedback was obtained from the patients about the strength of muscle stimulation in order to prevent the excessive current from the fatigue of wrist muscles.

*2.2. Participants.* Sixteen stroke patients in the sequela stage were randomly assigned to the BCI group ($n = 8$) and the control group ($n = 8$). The two groups received routine rehabilitation training, including limb dominance exercise, muscle tension, and limb control training, three times a week, for four weeks. On this basis, the BCI group underwent motor imagery rehabilitation training using the BCI-FES system. All participants signed a written consent form prior to this experiment. The local ethics committee approved the consent form and experimental procedure before any patient participated. All participants were right-handed, and they were diagnosed by computerized tomography (CT) or magnetic resonance imagining (MRI), without cognitive disorder and any unsuitable diseases for receiving the BCI-FES system. Table 1 shows the demographic information for all

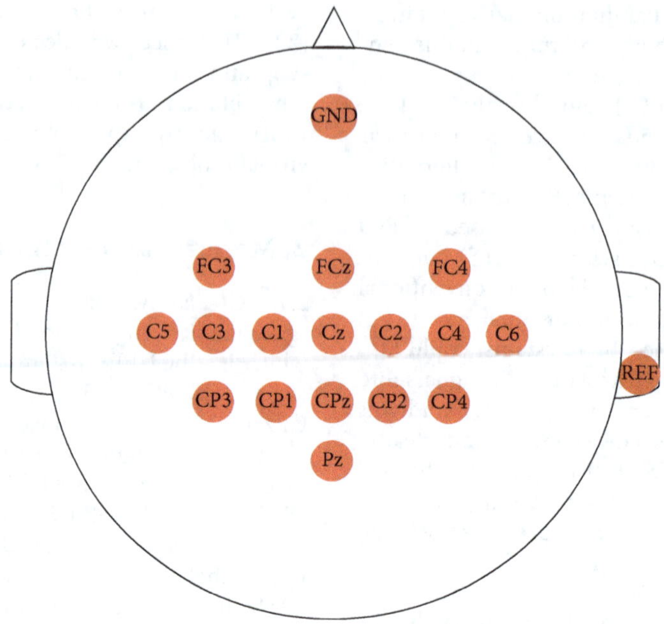


FIGURE 1: The electrode distribution used in this study.

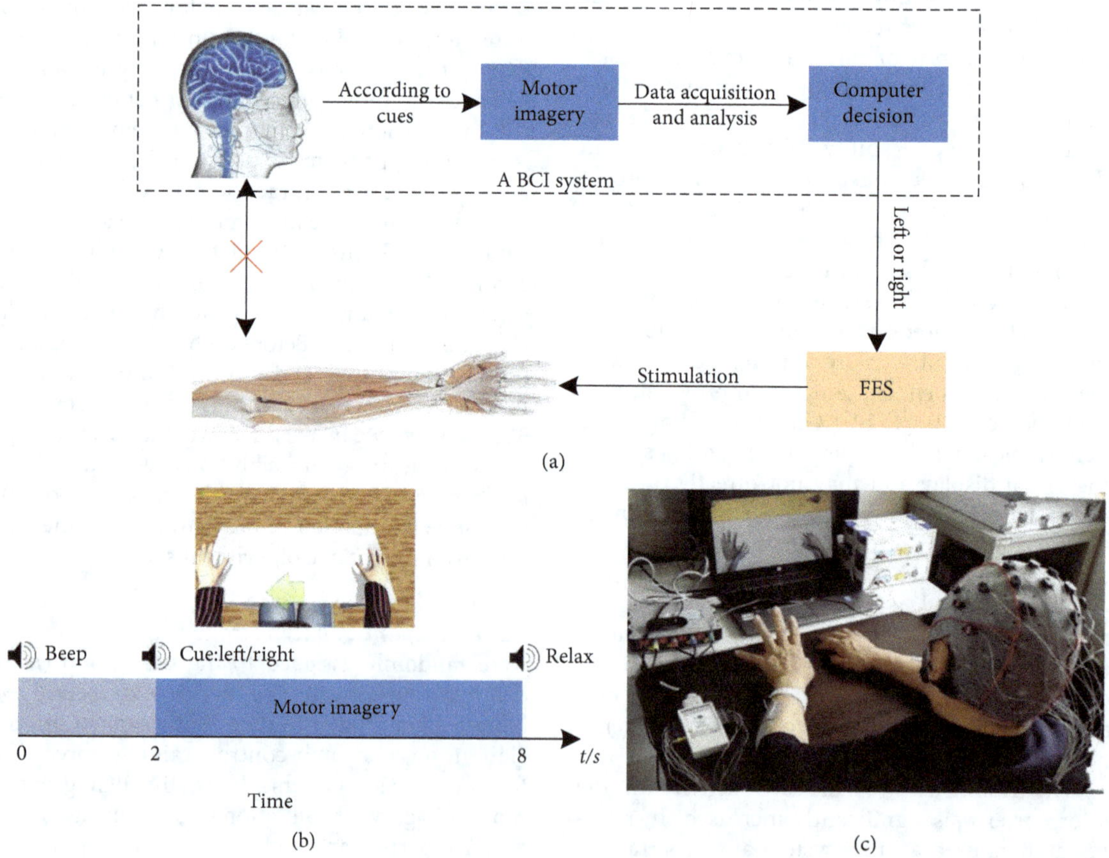


FIGURE 2: (a) The schematic of the BCI-FES system. (b) The timing of a trial of the motor imagery paradigm. Each trial consisted of task and rest periods. A patient started to execute motor imagery tasks upon the appearance of the cue ("left" or "right"). A virtual avatar of one patient's upper limbs was used to provide virtual reality feedback. (c) This picture shows the scene of BCI-FES rehabilitation training for one patient.

TABLE 1: Demographic information about the participants.

| Group | ID | Gender | Age | Stroke type | Paretic side | Stroke onset (months) |
|---|---|---|---|---|---|---|
| BCI | P1 | Male | 58 | Hemorrhage | Right | 6 |
| BCI | P2 | Female | 70 | Ischemic | Right | 8 |
| BCI | P3 | Female | 22 | Trauma | Left | 24 |
| BCI | P4 | Male | 65 | Ischemic | Right | 8 |
| BCI | P5 | Male | 44 | Hemorrhage | Right | 22 |
| BCI | P6 | Male | 45 | Hemorrhage | Left | 24 |
| BCI | P7 | Male | 30 | Trauma | Left | 38 |
| BCI | P8 | Male | 56 | Ischemic | Right | 16 |
| Control | P9 | Male | 52 | Infarction | Left | 14 |
| Control | P10 | Male | 64 | Infarction | Left | 6 |
| Control | P11 | Male | 65 | Infarction | Right | 13 |
| Control | P12 | Female | 54 | Infarction | Right | 9 |
| Control | P13 | Female | 25 | Trauma | Right | 20 |
| Control | P14 | Male | 72 | Hemorrhage | Left | 14 |
| Control | P15 | Male | 40 | Hemorrhage | Right | 6 |
| Control | P16 | Male | 30 | Infarction | Left | 7 |

participants (P1-P8 were in the BCI group and P9-P16 were in the control group).

*2.3. Experimental Procedure.* The participants sat in a comfortable chair in a shielded room after being prepared for EEG recording. During data acquisition, participants were asked to relax and avoid unnecessary movements. Instructions were delivered through both sounds and visual cues. The experimenter informed the participants that they would hear cues over a speaker that would instruct them to imagine either their left or their right wrist dorsiflexion. At the same time, the screen showed the hand avatar, which reflected the participants' movements to help them imagine. As shown in Figure 2(b), each trial lasts eight seconds and starts with a warning "beep." Two seconds later, the cue (the command to imagine a left or right wrist dorsiflexion) was played to ask participants to perform kinesthetic motor imagery. Six seconds later, a "relax" command was presented, informing participants that the trial was over. During the imagining time, the FES would be activated if the BCI system detected the user was imagining movement on the instructed side. The muscle contraction initiated by the FES was sufficient to cause dorsiflexion on the affected wrist. The feedback period lasted four seconds, and the intertrial interval lasted two seconds.

Figure 2(c) shows the scene of BCI-FES rehabilitation training for a sample patient. When the BCI detected the patient had performed the correct MI task upon the appearance of the cue ("left" or "right"), the avatar would give him/-her visual feedback and the FES would be activated to cause the wrist dorsiflexion of the corresponding side. Three rehabilitation sessions were carried out in a week (spaced evenly across the week). Each session contained two runs. Each patient participated in sixty trials within one recording run. Before each session, the participants needed to answer two questions: (1) Did you have a good rest last night? (2) Do you feel well now? After each session, the participants needed to answer two questions: (1) Are there any problems during this session? (2) How did you feel after this session?

*2.4. Pattern Recognition.* For motor imagery feature extraction, the EEG data were filtered using a fifth-order Butterworth band-pass filter from 8 to 30 Hz, since this frequency band included the range of frequencies that were mainly involved in performing motor imagery [22, 25].

We used the common spatial pattern (CSP) algorithm as a feature extraction method. CSP has been widely used in processing EEG data from motor imagery [26–30]. Consider the EEG signal $E_{i,c} \in \mathbb{R}^{N\times S}$ of the $i$-th trial in class $c$, where $N$ and $S$, respectively, represent the number of channels and the number of sampling points. The spatial covariance matrix of the class $c$ is computed as follows:

$$\Sigma_c = \frac{1}{n_c}\sum_{i=1}^{n_c} \frac{E_{i,c}E_{i,c}^T}{\operatorname{trace}\left(E_{i,c}E_{i,c}^T\right)}, \tag{1}$$

where $n_c$ represents the number of trials in class $c$.

CSP is based on the simultaneous diagonalization of two covariance matrices. It finds a spatial filter $w$ to maximize variance for one class and minimize variance for the other class at the same time:

$$\max_w J(w) = \frac{w^T\Sigma_1 w}{w^T\Sigma_2 w} \quad \text{s.t.}\|w\|_2 = 1. \tag{2}$$

Using the Lagrange multiplier method, Eq. (2) is transformed into the generalized eigenvalue problem:

$$\Sigma_1 w = \lambda\Sigma_2 w. \tag{3}$$

where $\lambda$ and $w$ are the generalized eigenvalue and eigenvector, respectively.

The spatial filters of CSP $W \in \mathbb{R}^{N\times 2m}$ are formed by eigenvectors which are corresponding to $m$ maximum and minimum eigenvalues. This study used the first three and last three columns (eigenvectors) of the projection matrix as the spatial filter to compute the features. The EEG data of the single trial $E$ can be transformed into:

$$Z = W^T E. \tag{4}$$

The feature $f_p$ can be obtained from $Z_p$ $(p = 1,\cdots,2m)$:

$$f_p = \log\left(\frac{\operatorname{var}(Z_p)}{\sum_{i=1}^{2m}\operatorname{var}(Z_i)}\right). \tag{5}$$

In the classification scheme, we applied linear discriminant analysis (LDA) as the classifier. It finds a linear combination of features that characterizes or separates two classes [31–34]. Discriminant scores are calculated by a discriminant function:

$$L_p = \arg \max_{L_p} \frac{L_p^T S_B L_p}{L_p^T S_W L_p}, \tag{6}$$

where $S_B$ and $S_W$ are, respectively, the between-class and within-class scatter matrices.

$$S_B = \sum_{i=1}^{2} N_i (m_i - m)(m_i - m)^T,$$
$$S_W = \sum_{i=1}^{2} \sum_{f_p \in C_i} \left(f_p - m_i\right)\left(f_p - m_i\right)^T, \tag{7}$$

where $N_i$ is the number of the samples in class $C_i$ $(i = 1, 2)$, $N$ is the number of all samples, $m_i = (1/N_i)\sum_{f_p \in C_i} f_p$ is the mean of the samples in class $C_i$, and $m = (1/N)\sum_{f_p} f_p$ is the mean of all the samples. This study used the data in the first run to train the LDA classifier, and then, the classifier could be used in a subsequent online run.

*2.5. Functional Assessment.* This study used the Fugl-Meyer Assessment (FMA) to evaluate the motor function of the upper limb control in the participants. This scale is an index to assess the sensorimotor impairment in individuals who have had a stroke. It was first proposed by Axel Fugl-Meyer and his colleagues as a standardized assessment test for post-stroke recovery [35]. It has been tested several times and is found to have excellent consistency, responsivity, and good accuracy [36–38]. It is now widely used for clinical assessment of motor function. The FMA assesses several impairment dimensions using a 3-point ordinal scale (0 = cannot perform; 1 = can perform partially; 2 = can perform fully).

## 3. Results

*3.1. Classification Performance Comparison.* Figure 3 presents the BCI classification performance (as measured by accuracy) across 12 training sessions for the eight participants in the BCI group. Results showed that most of the participants could get better performance in the last session than in the first session. The average motor imagery accuracy of the eight participants in the last session was 72.9%, an improvement of 5.0% from the first session.

Specifically, for participants P1, P2, and P7, the average accuracies in the last session were, respectively, 100%, 88.3%, and 73.3%; their performances were visibly improved from the first session (95%, 73.3%, and 61.7%). P1 achieved the best and most stable performance of all participants. An interesting observation is that, before motor imagery-based rehabilitation training, P1 had usually imagined the hand movements according to his report. In fact, P1 is clinically diagnosed with minor depression and often imagines his body parts. Hence, he is good at concentrating on motor imagery tasks and achieved the best performance of all participants.

Interestingly, the performance of participants P3, P4, P5, and P8 showed relatively large fluctuations. In particular, the performance of participant P3 in the last session was worse than in the first session. This may be because the young participant P3 felt the training boring after too many repeated sessions, and thus, she was not very motivated and dedicated in the later part of the training. For other participants, the undulating accuracies may be related to emotional fluctuations or normal intersession variability (nonstationarity) in EEG signals or noise causes. Hence, the average accuracies of them were lower than others in the two categories of motor imagery.

*3.2. Functional Improvement.* Table 2 shows the FMA scores before and after rehabilitation training over the two groups. Four participants' FMA scores have increased in the BCI group (the proportion is 50%), while three participants in the control group also exhibited increases in FMA (the proportion is 37.5%). Before rehabilitation training, the average score in the BCI group (19.5) was relatively lower than that in the control group (20.6). After 12 training sessions, the average score of the BCI group (23.0) was significantly higher than that of the control group (21.5). On the whole, the average score in the BCI group has been increased by 3.5, while the average score in the control group has been only raised by 0.9. The results also show that the BCI-FES rehabilitation training was significantly effective.

In terms of individual performance, the scores for participants P1, P6, P7, and P8 in the BCI group were observed to increase throughout the experiments; the scores for participants P10, P11, and P15 in the control group were also observed to increase. The scores for the remainder of the participants did not change. In particular, for participants P6 and P7 in the BCI group, the period after stroke onset was over 2 years. The health condition of these participants should have tended to be stable and difficult to improve using routine rehabilitation training [39]. However, after the BCI-FES rehabilitation training, certain motor functions were restored and the scores were also improved for them. Among the participants in the BCI group, P4 achieved the lowest score (8) after rehabilitation training, which is consistent with the former result that he got the worst average accuracy.

Paired one-tailed $t$-tests were used to show the differences between FMA scores before and after the rehabilitation for the two groups, respectively. After four weeks of rehabilitation training, the scores in the BCI group have been increased (mean = 3.5, $p = 0.049$), while the scores in the control group have been increased a little (mean = 0.9, $p = 0.044$).

In summary, improvements in motor functions have been achieved for some of the participants. The participants in the BCI group obtained more improvements than those in the control group (3.5 vs. 0.9).

*3.3. EEG Patterns.* This study used power spectral densities and topographic maps extracted by CSP to detect motor imagery EEG patterns.

Figure 4 shows the power spectral density (PSD) maps from electrodes C3 and C4 for the four participants in the

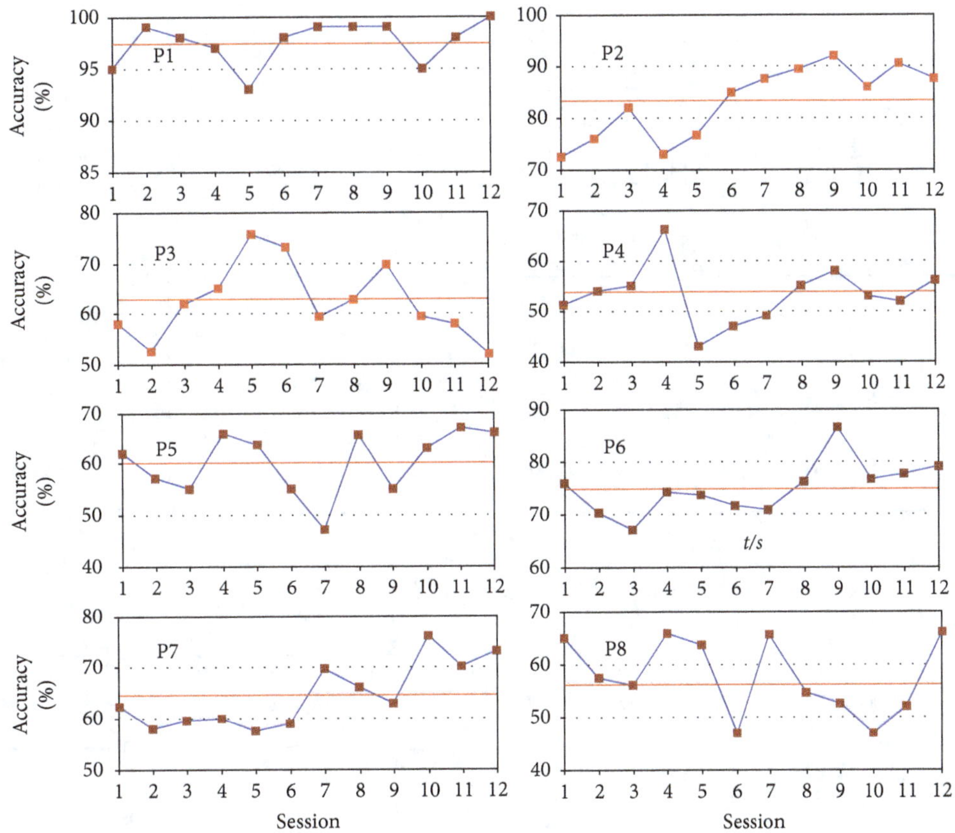


FIGURE 3: The accuracies across 12 sessions for all participants in the BCI group. The red line indicates the average accuracy.

TABLE 2: FMA score comparison before and after rehabilitation training over the two groups.

| BCI | Pre-FMA | Post-FMA | Stroke onset (months) | Control | Pre-FMA | Post-FMA | Stroke onset (months) |
|---|---|---|---|---|---|---|---|
| P1 | 24 | 27 | 6 | P9 | 20 | 20 | 14 |
| P2 | 10 | 10 | 8 | P10 | 30 | 32 | 6 |
| P3 | 39 | 39 | 24 | P11 | 21 | 24 | 13 |
| P4 | 8 | 8 | 8 | P12 | 14 | 14 | 9 |
| P5 | 14 | 14 | 22 | P13 | 36 | 36 | 20 |
| P6 | 20 | 35 | 24 | P14 | 4 | 4 | 14 |
| P7 | 24 | 28 | 38 | P15 | 18 | 20 | 6 |
| P8 | 17 | 23 | 16 | P16 | 22 | 22 | 7 |
| AVG | 19.5 ± 9.9 | 23.0 ± 11.4 | 18.3 ± 10.9 | AVG | 20.6 ± 9.7 | 21.5 ± 10.0 | 11.1 ± 5.0 |

BCI group, whose FMA scores were increased throughout the experiments. These two electrodes have been shown to record important characteristics of motor imagery [40, 41]. The PSDs in session 1 and session 12 were averaged over multiple trials (60 left-wrist dorsiflexion trials and 60 right-wrist dorsiflexion trials).

For participant P1, the PSD maps were consistent with the theory presented by Pfurtscheller and colleagues [11, 42] in both session 1 and session 12. At electrode C3, the EEG energy during right motor imagery was higher than the EEG energy during the left motor imagery, while at electrode C4, the situation was the opposite. For participants P6, P7, and P8, there were no significant differences in the EEG energy at electrodes C3 and C4 in session 1. It was thus difficult to distinguish the two motor imagery tasks. In session 12 of BCI-FES rehabilitation training, the EEG energy for these participants became similar to that observed for participant P1.

Figure 5 showed the topographic maps from the paretic side of the previously mentioned participants illustrating the first and last spatial patterns extracted by the CSP method (P1 and P8: right motor imagery; P6 and P7: left motor imagery). In CSP, $W$ is the projection matrix, and $W^{-1}$ is the inverse matrix of $W$. The columns of $W^{-1}$ are the time-

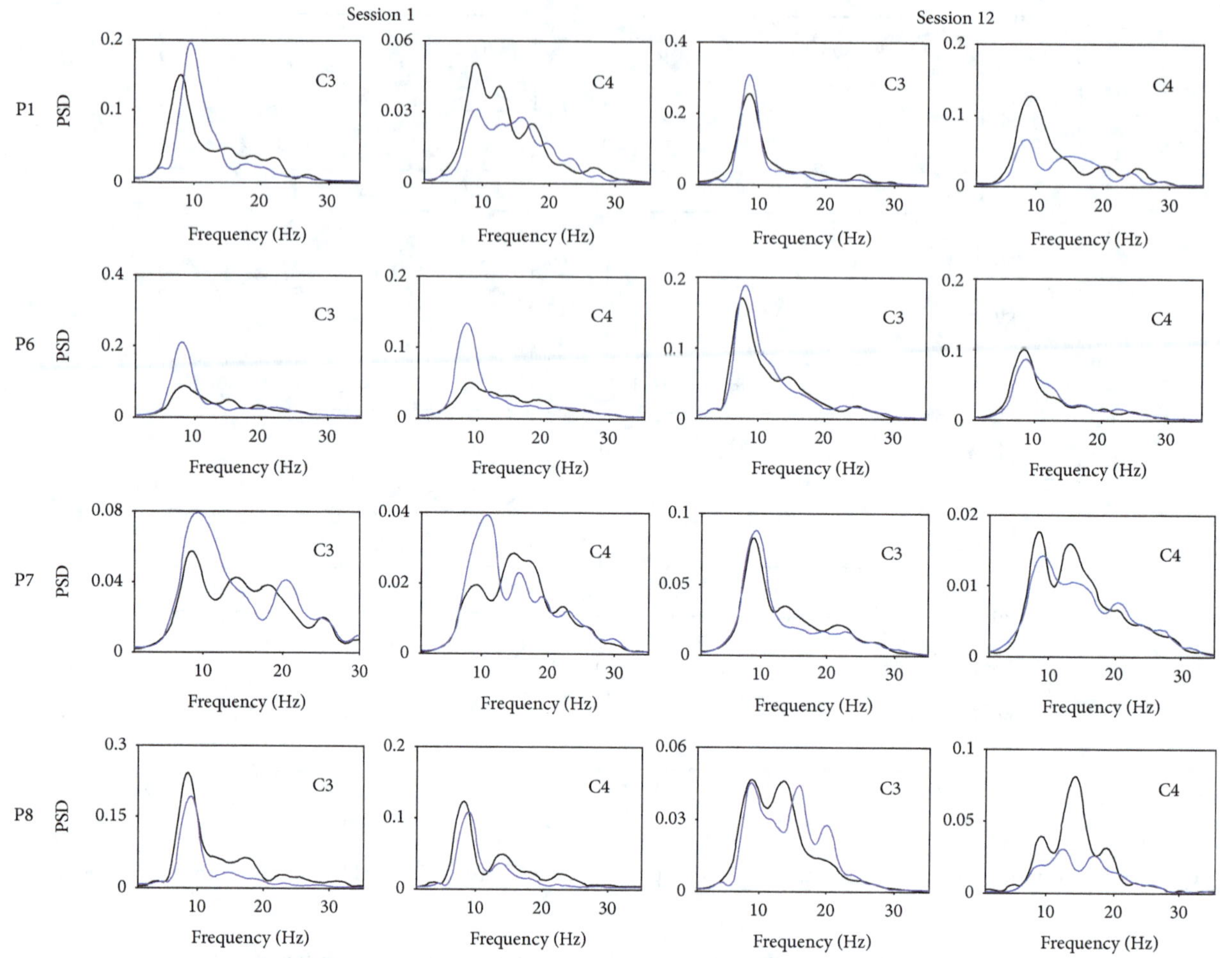


FIGURE 4: The power spectral density maps from electrodes C3 and C4 for four participants in the BCI group (blue: right motor imagery, black: left motor imagery).

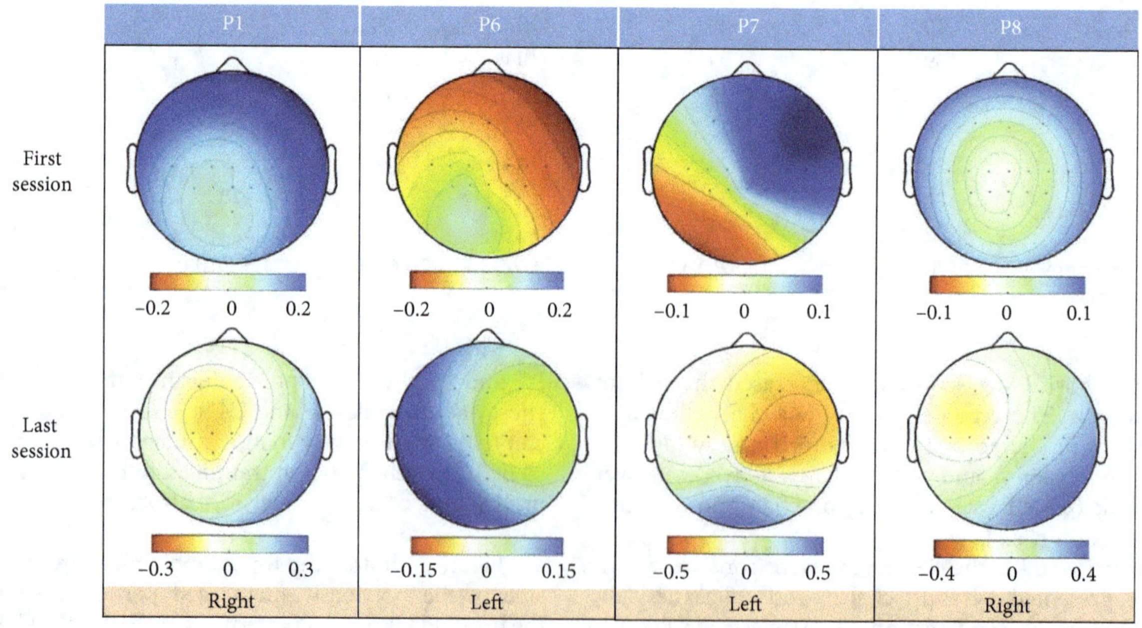


FIGURE 5: Topographic maps from four participants illustrating the first and last spatial patterns extracted by the CSP method.

invariant vectors of EEG source distribution vectors called common spatial patterns. The first pattern was obtained by maximizing the variance of the right motor imagery, which was associated with the ERD phenomenon over the left sensorimotor area of the cortex. Accordingly, the ERD phenomenon over the right motor area was associated with the last pattern, corresponding to the left motor imagery.

The results for participant P1 showed a clear ERD phenomenon in the left cerebral cortex during the right motor imagery. For participant P6, larger regions were initially active in session 1: the ERD phenomenon almost occupied the whole contralateral hemisphere. However, the ERD phenomenon became more centralized and was mainly distributed around electrode C4 in the last session, and the ERS phenomenon was observed in the left cerebral cortex. The results for participant P7 did not show a clear pattern from the contralateral hemisphere for left motor imagery in the first session. However, the map of the last session showed a clear ERD phenomenon in the right cerebral cortex. For participant P8, in both the first and last session, the ERD phenomenon was not particularly strong and occurred to the left of the central area for the first session and the upper left cerebral cortex for the last session.

By tracking the changes in the motor imagery EEG patterns during rehabilitation, we tried to explore cortical reorganization. Study results suggested that after rehabilitation, the sensorimotor cortex in the contralateral hemisphere could be activated. Figure 5 also indicated that areas around electrodes C3 and C4 were strongly associated with the left- and right-hand motor imageries, which was consistent with the neurophysiology phenomenon reported in [25, 41].

## 4. Discussion

In the experimental procedures of many studies, an arrow pointing left or right was used as the cue. However, some evidence suggests that viewing real or artificial body parts results in a stronger desynchronization in the EEG during attempted movement/motor imagery [22, 23]. Hence, this study used both virtual limbs and FES as feedback, which, we hypothesize, could help participants perform the motor imagery tasks better.

In data analysis, researchers have used the functional Magnetic Resonance Imaging (fMRI) approach to assess brain function after BCI therapy [43–46]. This study, instead, used EEG signals. Unfortunately, we have to note that not all participants were able to gain appreciable improvements in classification performance. Such results are in line with the literature [47]. Besides, classification performance did not exactly correspond with FMA scores. For example, although the average classification performance was poor (<60%) for participant P8, his FMA score was increased by 5. The reasons that half of the participants in the BCI group had not made any progress may be as follows: (1) Participants felt fidgety and bored after too many repeated sessions of the rehabilitation training and could not concentrate on motor imagery (for P4 and P5). (2) The original score was so high that it was difficult to improve (for P3). (3) Another possible reason could be the small sample sizes used and the short training time. Adding more participants or increasing the training time was difficult. On the one hand, most participants are reluctant to use systems that are not yet widely applied. On the other hand, if the training time becomes longer, it is hard for participants to stick with it.

This study also explored the changes in the EEG patterns as an index to objectively assess the efficacy of the BCI-FES rehabilitation training. After 12 sessions of the training, PSD maps for four of the participants became sufficiently distinct to allow our BCI classifier to differentiate the two motor imagery tasks; the active patterns in the topographic maps gradually became more centralized and shifted to the sensorimotor areas (around channels C3 and C4) and the premotor areas (around channels FC3 and FC4). Some literature has reported a similar phenomenon. For example, Tam et al. reported that some stroke patients were not able to produce focal ERD patterns in sensorimotor areas and that the active patterns were produced in frontal premotor areas and parietal areas [48]. This observation reveals the rehabilitation mechanism: functionality initially occurs in larger regions but gradually returns to the motor or nearby cortical regions during recovery. This could be a sign of cortical reorganization or neuroplasticity in the affected hemisphere.

Several limitations of our study merit further discussion. First, as to EEG signal analysis, this study may ignore the effect of nonstroke factors on the classification performance, such as fatigue [49–52] during rehabilitation. In future work, we seek to improve the experimental design to enhance the enthusiasm of the participants. For instance, we can design some simple games like the literature [53] and also can give the participants additional bonus based on their success rate in the experiment. Second, this study was unable to explain why four of the eight participants in the BCI group did not improve. The same situation also appeared in the literature [54], and none of the previous studies was able to explain the exceptions. Third, the number of training sessions (12) is low. However, we could not increase the session number due to the limited hospital stay duration of the participants. Last but not least, the FES muscle stimulators were only placed to trigger wrist dorsiflexion. They also could be placed in other muscle groups in order to help motor functional rehabilitation of other body parts such as the elbow, knee, and ankle. Their rehabilitation effect is still unknown, pending further research.

## 5. Conclusion

This study combined a motor imagery-based BCI and an FES system to provide stroke patients with closed-loop sensorimotor integration for motor rehabilitation. Both virtual limbs and FES were used as feedback, which could help patients improve their training through visual and sensory pathways. Our results showed that participants in the BCI group obtained more improvements than the participants in the control group. This study provides a more autonomous approach than traditional treatments for stroke rehabilitation. Additional research is needed to enhance the portability of the BCI-FES system.

## Conflicts of Interest

The authors confirm that there are no known conflicts of interest.

## Authors' Contributions

Yangyang Miao and Shugeng Chen contributed equally to this work.

## Acknowledgments

We are grateful to the patients, and their caregivers, who participated in this study. This work was supported by the National Key Research and Development Program (2017YFB13003002, 2018YFC2002300, and 2018YFC2002301). This work was also supported in part by the National Natural Science Foundation of China under Grant Nos. 61573142, 61773164, and 91420302, the Programme of Introducing Talents of Discipline to Universities (the 111 Project) under Grant B17017, and the "ShuGuang" Project supported by Shanghai Municipal Education Commission and Shanghai Education Development Foundation under Grant 19SG25.

## References

[1] A. Pollock, B. S. George, M. Fenton, and L. Firkins, "Top ten research priorities relating to life after stroke," *Lancet Neurology*, vol. 11, no. 3, p. 209, 2012.

[2] L. Brewer, F. Horgan, A. Hickey, and D. Williams, "Stroke rehabilitation: recent advances and future therapies," *QJM*, vol. 106, no. 1, pp. 11–25, 2012.

[3] W. H. Chang and Y.-H. Kim, "Robot-assisted therapy in stroke rehabilitation," *Journal of Stroke*, vol. 15, no. 3, pp. 174–181, 2013.

[4] D. Irimia, N. Sabathiel, R. Ortner et al., "recoveriX: a new BCI-based technology for persons with stroke," in *2016 38th Annual International Conference of the IEEE Engineering in Medicine and Biology Society (EMBC)*, pp. 1504–1507, Orlando, FL, USA, 2016.

[5] H. Sun, J. Jin, W. Kong, C. Zuo, S. Li, and X. Wang, "Novel channel selection method based on position priori weighted permutation entropy and binary gravity search algorithm," *Cognitive Neurodynamics*, pp. 1–16, 2020.

[6] Y. Y. Miao, E. Yin, B. Z. Allison et al., "An ERP-based BCI with peripheral stimuli: validation with ALS patients," *Cognitive Neurodynamics*, vol. 14, no. 1, pp. 21–33, 2020.

[7] C. L. Zuo, J. Jin, E. Yin et al., "Novel hybrid brain-computer interface system based on motor imagery and P300," *Cognitive Neurodynamics*, vol. 14, no. 2, pp. 253–265, 2020.

[8] M. Q. Huang, I. Daly, J. Jin, Y. Zhang, X. Y. Wang, and A. Cichocki, "An exploration of spatial auditory BCI paradigms with different sounds: music notes versus beeps," *Cognitive Neurodynamics*, vol. 10, no. 3, pp. 201–209, 2016.

[9] M. Q. Huang, J. Jin, Y. Zhang, D. W. Hu, and X. Y. Wang, "Usage of drip drops as stimuli in an auditory P300 BCI paradigm," *Cognitive Neurodynamics*, vol. 12, no. 1, pp. 85–94, 2018.

[10] X. G. Chen, Y. J. Wang, S. K. Gao, T. P. Jung, and X. R. Gao, "Filter bank canonical correlation analysis for implementing a high-speed SSVEP-based brain-computer interface," *Journal of Neural Engineering*, vol. 12, no. 4, p. 046008, 2015.

[11] G. Pfurtscheller, "Graphical display and statistical evaluation of event-related desynchronization (ERD)," *Electroencephalography and Clinical Neurophysiology*, vol. 43, no. 5, pp. 757–760, 1977.

[12] G. Pfurtscheller, "Event-related synchronization (ERS): an electrophysiological correlate of cortical areas at rest," *Electroencephalography and Clinical Neurophysiology*, vol. 83, no. 1, pp. 62–69, 1992.

[13] M. Jeannerod, "The representing brain: neural correlates of motor intention and imagery," *The Behavioral and Brain Sciences*, vol. 17, no. 2, pp. 187–202, 1994.

[14] V. Kaiser, I. Daly, F. Pichiorri, D. Mattia, G. R. Müller-Putz, and C. Neuper, "Relationship between electrical brain responses to motor imagery and motor impairment in stroke," *Stroke*, vol. 43, no. 10, pp. 2735–2740, 2012.

[15] K. K. Ang and C. Guan, "Brain-computer interface in stroke rehabilitation," *Journal of Computing Science and Engineering*, vol. 7, no. 2, pp. 139–146, 2013.

[16] N. Sharma, V. M. Pomeroy, and J. C. Baron, "Motor imagery - a backdoor to the motor system after stroke?," *Stroke*, vol. 37, no. 7, pp. 1941–1952, 2006.

[17] A. Ramos-Murguialday, D. Broetz, M. Rea et al., "Brain-machine interface in chronic stroke rehabilitation: a controlled study," *Annals of Neurology*, vol. 74, no. 1, pp. 100–108, 2013.

[18] A. Vourvopoulos, C. Jorge, R. Abreu, P. Figueiredo, J. C. Fernandes, and S. B. I. Badia, "Efficacy and brain imaging correlates of an immersive motor imagery BCI-driven VR system for upper limb motor rehabilitation: a clinical case report," *Frontiers in Human Neuroscience*, vol. 13, 2019.

[19] E. Buch, C. Weber, L. G. Cohen et al., "Think to move: a neuromagnetic brain-computer interface (BCI) system for chronic stroke," *Stroke*, vol. 39, no. 3, pp. 910–917, 2008.

[20] D. C. Irimia, W. Cho, R. Ortner et al., "Brain-computer interfaces with multi-sensory feedback for stroke rehabilitation: a case study," *Artificial Organs*, vol. 41, no. 11, pp. E178–E184, 2017.

[21] M. S. Christensen and M. J. Grey, "Modulation of proprioceptive feedback during functional electrical stimulation: an fMRI study," *The European Journal of Neuroscience*, vol. 37, no. 11, pp. 1766–1778, 2013.

[22] G. Pfurtscheller, R. Scherer, R. Leeb et al., "Viewing moving objects in virtual reality can change the dynamics of sensorimotor EEG rhythms," *Presence Teleoperators and Virtual Environments*, vol. 16, no. 1, pp. 111–118, 2007.

[23] P. Boord, A. Craig, Y. Tran, and H. Nguyen, "Discrimination of left and right leg motor imagery for brain–computer interfaces," *Medical & Biological Engineering & Computing*, vol. 48, no. 4, pp. 343–350, 2010.

[24] W. Kahle and M. Frotscher, "Color atlas of human anatomy," *Synapse*, vol. 20, p. 22, 2003.

[25] G. Pfurtscheller and F. L. Da Silva, "Event-related EEG/MEG synchronization and desynchronization: basic principles,"

*Clinical Neurophysiology*, vol. 110, no. 11, pp. 1842–1857, 1999.

[26] C. Guger, H. Ramoser, and G. Pfurtscheller, "Real-time EEG analysis with subject-specific spatial patterns for a brain-computer interface (BCI)," *IEEE Transactions on Rehabilitation Engineering*, vol. 8, no. 4, pp. 447–456, 2000.

[27] F. Lotte and C. Guan, "Regularizing common spatial patterns to improve BCI designs: unified theory and new algorithms," *IEEE Transactions on Biomedical Engineering*, vol. 58, no. 2, pp. 355–362, 2011.

[28] K. K. Ang, Z. Y. Chin, C. Wang, C. Guan, and H. Zhang, "Filter bank common spatial pattern algorithm on BCI competition IV datasets 2a and 2b," *Frontiers in Neuroscience*, vol. 6, p. 39, 2012.

[29] Z. Qiu, J. Jin, H.-K. Lam, Y. Zhang, X. Wang, and A. Cichocki, "Improved SFFS method for channel selection in motor imagery based BCI," *Neurocomputing*, vol. 207, pp. 519–527, 2016.

[30] J. Feng, E. Yin, J. Jin et al., "Towards correlation-based time window selection method for motor imagery BCIs," *Neural Networks*, vol. 102, pp. 87–95, 2018.

[31] R. A. Fisher, "The use of multiple measurements in taxonomic problems," *Annals of Eugenics*, vol. 7, no. 2, pp. 179–188, 1936.

[32] G. McLachlan, *Discriminant analysis and statistical pattern recognition*, vol. 544, John Wiley & Sons, 2004.

[33] S. Kumar, K. Mamun, and A. Sharma, "CSP-TSM: optimizing the performance of Riemannian tangent space mapping using common spatial pattern for MI-BCI," *Computers in Biology and Medicine*, vol. 91, pp. 231–242, 2017.

[34] J. K. Feng, J. Jin, I. Daly et al., "An Optimized Channel Selection Method Based on Multifrequency CSP-Rank for Motor Imagery-Based BCI System," vol. 2019, Article ID 8068357, 10 pages, 2019, Computational Intelligence and Neuroscience.

[35] A. R. Fugl-Meyer, L. Jääskö, I. Leyman, S. Olsson, and S. Steglind, "The post-stroke hemiplegic patient. 1. A method for evaluation of physical performance," *Scandinavian Journal of Rehabilitation Medicine*, vol. 7, no. 1, pp. 13–31, 1975.

[36] J. H. van der Lee, H. Beckerman, G. J. Lankhorst, and L. M. Bouter, "The responsiveness of the action research arm test and the Fugl-Meyer assessment scale in chronic stroke patients," *Journal of Rehabilitation Medicine*, vol. 33, no. 3, pp. 110–113, 2001.

[37] D. J. Gladstone, C. J. Danells, and S. E. Black, "The Fugl-Meyer assessment of motor recovery after stroke: a critical review of its measurement properties," *Neurorehabilitation and Neural Repair*, vol. 16, no. 3, pp. 232–240, 2002.

[38] K. J. Sullivan, J. K. Tilson, S. Y. Cen et al., "Fugl-Meyer assessment of sensorimotor function after stroke: standardized training procedure for clinical practice and clinical trials," *Stroke*, vol. 42, no. 2, pp. 427–432, 2011.

[39] N. Takeuchi and S.-I. Izumi, "Rehabilitation with poststroke motor recovery: a review with a focus on neural plasticity," *Stroke Research and Treatment*, vol. 2013, Article ID 128641, 13 pages, 2013.

[40] G. Pfurtscheller, C. Brunner, A. Schlögl, and F. L. Da Silva, "Mu rhythm (de) synchronization and EEG single-trial classification of different motor imagery tasks," *NeuroImage*, vol. 31, no. 1, pp. 153–159, 2006.

[41] S. Ge, R. Wang, and D. Yu, "Classification of four-class motor imagery employing single-channel electroencephalography," *PLoS One*, vol. 9, no. 6, article e98019, 2014.

[42] Y. Liu, H. Zhang, M. Chen, and L. Zhang, "A boosting-based spatial-spectral model for stroke patients' EEG analysis in rehabilitation training," *IEEE Transactions on Neural Systems and Rehabilitation Engineering*, vol. 24, no. 1, pp. 169–179, 2016.

[43] A. Caria, C. Weber, D. Brötz et al., "Chronic stroke recovery after combined BCI training and physiotherapy: a case report," *Psychophysiology*, vol. 48, no. 4, pp. 578–582, 2011.

[44] B. Várkuti, C. Guan, Y. Pan et al., "Resting state changes in functional connectivity correlate with movement recovery for BCI and robot-assisted upper-extremity training after stroke," *Neurorehabilitation and Neural Repair*, vol. 27, no. 1, pp. 53–62, 2013.

[45] B. M. Young, Z. Nigogosyan, A. Remsik et al., "Changes in functional connectivity correlate with behavioral gains in stroke patients after therapy using a brain-computer interface device," *Frontiers in Neuroengineering*, vol. 7, p. 25, 2014.

[46] C. Grefkes and G. R. Fink, "Connectivity-based approaches in stroke and recovery of function," *Lancet Neurology*, vol. 13, no. 2, pp. 206–216, 2014.

[47] R. Leeb, S. Perdikis, L. Tonin et al., "Transferring brain–computer interfaces beyond the laboratory: successful application control for motor-disabled users," *Artificial Intelligence in Medicine*, vol. 59, no. 2, pp. 121–132, 2013.

[48] W.-K. Tam, K.-y. Tong, F. Meng, and S. Gao, "A minimal set of electrodes for motor imagery BCI to control an assistive device in chronic stroke subjects: a multi-session study," *IEEE Transactions on Neural Systems and Rehabilitation Engineering*, vol. 19, no. 6, pp. 617–627, 2011.

[49] H. T. Wang, A. Dragomir, N. I. Abbasi, J. H. Li, N. V. Thakor, and A. Bezerianos, "A novel real-time driving fatigue detection system based on wireless dry EEG," *Cognitive Neurodynamics*, vol. 12, no. 4, pp. 365–376, 2018.

[50] H. A. Lamti, M. M. Ben Khelifa, and V. Hugel, "Mental fatigue level detection based on event related and visual evoked potentials features fusion in virtual indoor environment," *Cognitive Neurodynamics*, vol. 13, no. 3, pp. 271–285, 2019.

[51] G. Li, Y. Luo, Z. Zhang et al., "Effects of mental fatigue onSmall-WorldBrain functional network organization," *Neural Plasticity*, vol. 2019, Article ID 1716074, 10 pages, 2019.

[52] R. Foong, K. K. Ang, C. Quek et al., "Assessment of the efficacy of EEG-based MI-BCI with visual feedback and EEG correlates of mental fatigue for upper-limb stroke rehabilitation," *IEEE Transactions on Biomedical Engineering*, vol. 67, no. 3, pp. 786–795, 2020.

[53] M. de Castro-Cros, M. Sebastian-Romagosa, J. Rodríguez-Serrano et al., "Effects of gamification in BCI functional rehabilitation," *Frontiers in Neuroscience*, vol. 14, 2020.

[54] A. Biasiucci, R. Leeb, I. Iturrate et al., "Brain-actuated functional electrical stimulation elicits lasting arm motor recovery after stroke," *Nature Communications*, vol. 9, no. 1, p. 2421, 2018.

# 38

# Systematic Review of Hospital Readmissions in Stroke Patients

**Ahsan Rao,[1] Emily Barrow,[2] Sabine Vuik,[2] Ara Darzi,[2] and Paul Aylin[1]**

[1]*School of Public Health, Faculty of Medicine, Dr. Foster Unit, 3 Dorset Rise, London EC4Y 8EN, UK*
[2]*Centre for Health Policy, Institute for Global Health Innovation, Imperial College London, QEQM, St Mary's Hospital, Floor 10, Praed Street, London W2 1NY, UK*

Correspondence should be addressed to Ahsan Rao; a.rao@imperial.ac.uk

Academic Editor: Graeme J. Hankey

*Background.* Previous evidence on factors and causes of readmissions associated with high-impact users of stroke is scanty. The aim of the study was to investigate common causes and pattern of short- and long-term readmissions stroke patients by conducting a systematic review of studies using hospital administrative data. Common risk factors associated with the change of readmission rate were also examined. *Methods.* The literature search was conducted from 15 February to 15 March 2016 using various databases, such as Medline, Embase, and Web of Science. *Results.* There were a total of 24 studies ($n$ = 2,126,617) included in the review. Only 4 studies assessed causes of readmissions in stroke patients with the follow-up duration from 30 days to 5 years. Common causes of readmissions in majority of the studies were recurrent stroke, infections, and cardiac conditions. Common patient-related risk factors associated with increased readmission rate were age and history of coronary heart disease, heart failure, renal disease, respiratory disease, peripheral arterial disease, and diabetes. Among stroke-related factors, length of stay of index stroke admission was associated with increased readmission rate, followed by bowel incontinence, feeding tube, and urinary catheter. *Conclusion.* Although risk factors and common causes of readmission were identified, none of the previous studies investigated causes and their sequence of readmissions among high-impact stroke users.

## 1. Introduction

Stroke is one of the leading causes of morbidity and mortality in the world and the cost of management of stroke has vastly increased [1]. Most cases occur in people over the age of 65 years [2]. Approximately 80% of stroke cases are ischaemic in nature, while the remainder are haemorrhagic [2]. Ischaemic stroke (IS) is caused by a thromboembolic event in the diseased artery resulting in acute blockage of the blood supply to a region of the brain [2, 3]. Haemorrhagic stroke results from rupture of a blood vessel or an abnormal vascular structure [3]. This results in bleed in the brain. Subarachnoid haemorrhage (SAH) is a subtype of haemorrhagic stroke that is caused by bleeding on the surface of the brain, whereas in intracerebral haemorrhage (ICH) bleeding occurs within the brain tissue [4].

Various aspects of stroke management have evolved in recent years [5]. Regional programs took a range of initiatives to improve outcomes of stroke, including quicker paramedic services to reach specialised stroke units early, rapid scanning, increased use of thrombolysis within 4 hours of stroke onset, and early rehabilitative program [2]. Previous clinical trials and observational studies have not thoroughly analysed the impact of new management strategies on outcomes of stroke due to small patient cohorts and limited follow-up [6].

Hospital administrative data provides an alternative method to evaluate outcomes of stroke [7]. The initial care of stroke is hospital-based and most complications require hospital reviews, admissions, and regular follow-up [6]. This piece of information is recorded in hospital administrative data and can be used to analyse readmissions [7]. Hospital administrative data has been used in recent years to study various aspects of stroke care [8]. It has the advantage of providing a large cohort of patients, which can be followed up for a long period because the data are generally linked by individual identifier [8].

Hospitalisation and readmission are commonly available information in hospital administrative data [9]. The World

Table 1: MESH terms used for literature search.

| | |
|---|---|
| 1 | exp stroke/ |
| 2 | Brain Ischemia/ or Stroke/ or ischaemic stroke.mp. or Cerebrovascular Disorders/ or Cerebral Infarction/ |
| 3 | haemorrhagic stroke.mp. |
| 4 | Intracranial Hemorrhages/ or hemorrhagic stroke.mp. |
| 5 | ischemic stroke.mp. |
| 6 | exp hospitalization/ |
| 7 | hospitalisation.mp. |
| 8 | Patient Readmission/ or readmission.mp. |
| 9 | readmission rate.mp. |
| 10 | Treatment Outcome/ or complication rate.mp. |
| 11 | 6 or 7 or 8 or 9 or 10 |
| 12 | 1 or 2 or 3 or 4 or 5 |
| *13* | *11 and 12* |

Health Organisation suggested that the use of imaging, thrombolysis, length of stay in hospital, and duration of rehabilitation vary in different regions giving rise to variation in mortality and readmission rate of stroke patients [10]. The Patient Protection and Affordable Care Act (PPACA) in US penalizes healthcare for increased RR but it is still not clear what proportion of these readmissions are preventable [11]. The patient population has been categorised into two groups, "high-impact" and "low-impact" users, based on the use of healthcare resources [12]. High-impact users form a small subgroup of patients who utilise the majority of healthcare resources with repeated and persistent readmissions to hospital [12]. The evidence on factors and causes of readmissions associated with high-impact users is scanty [9]. Moreover, most of the readmissions are measured within 30 days of a stroke event; hence, it is still to be discovered if the reasons for long-term readmissions are common in different regions [13]. The aim of the study was to review the evidence on common causes and patterns of short- and long-term readmissions in stroke patients by conducting a systematic review of studies using hospital administrative data. Common risk factors associated with changes in readmission rates were also examined.

## 2. Methods

The literature search was conducted from 15 February to 15 March 2016. The following literature databases were used: Embase (1947–2016), Medline (1946–2016), and Web of Science (1950–2016). Various MESH terms were used to identify studies that evaluated outcomes of stroke patients (Table 1). Alternative spellings for the terms were also included in the search, such as "hemorrhage", "haemorrhagic", "ischemia", and "ischemic". All the terms were combined with option "OR" to include all search titles. All the subheadings were included in the search. Further studies were identified through cross-referencing of studies reviewed initially. Once, various search terms were explored for stroke and readmission, they were combined with "AND" to include relevant studies for review.

The following inclusion criteria were used:

(1) Studies looking at an adult patient population over the age of 18 years diagnosed with nontraumatic ischaemic or haemorrhagic stroke.

(2) Studies utilising hospital administrative data to assess clinical outcomes following an event of stroke.

(3) Studies evaluating readmission of stroke patients due to any cause.

The following exclusion criteria were used:

(1) Studies that reported stroke as a complication or adverse event of another disease.

(2) Studies that reported cost-effectiveness rather than clinical outcomes of stroke.

The search strategy for the selection of studies was based on PRISMA protocol, which is primarily used to conduct systematic reviews [14] (Figure 1). Further studies were identified through the cross-referencing of initial studies reviewed. Two independent researchers, EB and AR, reviewed the selected studies separately. Basic demographics were obtained from each study included in the review. Year of study, place of data collection, administrative databases used, and aims and objectives of studies were recorded. Information on methodology of each study was collected, such as number of patients, types of stroke, kinds of readmission rate, and follow-up period. Significant effect of risk factor associated with change in readmission rate was measured as odds ratio (OR), hazards ratio (HR), percentage change, or relative risk (RR), with the confidence interval (CI) of 95%. Ratios and risks adjusted for other confounding factors and having significant impact on RR, $p < 0.05$, were mentioned in the review.

The Newcastle-Ottawa scale was used to assess bias in the studies [15]. The scale uses a star ranking system based on 3 major criteria: selection of participants, comparability, and definition of outcome. A maximum of 8 stars can be obtained by a study and would indicate a low degree of bias. The scale is validated and recommended by Cochrane

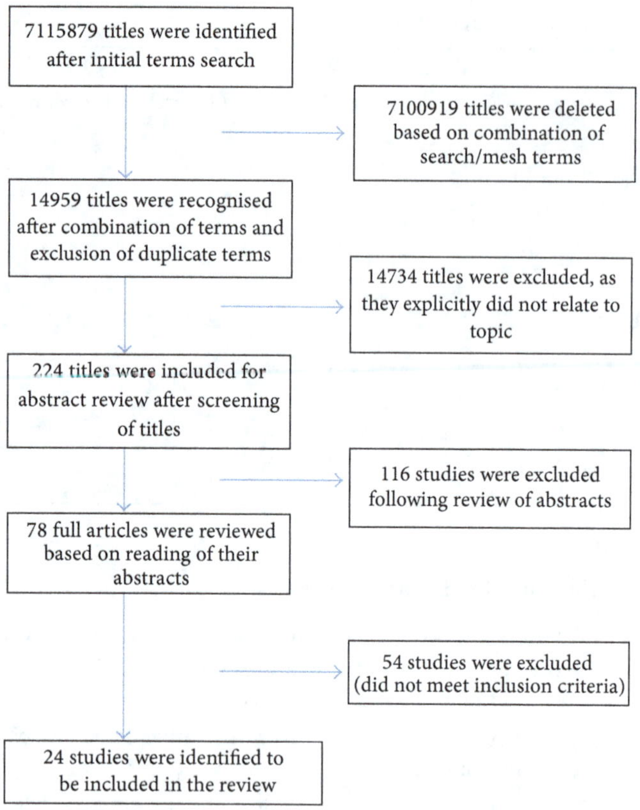


FIGURE 1: PRISMA diagram for the selection of studies included in the review.

review methodological guidelines for nonrandomised cohort studies.

## 3. Results

There were a total of 24 studies included in the review (Table 2). Eleven studies selected patients over the age of 65 [9, 13, 16–21], while the rest of the studies included all adult patients. The majority of the studies only included patients with ischaemic stroke. Few studies assessed outcomes in both haemorrhagic and ischaemic stroke patients [4, 6, 18, 21–25]. Eleven studies had high rating on the Newcastle-Ottawa scoring system, 6 and above, suggesting a low risk of bias associated with them [9, 13, 16–19, 22, 23, 25–28]. These studies benefitted from large population-based cohort of stroke patients, selection of a comparison group from the same population, clearly defined outcome measure, comparison of readmission rates between groups, and adequate follow-up. Other studies with low scoring lacked a well-demarcated control group, comparison of outcomes between groups, and complete long-term follow-up.

*3.1. Causes of Readmission.* Four studies evaluated causes of readmissions in stroke patients (Table 3). Common disease-related groups for all-cause 30-day readmission in all types of stroke patients were as follows: kidney and urinary tract infections, simple pneumonia and pleurisy, heart failure and shock, oesophagitis, gastritis, and other gastrointestinal disorders, and, lastly, nutritional and other metabolic disorders [21]. Common causes of 30-day unplanned readmissions in ischaemic stroke patients were recurrent stroke (33%), infections (septicaemia, aspiration pneumonia, pneumonia, and urinary tract infections, collectively 14.5%), and cardiac conditions (dysrhythmia, congestive heart failure, chest pain, and acute myocardial infarction, collectively 10.4%) [11]. Common causes of all-cause 1-year readmissions for haemorrhagic and ischaemic stroke were recurrent stroke (26.3%), infections (15.1%), accidents (9.5%), cardiopulmonary disease (9.1%), cancer (3.5%), diabetes (2.2%), and other causes (32.7%) [6]. In a study with a 5-year follow-up, the causes of readmissions were as follows: pneumonia and respiratory causes (8.6%), acute MI (5%), recurrent stroke (4.9%), gastrointestinal disorders (3.9%), congestive heart failure (3%), other vascular diagnoses (2.9%), cardiothoracic procedures (1.8%), psychiatric disorders (0.4%), hip fractures (0.2%), and other diagnoses (21.8%) [9].

*3.2. Factors Associated with the Change in the Readmission Rate.* Based on the net number of studies mentioning risk factors impacting the readmission rate, common patient-related risk factors associated with increased readmission rate were age and history of coronary heart disease, heart failure, renal disease, respiratory disease, peripheral arterial disease, and diabetes (Table 4). Among stroke-related factors, length of stay of index stroke admission was associated with increased readmission rate, followed by bowel incontinence, feeding tube, and urinary catheter.

Increased age, past medical history of vascular conditions, heart failure, and renal disease were common risk factors associated with the increase in the readmission rate of various types based on studies that reported factors with positive impact on readmission rate (Table 5).

Certain risk factors were found to be associated with reduction in the readmission rate. All-cause 30-day readmission rate was significantly reduced by early decision of not to resuscitate [29], social engagement [29], and higher use of occupational therapy [11]. All-cause 90-day readmission rate was significantly reduced by the use of inpatient rehabilitation [24] and all-cause 1-year readmission rate was declined by the persistent use of antiplatelet therapy [26].

Care of patients in the certified stroke centres [18] and critical access hospitals [19] had no impact on readmission rate. Two studies evaluated 1-year all-cause readmission rate and 1-year readmission for fractures in stroke patients but did not assess risk factors associated with change in readmission rate [30, 31].

## 4. Discussion

This review was based on 24 studies that identified various risk factors and causes of readmission. Prominent causes of readmissions were recurrent stroke, respiratory and urinary infections, acute cardiac conditions, and diabetes. In general, elderly patients with a background of cardiovascular conditions had increased short- and long-term readmission rate. None of the studies evaluated factors and causes of

TABLE 2: List and characteristics of all studies included in the review.

| Study | Year | Place (country) | Population ($n$) | Database source | Type of readmission measure | Bias assessment of study |
|---|---|---|---|---|---|---|
| Sacco et al. [22] | 1991 | USA | 1,034 | Statewide Planning and Research Cooperative System (SPARCS) | 2-year all-cause readmission | * * * * * * |
| Smith et al. [13] | 2006 | USA | 44,099 | Medicare and Medicaid Databases | 30-day cause-specific and all-cause readmission | * * * * * * |
| Smith et al. [16] | 2005 | USA | 9003 | Medicare | 30-day all-cause readmission | * * * * * * |
| Ghose et al. [23] | 2005 | USA | 51,119 | Veterans Affair Administrative databases | 3-year all-cause readmission and cumulative LOS | * * * * * * * * |
| Johansen et al. [30] | 2006 | Canada | 32,107 | Canadian Institute for Health Information | 1-year all-cause readmission | * * * * |
| Caro et al. [8] | 2006 | Canada | 18,704 | Saskatchewan Health database | 5-year all-cause and readmission for cardiovascular | * * * * * |
| McGuire et al. [4] | 2007 | Scotland | 9,598 | Scottish Medical Record Linkage System | 1-yr, 5-yr, and 11-yr readmission | * * * * * |
| Bravata et al. [9] | 2007 | USA | 2,603 | Medicare and Medicaid Services | 5-yr all-cause readmission | * * * * * * |
| Brown et al. [31] | 2008 | USA | 642 | Medicaid | Readmission for fractures | * * * * * |
| Tseng and Lin [6] | 2009 | Taiwan | 515 | Universal National Health Insurance | 1-year cause-specific readmission | * * * * * |
| Allen et al. [17] | 2010 | USA | 895,916 | Medicare | 1-year readmission for recurrent stroke | * * * * * * |
| Burke et al. [26] | 2010 | USA | 1413 | Medicare and Medicaid Services | 1-year readmission (time to recurrent stroke) | * * * * * * |
| Howrey et al. [27] | 2011 | USA | 9185 | Medicare | 30-day all-cause readmission | * * * * * * * |
| Gattellari et al. [28] | 2011 | Australia | 26,960 | Admitted Patient Data Collection | 90-day readmission to calculate cumulative LOS | * * * * * * |
| Lichtman et al. [18] | 2011 | USA | 37,469 | Medicare and Medicaid Services | 30-day all-cause readmission | * * * * * * * |
| Lichtman et al. [19] | 2012 | USA | 10,267 | Medicare and Medicaid Services | 30-day risk-standardised readmission | * * * * * * * |
| Palmer et al. [32] | 2013 | England | 91,936 | HES (Hospital Episode Statistics) | 30-day all-cause readmission | * * * * |
| Lichtman et al. [20] | 2013 | USA | 307,887 | Medicare | 30-day cause-specific readmission | * * * * * |
| Ottenbacher et al. [21] | 2014 | USA | 155,476 | Medicare and Medicaid Services | 30-day cause-specific readmission | * * * * |
| Burke et al. [11] | 2014 | USA | 129,676 | State Inpatient Database (SID) | Unplanned 30-day readmission | * * * * * |
| Chu et al. [33] | 2015 | USA | 17,3966 | California State Inpatient Database and State Emergency Department Database | 14-day readmission for infective endocarditis | * * * * |
| Andrews et al. [24] | 2015 | USA | 64,065 | State Inpatient database from Arkansas and Florida | 90-day all-cause readmission | * * * * |
| Lewsey et al. [25] | 2010 | Scotland | 51,182 | Scottish Morbidity Record Scheme | 1-year readmission rate for infective, gastrointestinal, and immobility complications | * * * * * * |
| Fehnel et al. [29] | 2015 | USA | 39,178 | Medicare linked to MDS (Minimum Data Set) | 30-day all-cause readmission | * * * * * |

Table 3: Studies evaluating causes of readmission in stroke patients.

| Studies | Primary aim of the study | Type of outcome measure | Type of stroke | Categorisation of causes | Common causes |
|---|---|---|---|---|---|
| Bravata et al. 2007 [9] | To examine rates and reasons for 5-year readmission following stroke | 5-year all-cause readmissions | Ischaemic stroke | DRG diagnosis | Pneumonia, acute MI, recurrent stroke, gastrointestinal disorders, congestive heart failure, other vascular diagnoses, cardiothoracic procedures, psychiatric disorders, and hip fractures. |
| Tseng and Lin 2009 [6] | To evaluate population-based readmission rate after stroke | 1-year all-cause readmissions | All types (haemorrhagic and ischaemic) | Not mentioned | Recurrent stroke, infections, accidents, cardiopulmonary disease, cancer, and diabetes. |
| Burke et al. 2014 [11] | To find association between hospital-level practices and readmission rate | 30-day unplanned readmissions | Ischaemic stroke | Not mentioned | Recurrent stroke, infections, and cardiac conditions. |
| Ottenbacher et al. 2014 [21] | To assess readmission rate following postacute inpatient rehabilitation discharge | 30-day all-cause readmissions | All types (haemorrhagic and ischaemic) | DRG diagnosis | Urinary tract infection, pneumonia, heart failure and shock, oesophagitis, and gastritis. |

TABLE 4: Risk factors and their impact on all-cause, preventable, and cerebrovascular readmission rate.

| Risk factors | Number of studies with positive association | Number of studies with negative association | Number of studies with no significant association |
|---|---|---|---|
| *Patient-related factors* | | | |
| Age | 8 | 1 | |
| Coronary heart disease | 4 | | |
| Female gender | 4 | 3 | |
| Heart failure | 4 | 1 | |
| Renal disease | 4 | | |
| Diabetes | 3 | 1 | |
| Peripheral arterial disease | 3 | | |
| Respiratory disease | 3 | | |
| Atrial fibrillation | 2 | 1 | |
| Cancer | 2 | 1 | |
| Comorbidity score | 2 | | |
| Depression | 2 | 1 | |
| Prior hospitalisations | 2 | | |
| Socioeconomic status | 2 | | |
| Alcohol misuse | 1 | | |
| Anaemia | 1 | | |
| C difficile infection | 1 | | |
| Dementia | 1 | 2 | |
| Hypertension | 1 | 3 | |
| Hypotension | 1 | | |
| Immobility | 1 | | |
| Marital status, married | 1 | | |
| Non-Caucasian ethnicity | 1 | 1 | 1 |
| Parkinson's disease | 1 | | |
| Pressure ulcers | 1 | | |
| TIA | 1 | | |
| Valvular heart disease/prosthetic valves | 1 | | |
| Do not resuscitate order | | 1 | |
| Hypercholesterolemia | | | 1 |
| Obesity | | 1 | |
| Previous stroke | | 1 | |
| Rheumatic disorders | | 1 | |
| Smoking | | 1 | |
| *Stroke-related factors* | | | |
| Length of stay | 3 | | |
| Feeding tube | 1 | | |
| Bowel incontinence | 1 | | |
| Urinary catheter | 1 | | |
| Bladder incontinence | | 1 | |
| Signs and symptoms score | | 1 | |
| Aphasia | | | 1 |
| Hemiparesis | | | 1 |
| Aspiration pneumonia | | | 1 |
| *Hospital care related factors* | | | |
| District hospitals with critical care access | 1 | | 1 |

Table 4: Continued.

| Risk factors | Number of studies with positive association | Number of studies with negative association | Number of studies with no significant association |
|---|---|---|---|
| Treatment by neurologist | 1 | 1 | |
| Discharge to nursing home | | 1 | 1 |
| Specialised stroke centres | | | 1 |
| Inpatient rehabilitation facility | | 1 | 1 |
| Use of ICU/HDU | | | 2 |
| Endarterectomy | | | 1 |
| Stenting | | | 1 |
| Gastrostomy | | | 1 |
| Intubation | | | 1 |
| Dialysis | | | 1 |
| Occupational therapy | | 1 | |
| Thrombolysis | | | 2 |
| Urgent scanning | | | 1 |

readmission in different subgroups of stroke patients, in particular high-impact users. Studies used different definitions of readmission rate, which made it difficult to compare the data and perform meta-analysis.

The review has focused on studies using administrative data to analyse significant factors and causes of readmission at population level. This may help health policy makers to develop accurate prediction models and management plans at regional level for patients at high risk of readmissions. Previous clinical studies have assessed similar risk factors but they had the disadvantage of limited number of patients and a shorter follow-up period [7, 32]. Calculation of cause-specific readmission rates required a larger sample of patients, possibly with the use of hospital administrative data [25, 33].

The long-term pattern of readmissions in different subgroups of stroke patients could not be deduced from the review. Most of the studies calculated readmission rate with a follow-up of less than one year [13, 16, 27, 28]. Studies with long-term follow-up period merely focused on risk factors associated with higher readmission rate [4, 31]. A minority of studies evaluated common causes of readmission with crude cross-sectional analysis of whole population. No effort was made to categorise patients into subgroups based on rate of readmission and cumulative LOS. This would have been particularly helpful to identify patients with a high-impact use of hospital care or those who have the potential to become high impact [12, 34]. None of the studies investigated the sequence of hospitalisations in stroke patients. Although common causes of readmission were identified, further investigation is needed to find out the timing of occurrence of causes of readmission. If there is a difference in the timing of occurrence of causes of readmission or pattern of hospital care use in subgroups of stroke patients is still uncertain. This could provide vital information as it has been shown that subgroups of pneumonia patients had variable prognosis and time to recovery based on timing of occurrence of complications [35].

The readmission rate was shown to provide relevant and detailed information on the outcome of stroke when the metric was cause-specific, risk-standardised, and assessed unplanned readmissions for preventable causes [6, 9]. Cause-specific readmission rates were mostly calculated for preventable complications, for example, sepsis, recurrent stroke, and fracture [25, 26, 31]. Recurrence rate was a cause-specific readmission rate that measured rate of another stroke event after first stroke. In another study, time to first recurrent stroke was also analysed [26]. The identification of specific causes of readmission based on ICD discharge coding has been shown to be validated and highly sensitive [32].

Measurement of 30-day all-cause readmission to assess the quality of care was recommended by the Affordable Care Act and the Agency of Healthcare Research and Quality (AHRQ) in the US [26]. Hospitals with higher 30-day readmission rates were penalized, with the aim of improving the quality of care by reducing readmission rate. However, a significant proportion of patients after stroke get readmitted for planned procedures, on-going care follow-up, and rehabilitation [11, 29]. The measurement of cause-specific 30-day readmission rate would be better instead, because it can be used to calculate readmission rates due to preventable causes. For example, compliance with antiplatelet therapy was shown to reduce readmission rates for recurrent stroke [29].

Studies have used readmission rate as an outcome measure to assess morbidity in the patients after they had stroke [4, 13, 17–19, 22, 23, 27, 30]. It has been used along with other outcome metrics, such as length of stay, discharge destination, and mortality rate. They have performed separate analysis to evaluate factors impacting the mortality rate of the patients. They mainly focused on assessing annual trends and the impact of various factors on the overall outcome and prognosis of the stroke patients. Hence, factors were recognized which impacted both readmission and mortality rate or just one of them. Since hospitals are penalized for higher readmission rate in some regions, certain studies have only focused on measuring factors associated with higher

Table 5: Studies demonstrating risk factors that increased readmission rate. The rate of increase was described as hazard ratio (HR), odds ratio (OR), relative risk (RR), or increase in the percentage.

| Studies | Outcome measured | Risk factors |
|---|---|---|
| Chu et al. 2015 [33] | 14 d readmission for infective endocarditis | Valvular heart disease (OR 1.5; 95% CI, 0.2–10.8)<br>Prosthetic heart valve (OR 15.8; 95%CI, 1.9–129.0)<br>Urinary tract infection (OR 3.5; 95% CI, 1.0–12.3) |
| Lichtman et al. 2013 [20] | All-cause 30 d readmission | Female sex (HR 1.14; 95% CI, 1.08–1.21)<br>Age (per year increase) (HR 1.02; 95% CI, 1.01–1.02)<br>Diabetes (HR 1.43; 95% CI, 1.35–1.51)<br>Congestive heart failure (HR 2.29; 95% CI, 2.15–2.43)<br>Myocardial infarction (HR 1.54; 95% CI, 1.29–1.85)<br>Peripheral vascular disease (HR 1.14; 95% CI, 1.05–1.24)<br>Unstable angina (HR 1.49; 95% CI, 1.11–1.98)<br>Protein malnutrition (HR 1.43; 95% CI, 1.23–1.67)<br>Dementia (HR 1.10; 95% CI, 1.02–1.20)<br>Anaemia (HR 1.43; 95% CI, 1.35–1.51)<br>Renal failure (HR 2.31; 95% CI, 2.14–2.48)<br>Pneumonia (HR 1.28; 95% CI 1.59–1.42) |
| Burke et al. 2014 [11] | All-cause 30 d readmission | Use of hospice care (OR 5.86; 95% CI, 1.13–30.3) |
| Howrey et al. 2011 [27] | All-cause 30 d readmission | Hospitalist care (versus nonhospitalist) (HR 1.30; 95% CI, 1.11–1.52) |
| Smith et al. 2005 [16] | All-cause 30 d readmission | Care by health maintenance organisation (HMO) compared to Fee-For-Service (FFS) health insurance (HR 1.45; 95%, 1.14–1.83) |
| Smith et al. 2006 [13] | 30 d readmission for atherosclerotic diseases | Care by neurologist (versus generalist) (HR 1.17; 95% CI, 1.02–1.34) |
| Fehnel et al. 2015 [29] | Unplanned 30-day readmission | Bowel incontinence (OR 1.16; 95% CI, 1.06–1.28)<br>Feeding tube (OR 1.21; 95% CI, 1.08–1.35)<br>Chronic obstruction pulmonary disease (OR 1.26; 95% CI, 1.16–1.38)<br>Renal disease (OR 1.26; 95% CI, 1.13–1.42)<br>Heart failure (OR 1.17; 95% CI, 1.08–1.27)<br>Pressure ulcer grade 4 (OR 1.33; 95% CI, 1.09–1.62) |
| Tseng and Lin 2009 [6] | 1 yr all-cause readmission | Care by nonneurologist (versus neurologist) (OR 1.81; 95% CI, 1.13–2.88) |

Table 5: Continued.

| Studies | Outcome measured | Risk factors |
|---|---|---|
| Allen et al. 2010 [17] | 1 yr readmission for recurrent stroke | Prior hospital admissions (RR 12.64; 95% CI, 9.24–17.29)<br>High comorbidity score (RR 2.28; 95% CI, 1.18–2.90) |
| Lewsey et al. 2010 [25] | 1-year readmissions for infections, gastrointestinal, and immobility complications | Heart failure (HR 1.19; 95% CI, 110–1.30)<br>Renal failure (HR 1.23; 95% CI, 1.10–1.38)<br>Respiratory disease (HR 1.24; 95% CI, 1.15–1.33)<br>Increased age (HR 2.08; 95% CI, 1.87–2.31)<br>Higher socioeconomic deprivation (HR 1.16; 95% CI, 1.08–1.26)<br>Prior complications of infections (HR 1.31; 95% CI, 1.24–1.38)<br>Prior gastrointestinal complications (HR 1.58; 95% CI, 1.51–1.66)<br>Prior immobility complications (HR 1.23; 95% CI, 1.16–1.30) |
| Ghose et al. 2005 [23] | 3 yr all-cause readmission rate | Depression during stroke (log-OR 2.09; 95% CI, 2.03–2.16) |
| Caro et al. 2006 [8] | 5 yr all-cause readmission rate | ↑36.2% (95% CI, 30.3%–42.4%) for age (>65 years)<br>↑18.1% (95% CI, 14.1%–22.2%) for male sex<br>↑20.9% (95% CI, 13.9%–28.4%) for atrial fibrillation<br>↑21.6% (95% CI, 16.6%–26.8%) for heart failure<br>↑12.1% (95% CI, 7.6%–17.8%) for angina<br>↑10.1% (95% CI, 2.7%–14.8%) for prior myocardial infarction<br>↑14.0% (95% CI, 9.7%–18.7%) for hypertension<br>↑4% (95% CI, 0.2%–8.1%) for transient ischaemic attack |

readmission rate and avoidable causes of readmission [8, 11, 21, 26, 29].

The review had a few limitations. The review only included those studies that used administrative data. The data is collected over a large patient population increasing its generalizability. Most of the studies evaluating causes of readmissions have used administrative data. Other studies using local observational or clinical data had a small patient sample and mainly focused on assessing risk factors associated with the change in the readmission rate. By reviewing studies using administrative data, we have tried to reduce heterogeneity between the studies. However, the selection of stroke patients is based on coding system used by the researchers, which can introduce selection bias and impair its validity. The use of diagnostic coding is prone to errors when used to select cohort of the stroke patients and identifying causes of readmissions. This can lead to bias in the effect measure estimates, such as odds ratio and relative risk. Very few studies evaluated long-term outcomes of stroke. Some studies used the same database; common databases used were Medicare, Medicaid, and Veterans Affairs (VA) administrative data [9, 13, 16, 17, 23, 26, 32]. Readmission rates with multiple definitions were used in the studies, making it difficult for homogenous international comparison. The studies analysing hospital administrative data are prone to selection bias as specific codes are used to identify the cohort of patients from retrospectively collected data and the comparison groups are not randomised [32]. Coding errors have been associated with the use of administrative data [12]. This may affect precise identification of stroke patients and calculation of incidence of complications. In some studies, comparison groups were not matched for confounding factors [4, 9]. Similarly, readmission rates were not risk-standardised to tackle a common problem with the use of administrative data, that is, patient case-mix [26, 33].

Common causes of readmission were identified, but further research is required to find out the sequence and pattern of causes of long-term readmission in stroke patients. Previous studies have evaluated risk factors and causes of readmission for stroke population as a whole [12]. However, it will be more beneficial to investigate risk factors and pattern of readmission in subgroups of patients based on their readmission rate [12].

## Abbreviations

RR: Relative risk
OR: Odds ratio
HR: Hazards ratio
NOS: Newcastle-Ottawa scale
CI: Confidence interval
LOS: Length of stay
cLOS: Cumulative length of stay
CHF: Congestive heart failure
MI: Myocardial infarction
RF: Renal failure
AF: Atrial fibrillation
COPD: Chronic obstructive pulmonary disease
TIA: Transient ischaemic attack
SAH: Subarachnoid haemorrhage
ICH: Intracerebral haemorrhage
CAH: Critical access hospital
AHRQ: Agency of Healthcare Research and Quality
ICD: International classification of diseases
VA: Veterans affairs.

## Additional Points

*Availability of Data and Materials.* The study was review of previously published studies.

## Competing Interests

The authors declare that they have no competing interests.

## Authors' Contributions

Ahsan Rao and Emily Barrow made significant contribution to concept and design and analysis and acquisition of data. Ahsan Rao and Sabine Vuik were involved in analysis and interpretation of data, as well as drafting the manuscript. Paul Aylin and Ara Darzi critically revised the manuscript and gave final approval for it to be published.

## References


[1] M. Rahman, D. Neal, K. M. Fargen, and B. L. Hoh, "Establishing standard performance measures for adult stroke patients: a nationwide inpatient sample database study," *World Neurosurgery*, vol. 80, no. 6, pp. 699–708.e2, 2013.

[2] L. S. Williams, G. J. Eckert, G. J. L'italien, P. Lapuerta, and M. Weinberger, "Regional variation in health care utilization and outcomes in ischemic stroke," *Journal of Stroke and Cerebrovascular Diseases*, vol. 12, no. 6, pp. 259–265, 2003.

[3] A. A. Divani, G. Vazquez, M. Asadollahi, A. I. Qureshi, and P. Pullicino, "Nationwide frequency and association of heart failure on stroke outcomes in the United States," *Journal of Cardiac Failure*, vol. 15, no. 1, pp. 11–16, 2009.

[4] A. J. McGuire, M. Raikou, I. Whittle, and M. C. Christensen, "Long-term mortality, morbidity and hospital care following intracerebral hemorrhage: an 11-year cohort study," *Cerebrovascular Diseases*, vol. 23, no. 2-3, pp. 221–228, 2007.

[5] H. F. Zhu, N. N. Newcommon, M. E. Cooper et al., "Impact of a stroke unit on length of hospital stay and in-hospital case fatality," *Stroke*, vol. 40, no. 1, pp. 18–23, 2009.

[6] M.-C. Tseng and H.-J. Lin, "Readmission after hospitalization for stroke in Taiwan: results from a national sample," *Journal of the Neurological Sciences*, vol. 284, no. 1-2, pp. 52–55, 2009.

[7] O. Groene, S. Kristensen, O. A. Arah et al., "Feasibility of using administrative data to compare hospital performance in the EU," *International Journal for Quality in Health Care*, vol. 26, pp. 108–115, 2014.

[8] J. J. Caro, K. Migliaccio-Walle, K. J. Ishak, I. Proskorovsky, and J. A. O'Brien, "The time course of subsequent hospitalizations and associated costs in survivors of an ischemic stroke in Canada," *BMC Health Services Research*, vol. 6, article 99, 2006.

[9] D. M. Bravata, S.-Y. Ho, T. P. Meehan, L. M. Brass, and J. Concato, "Readmission and death after hospitalization for acute

ischemic stroke—5-year follow-up in the medicare population," *Stroke*, vol. 38, no. 6, pp. 1899–1904, 2007.

[10] S. Chatterji, "World health Organization's (WHO) study on global ageing and adult health (SAGE)," *BMC Proceedings*, vol. 7, supplement 4, article S1, 2013, Proceedings of the European Workshop on Health and Disability Surveillance in Ageing Populations.

[11] J. F. Burke, L. E. Skolarus, E. E. Adelman, M. J. Reeves, and D. L. Brown, "Influence of hospital-level practices on readmission after ischemic stroke," *Neurology*, vol. 82, no. 24, pp. 2196–2204, 2014.

[12] A. Bottle, P. Aylin, and A. Majeed, "Identifying patients at high risk of emergency hospital admissions: a logistic regression analysis," *Journal of the Royal Society of Medicine*, vol. 99, no. 8, pp. 406–414, 2006.

[13] M. A. Smith, J.-I. Liou, J. R. Frytak, and M. D. Finch, "30-Day survival and rehospitalization for stroke patients according to physician specialty," *Cerebrovascular Diseases*, vol. 22, no. 1, pp. 21–26, 2006.

[14] D. Moher, L. Shamseer, M. Clarke et al., "Preferred reporting items for systematic review and meta-analysis protocols (PRISMA-P) 2015 statement," *Systematic Reviews*, vol. 4, no. 1, p. 1, 2015.

[15] J. P. T. Higgins, D. G. Altman, P. C. Gøtzsche et al., "The cochrane collaboration's tool for assessing risk of bias in randomised trials," *The British Medical Journal*, vol. 343, article d5928, 2011.

[16] M. A. Smith, J. R. Frytak, J.-I. Liou, and M. D. Finch, "Rehospitalization and survival for stroke patients in managed care and traditional medicare plans," *Medical Care*, vol. 43, no. 9, pp. 902–910, 2005.

[17] N. B. Allen, T. R. Holford, M. B. Bracken et al., "Geographic variation in one-year recurrent ischemic stroke rates for elderly medicare beneficiaries in the USA," *Neuroepidemiology*, vol. 34, no. 2, pp. 123–129, 2010.

[18] J. H. Lichtman, S. B. Jones, E. C. Leifheit-Limson, Y. Wang, and L. B. Goldstein, "30-Day mortality and readmission after hemorrhagic stroke among medicare beneficiaries in Joint Commission Primary Stroke Center-certified and noncertified hospitals," *Stroke*, vol. 42, no. 12, pp. 3387–3391, 2011.

[19] J. H. Lichtman, E. C. Leifheit-Limson, S. B. Jones, Y. Wang, and L. B. Goldstein, "30-Day risk-standardized mortality and readmission rates after ischemic stroke in critical access hospitals," *Stroke*, vol. 43, no. 10, pp. 2741–2747, 2012.

[20] J. H. Lichtman, E. C. Leifheit-Limson, S. B. Jones, Y. Wang, and L. B. Goldstein, "Preventable readmissions within 30 days of ischemic stroke among medicare beneficiaries," *Stroke*, vol. 44, no. 12, pp. 3429–3435, 2013.

[21] K. J. Ottenbacher, A. Karmarkar, J. E. Graham et al., "Thirty-day hospital readmission following discharge from postacute rehabilitation in fee-for-service medicare patients," *The Journal of the American Medical Association*, vol. 311, no. 6, pp. 604–614, 2014.

[22] R. L. Sacco, W. A. Hauser, and J. P. Mohr, "Hospitalized stroke in blacks and hispanics in northern manhattan," *Stroke*, vol. 22, no. 12, pp. 1491–1496, 1991.

[23] S. S. Ghose, L. S. Williams, and R. W. Swindle, "Depression and other mental health diagnoses after stroke increase inpatient and outpatient medical utilization three years poststroke," *Medical Care*, vol. 43, no. 12, pp. 1259–1264, 2005.

[24] A. W. Andrews, D. Li, and J. K. Freburger, "Association of rehabilitation intensity for stroke and risk of hospital readmission," *Physical Therapy*, vol. 95, no. 12, pp. 1660–1667, 2015.

[25] J. Lewsey, P. S. Jhund, M. Gillies et al., "Temporal trends in hospitalisation for stroke recurrence following incident hospitalisation for stroke in Scotland," *BMC Medicine*, vol. 8, article 23, 2010.

[26] J. P. Burke, S. Sander, H. Shah, V. Zarotsky, and H. Henk, "Impact of persistence with antiplatelet therapy on recurrent ischemic stroke and predictors of nonpersistence among ischemic stroke survivors," *Current Medical Research and Opinion*, vol. 26, no. 5, pp. 1023–1030, 2010.

[27] B. T. Howrey, Y.-F. Kuo, and J. S. Goodwin, "Association of care by hospitalists on discharge destination and 30-day outcomes after acute ischemic stroke," *Medical Care*, vol. 49, no. 8, pp. 701–707, 2011.

[28] M. Gattellari, C. Goumas, R. Aitken, and J. M. Worthington, "Outcomes for patients with ischaemic stroke and atrial fibrillation: the PRISM study (A program of research informing stroke management)," *Cerebrovascular Diseases*, vol. 32, no. 4, pp. 370–382, 2011.

[29] C. R. Fehnel, Y. Lee, L. C. Wendell, B. B. Thompson, N. S. Potter, and V. Mor, "Post-acute care data for predicting readmission after ischemic stroke: a nationwide cohort analysis using the minimum data set," *Journal of the American Heart Association*, vol. 4, no. 9, Article ID e002145, 2015.

[30] H. L. Johansen, A. T. Wielgosz, K. Nguyen, and R. N. Fry, "Incidence, comorbidity, case fatality and readmission of hospitalized stroke patients in Canada," *Canadian Journal of Cardiology*, vol. 22, no. 1, pp. 65–71, 2006.

[31] D. L. Brown, L. B. Morgenstern, J. J. Majersik, M. Kleerekoper, and L. D. Lisabeth, "Risk of fractures after stroke," *Cerebrovascular Diseases*, vol. 25, no. 1-2, pp. 95–99, 2008.

[32] W. L. Palmer, A. Bottle, C. Davie, C. A. Vincent, and P. Aylin, "Meeting the ambition of measuring the quality of hospitals' stroke care using routinely collected administrative data: a feasibility study," *International Journal for Quality in Health Care*, vol. 25, no. 4, pp. 429–436, 2013.

[33] S. Y. Chu, A. E. Merkler, N. T. Cheng, and H. Kamel, "Readmission for infective endocarditis after ischemic stroke or transient ischemic attack," *The Neurohospitalist*, vol. 5, no. 2, pp. 55–58, 2015.

[34] K. Tilling, J. A. C. Sterne, A. G. Rudd, T. A. Glass, R. J. Wityk, and C. D. A. Wolfe, "A new method for predicting recovery after stroke," *Stroke*, vol. 32, no. 12, pp. 2867–2873, 2001.

[35] G. W. Hougham, S. A. Ham, G. W. Ruhnke et al., "Sequence patterns in the resolution of clinical instabilities in community-acquired pneumonia and association with outcomes," *Journal of General Internal Medicine*, vol. 29, no. 4, pp. 563–571, 2014.

# Determinants of Stroke Mortality through Survival Models: The Case of Mettu Karl Referral Hospital, Mettu, Ethiopia

**Dereje Gebeyehu Ababu and Azmeraw Misganaw Getahun**

*Department of Statistics, Faculty of Natural & Computational Science, Mettu University, Ethiopia*

Correspondence should be addressed to Dereje Gebeyehu Ababu; derejegebe@gmail.com

Academic Editor: Augusto Fusco

*Introduction.* Every year worldwide, between five to six million deaths are associated with stroke; on average, one stroke-related death occurs every four minutes. In Ethiopia, stroke is a frequent cause of mortality and morbidity from noncommunicable diseases. Therefore, this study was aimed at determining factors associated to stroke mortality through survival models in Mettu Karl Referral Hospital. *Methods.* This study was conducted from September 1, 2014, to April 1, 2017, and encompassed 202 stroke patients at Mettu Karl Referral Hospital. The Cox semiparametric regression was used for analyzing survival analysis of stroke patients using R software. *Results.* A total of 202 stroke patients were included in the study, and among those patients, 72.8% and 27.2% were censored and died, respectively. According to the result of Cox semiparametric regression model, sex of patients, hypertension, baseline complication, and stroke type had significant effect on survival of the stroke patient at 5% significance level. *Conclusion.* The results from Cox semiparametric regression model indicated that sex of patients, hypertension, baseline complication, and stroke type were major factors related to the survival time of stroke patients. The researcher recommends that the people should be aware on the burden of those risk factors and well informed about the disease.

## 1. Introduction

Globally, stroke is the second leading cause of death above the age of 60 years and about 16 million new cases of stroke and 62 million stroke survivors were estimated in 2005, with deaths from stroke accounting for 9.7% of all global deaths, and this is expected to increase to over 23 million new stroke cases and 7.8 million stroke deaths by 2030 in the absence of significant global public health response [1].

The study conducted in south western Saudi Arabia showed that prestroke smoking, prestroke hypertension, poststroke disturbed consciousness poor mobility, and developing pulmonary embolism as significant predictors of in-hospital stroke mortality [2].

In Africa, the impact of stroke is increasing due to a rising prevalence of hypertension associated with a very poor level of awareness and control. African countries are undergoing an epidemiological transition driven by socio-demographic and lifestyle changes [3]. The burden of noncommunicable diseases (NCD), including cardiovascular risk factors, is increasing. Consequently, the incidence of stroke, a cardinal complication of cardiovascular risk factors, appears to be rising in Africa [4].

In Ethiopia, hypertension was the most important risk factor identified in 1990. However, during that time, computed tomography (CT) scan was not available to differentiate stroke subtypes and the modern approach in treating patients with strokes requires early CT scan as it is imperative to diagnose whether the stroke is ischemic or hemorrhagic [5].

Although Ethiopia is progressing towards universal health coverage, the country faces the double burden of both communicable and noncommunicable diseases [6]. According to the report of WHO in 2017, stroke deaths in Ethiopia reached 6.23%. Moreover, the age-adjusted death rate of stroke in Ethiopia was 89.82 per 100,000 of the population.

TABLE 1: Baseline covariate characteristics with their time-to-death status.

| Variables | Categories | Frequency | Death (%) | Censored (%) | Mean (days) | [95% CI] |
|---|---|---|---|---|---|---|
| Gender | Male | 120 (59.4%) | 34 (55.7%) | 86 (61%) | 9.179131 | [8.04889, 10.3094] |
| | Female | 82 (40.6%) | 27 (44.3%) | 55 (39%) | 5.150107 | [4.22813, 6.07208] |
| Blood pressure | Yes | 123 (60.9%) | 44 (72.13%) | 77 (54.6%) | 5.761887 | [5.15259, 6.37119] |
| | No | 79 (39.1%) | 17 (27.87%) | 64 (45.4%) | 9.764186 | [8.30564, 11.2227] |
| Cardiac disease | Yes | 26 (12.9%) | 11 (20%) | 15 (10.2%) | 8.069148 | [5.14086, 10.9974] |
| | No | 176 (87.1%) | 44 (80%) | 132 (89.8%) | 7.770081 | [6.85184, 8.68832] |
| Diabetes mellitus | Yes | 15 (7.4%) | 3 (5.45%) | 12 (8.2%) | 6.289487 | [4.67067, 7.9083] |
| | No | 187 (92%) | 52 (94.54%) | 135 (91.8%) | 7.918552 | [6.98651, 8.8506] |
| Stroke type | Hemorrhagic | 70 (34.7%) | 29 (52.73%) | 41 (27.9%) | 6.137696 | [5.17646, 7.09893] |
| | Ischemic | 117 (57.9%) | 23 (41.82%) | 94 (63.9%) | 8.719683 | [7.5657, 9.87366] |
| | Both | 15 (7.4%) | 3 (5.45%) | 12 (8.2%) | 4.584416 | [3.25288, 5.91595] |
| Baseline complication | Yes | 115 (56.9%) | 37 (67.3%) | 78 (53%) | 5.391817 | [4.83329, 5.95035] |
| | No | 87 (43.1%) | 18 (32.7%) | 69 (47%) | 9.92229 | [8.54041, 11.3042] |

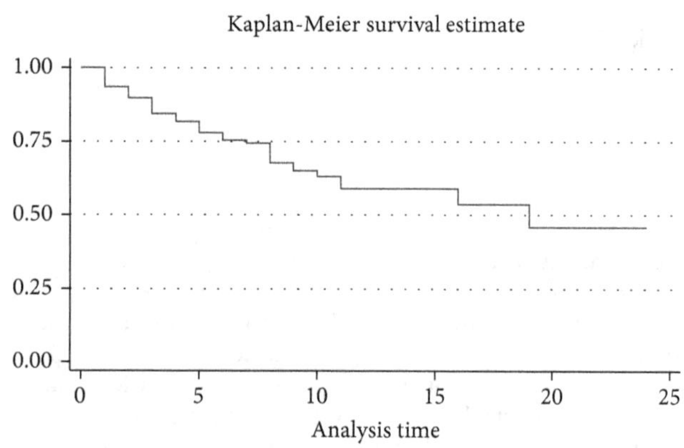


FIGURE 1: Overall Kaplan-Meier survivor function.

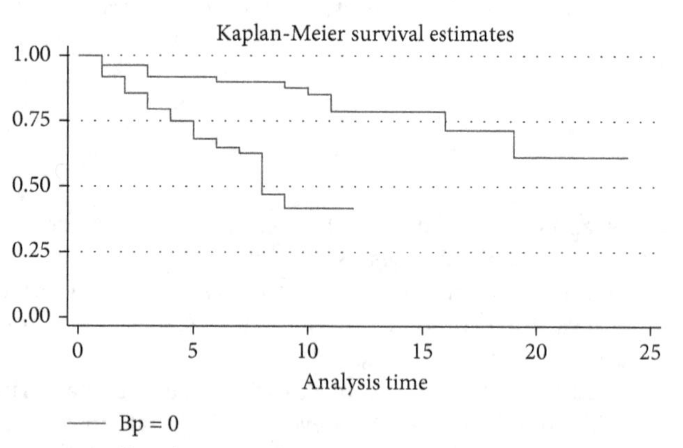


FIGURE 2: K-M plot survival of time-to-death by hypertension of stroke patients.

Earlier reports showed that the future trend of stroke in Sub-Sahara Africa will increase over the coming years owing to poor healthcare and poor neurologic interventions [7].

Therefore, chronic diseases become major global public health problems, mainly, in developing countries. However, there is limited evidence on the magnitude and factors of stroke in Ethiopia using survival models, particularly, in Mettu Karl Referral Hospital, which is the aim of this study. Findings of this study were important evidence to the studied hospital and Oromia Regional Health Bureau to know the burden of stroke and determinant factors and plan appropriate preventive methods against stroke.

TABLE 2: Log rank tests of each covariate.

| Variable | Log rank test | | |
|---|---|---|---|
| | Chi.sq | Df | *P* value |
| Gender | 27.4 | 1 | <0.001 |
| Age | 100 | 52 | <0.001 |
| Cardiac disease | 0 | 1 | 0.988 |
| Diabetes mellitus | 0.9 | 1 | 0.341 |
| Blood pressure (hypertension) | 22.3 | 1 | <0.001 |
| Drug type | 9.4 | 6 | 0.152 |
| Baseline complication | 31.4 | 1 | <0.001 |
| Stroke type | 8.1 | 2 | 0.150 |

## 2. Methodology

*2.1. Study Area.* This study was conducted in Mettu Karl Referral Hospital. This study was conducted from the 1st of September 2014 to the 1st of April 2017 in Mettu Karl Hospital.

*2.2. Study Design and Population.* Retrospective data were gathered from a total number of 202 stroke disease patients diagnosed with stroke case patients in the medical and surgical wards from the 1st of September 2014 to the 1st of April 2017 in MCRH.

*2.3. Variable in the Study.* The dependent (outcome) variable in this study was the survival time measured (in days) from the start date of stroke treatment until the date of the patient's death or censor. The following are covariate variables in the study: sex, age, hypertension, cardiac disease,

Table 3: Summary univariable (single covariate) Cox PH analysis.

| Covariate | Category | Coef ($\beta$) | HR | se ($\beta$) | Wald | Pr (>\|z\|) | 95% CI |
|---|---|---|---|---|---|---|---|
| Age | | 0.011662 | 1.011731 | 0.004634 | 6.33 | 0.012 | [1.003, 1.0210] |
| Gender | 0 female | Ref | | | | | |
| | 1 male | -0.8860 | 0.4123 | 0.1845 | 23.05 | <0.001 | [0.2872, 0.5920] |
| Cardiac disease | 0 no | Ref | | | | | |
| | 1 yes | -0.003844 | 0.996164 | 0.273690 | -0.014 | 0.989 | [0.5826, 1.7030] |
| Diabetes mellitus | 0 no | Ref | | | | | |
| | 1 yes | 0.2712 | 1.3116 | 0.3046 | 0.79 | 0.373 | [0.7219, 2.3830] |
| Hypertension | 0 no | Ref | | | | | |
| | 1 yes | 0.9365 | 2.5510 | 0.1986 | 22.24 | <0.001 | [1.7290, 3.7650] |
| Stroke type | 0 (hemorrhagic) | Ref | | | | | |
| | 1 (ischemic) | -0.4857 | 0.6152 | 0.1976 | -2.458 | 0.014 | [0.4177, 0.9062] |
| | 2 (both type) | 0.5496 | 1.7325 | 0.3303 | 13.44 | 0.096 | [0.9068, 3.3101] |
| Baseline complication | 0 no | Ref | | | | | |
| | 1 yes | 1.1220 | 3.0710 | 0.2056 | 29.78 | <0.001 | [2.052, 4.5950] |

Table 4: Summary multivariable Cox PH analysis to the stroke data set from the MCRH.

| Covariates | Category | Coef ($\beta$) | Haz. ratio | Std. Err. ($\beta$) | Wald | $P > \|z\|$ | [95% Conf. Interval HR] |
|---|---|---|---|---|---|---|---|
| Age | | 0.0051853 | 1.0051988 | 0.0052631 | 0.985 | 0.325 | [0.9949, 1.0156] |
| Gender | 0 female | Ref | | | | | |
| | 1 male | -0.7226692 | 0.4854547 | 0.1937196 | -3.730 | <0.001 | [0.3321, 0.7096] |
| Blood pressure (hypertension) | 0 no | Ref | | | | | |
| | 1 yes | 0.6713666 | 1.9569097 | 0.2145444 | 3.129 | 0.002 | [1.2851, 2.9798] |
| Baseline complication | 0 (no) | Ref | | | | | |
| | 1 (yes) | 0.5218596 | 1.6851584 | 0.2236382 | 2.333 | 0.020 | [1.0871, 2.6122] |
| Stroke type | 0 (hemo) | Ref | | . | | | . |
| | 1 (ische) | -0.2105377 | 0.8101485 | 0.2094069 | -1.005 | 0.315 | [0.5374, 1.2213] |
| | 2(both) | 0.6232302 | 1.8649425 | 0.3409207 | 1.828 | 0.068 | [0.9560, 3.6380] |

diabetes mellitus, stroke type, baseline complication, and drug type.

*2.4. Method of Data Analysis.* Survival analysis is a collection of statistical procedures for data analysis for which the outcome variable of interest is time until an event occurs. An initial step in the analysis of a set of survival data is to present numerical or graphical summaries of the survival times in a particular group. In summarizing survival data, the two common functions of applied are the survivor function and the hazard function [6].

The Kaplan-Meier estimator is a nonparametric statistic used to estimate the survival function from lifetime data.

The Kaplan-Meier estimator of the survivorship function (or survival probability) $S(t) = P(T \geq t)$ is defined as

$$\widehat{S}(t) = \prod_{t_i \leq t} \frac{n_i - d_i}{n_i} = \prod_{t_i \leq t} 1 - \frac{d_i}{n_i}, \quad (1)$$

where $t_1, t_2, \cdots, t_n$ a set of survival time of $n$ independent observations and $t_{(1)} \leq t_{(2)} \leq \cdots \leq t_{(m)}$, $m \leq n$ is the survival time of the $m$ distinct ordered death times; $d_i$ is the number of individuals who failed (died) at time $t_i$; and $n_i$ is the number of individuals who are at risk of dying at time $t_i$.

One of the most popular types of regression models used in survival analysis is the Cox proportional hazard model [8]. The authors proposed a semiparametric model for the hazard function that allows the addition of covariates, while keeping the baseline hazards unspecified, and only positive values with this parameterization the Cox hazard function are given by

$$h(t, x) = h_o(t) \exp(\beta x), \quad (2)$$

where$h_0(t)$ is the baseline hazard function and is called the baseline hazard function; $x = (x_1, x_2, \cdots, x_p)'$ is the values of the vector of explanatory variables; and $\beta' = (\beta_1, \beta_2, \cdots, \beta_p)$ is a vector of regression coefficients. The main assumption of the Cox proportional hazard model is proportional hazards that means that the hazard function of one individual is proportional to the hazard function of the other individual; i.e., the hazard ratio is constant over time.

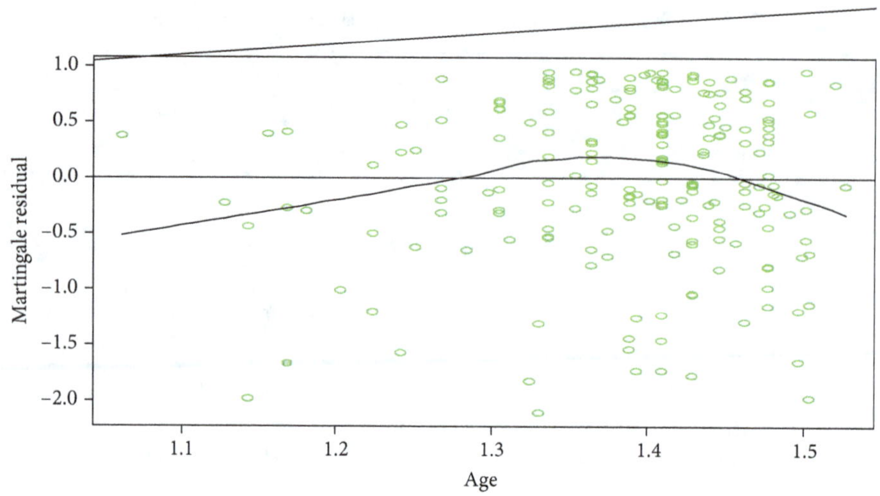


FIGURE 3: Plots of the martingale residuals against the covariate age.

## 3. Result and Discussion

*3.1. Descriptive Summaries.* A total of 295 stroke patients were treated in the hospital during the study period from the 1st of September 2014 to the 1st of April 2017. Of total population, this study included 202 stroke patients for whom data for variables of interest are complete. Of all 202 stroke patients, 147 (72.8%) were censored or did not experience the event and 55 (27.2%) died. Average time duration for all patients was 6.05 with a standard deviation of 4.698, and the median and mean survival time of age were 6 and 7.168 days, respectively. The mean and median age of stroke patient were 62.56 and 65 days, respectively. The mean and median survival time from stroke were found to be 15.596 and 19 days, respectively. The mean and median survival time from stroke were found to be 15.596 19 days, respectively. The mean survival time of male and female was 9.1 days and 5.1 days, respectively. The minimum and maximum survival times observed in the data were 1 day and 24 days, respectively. The median survival time of female and male was 3 days and 6 days, respectively. Patients with hypertension stayed for 4 days of which 72.13% were death. However, patients with no hypertension stayed for 9 days on average of which 27.87% were death. Patients with baseline complication stayed for 4 days on average of which 67.3% were death (Table 1).

*3.2. The Kaplan-Meier Estimate.* The estimate for overall Kaplan-Meier survivor function depicted that a relatively large number of the deaths occurred at the earlier days of antistroke treatment, and the same graph showed the decrement over a follow-up period (Figure 1).

Kaplan-Meier estimates represented by the survival curves for without hypertension diseases are above those of the patients' complications with hypertension. This implied that the patients without hypertension have more chances of survival than those with hypertension (Figure 2).

*3.3. Log-Rank Tests of Each Covariate.* The log-rank test indicates that statistically there is a significant difference of survival experience among groups of gender, age, blood pressure (hypertension), and baseline complication. On the other hand, there are statistically no significant differences in survival/death experience among groups of the categorical covariates cardiac disease, diabetes mellitus, stroke type, and drug type. Accordingly, the mean survival time of male patient to death had been 9.1 days greater than that of female patients (5.1 days with 95% CI [8.04889, 10.3094]) (Table 2).

*3.4. Univariable Analysis of Cox PH Regression Model.* From the outputs in univariable analysis, we can observe that the covariate age of stroke patient (HR = 1.011731, $P$ value = 0.0119), gender of patient (HR = 0.4123, $P$ value = $1.58e-06$), hypertension (HR = 2.5510, $P$ value = $2.40e-06$), stroke type (HR = 0.6152, 1.7325; $P$ value = 0.014, 0.0961), and drug type and baseline complication (HR = 3.0710, $P$ value = $4.84e-08$) are significant and hypertension, baseline complication, gender, and stroke type are highly significant in the univariable analysis. However, diabetes mellitus and cardiac are not significant factors for the death time at 5% level of significance (Table 3). This result is consistent with a previous study [3, 9] that age of patients was a significant factor in affecting the survival of stroke patients.

*3.5. Multivariable Analysis of Cox PH Regression Model.* Covariates which become insignificant in the multivariable analysis were removed from the model by using a stepwise elimination technique. Accordingly, cardiac disease and diabetes mellitus were excluded. In order to decide whether or not a variable is significant, the $P$ value associated with each parameter has been estimated and variables that have $P$ value less than 0.05 cut-point or 5% significance level are considered important variables and, hence, are included in the final model. Accordingly, sex, hypertension, baseline complication, and stroke type had significant effect on the survival of the stroke patient (Table 4). This result is supported by research conducted in China [5] in that hypertension was a significant factor in affecting the survival of stroke patients. The result is also consistent with that of a previous

TABLE 5: Schoenfeld residual for each covariate.

| Covariates | Categories | Rho | $\mathrm{Chi}^2$ | Prob > $\mathrm{chi}^2$ |
|---|---|---|---|---|
| Age | | 0.0462 | 0.2586 | 0.611 |
| Gender | Female ref | | | |
| | Male | 0.0304 | 0.1364 | 0.712 |
| Hypertension | No ref | | | |
| | Yes | 0.1115 | 2.3567 | 0.125 |
| Baseline complication | No ref | | | |
| | Yes | 0.0625 | 0.8123 | 0.367 |
| Drug type | Nondrug (ref) | | | |
| | Drug type 1 | -0.0974 | 1.3874 | 0.239 |
| | Drug type 2 | -0.0573 | 0.4887 | 0.485 |
| | Drug type 3 | -0.0111 | 0.0177 | 0.894 |
| | Drug type 4 | -0.0374 | 0.1989 | 0.656 |
| | Drug type 5 | -0.0445 | 0.2939 | 0.588 |
| Stroke type | 0 ref | | | |
| | Stroke type 1 | -0.0229 | 0.0874 | 0.768 |
| | Stroke type 2 | 0.0360 | 0.1898 | 0.663 |
| Global test | | | 8.4942 | 0.668 |

TABLE 6: The likelihood ratio and significance of the PH model.

| Covariate | Coef ($\beta$) | HR | se ($\beta$) | Wald | $P$ value |
|---|---|---|---|---|---|
| Factor (gender) 1 | -0.712 | 0.491 | 0.193 | -3.69 | <0.001 |
| Factor (BP) 1 | 0.654 | 1.923 | 0.208 | 3.15 | 0.002 |
| Factor (baseline) 1 | 0.666 | 1.947 | 0.218 | 3.06 | 0.002 |

Likelihood ratio test = 49.8 on 3 DF; $P = 8.87e - 11$; $n = 202$; number of events = 147.

study [10] that sex of patients was a significant factor in affecting the survival of stroke patients. The finding of the study is also consistent with that of a previous study [9] that stroke mortality increased with age of patients.

*3.6. Checking for the Linearity of Continuous Covariates in the Model.* For the age covariate, the plots show systematic patterns or trends and the resulting smoothed plots are not a straight line. Therefore, the plots of martingale residual confirm that age of a patient has no linear relationship with the survival time (Figure 3).

*3.7. Checking of Proportional Hazard Assumption.* The test of correlation (rho) is insignificant that indicates proportional hazards assumption is fulfilled. Variables including age, gender of patients, hypertension (blood pressure), baseline complication, drug type, and stroke type fulfilled the assumption because all the $P$ values are greater than 0.05. In Schoenfeld residual, if the $P$ value is greater than 0.05 it indicates that the Cox proportional hazard assumptions are fulfilled (Table 5).

*3.7.1. Diagnosis of the Model.* In the likelihood ratio and significance of the final Cox PH model from the likelihood ratio test, it can be seen that the PH model is significant since $P$ value is less than 5% (Table 6).

## 4. Conclusions and Recommendation

The objective of the study was to identify significant risk factors that affect survival of stroke patients who have been under follow-up at Mettu Karl Referral Hospital. For determining the risk factors for the survival time of stroke patients, a total of 202 patients were included in the study out of which 40.6% were females and 59.4% were males. Among those patients, 27.2% died and the rest were censored.

The Cox regression analysis showed that the major factors that affect the survival of stroke patients are hypertension, gender of the patients, and baseline complication which were strongly related to mortality, and based on the hospital outcome, the most common causes of death were hypertension and base line complication. However, there were variables that were significant at univariable stage of analysis but not at multivariate analysis stage. These were stroke type, drug type, and age of patients. Moreover, variables that were significant neither at univariable nor at multivariable analyses were gender, baseline complication, and hypertension. The result of this study also indicated that survival probability of a patient is not statistically different among groups classified by cardiac disease, diabetes mellitus, stroke type, and drug type.

The researchers recommend that the people should be aware on the burden of those risk factors and well informed about the disease. Finally, the researchers propose the concerned body special health management to improve the health of the society based on the result of the study.

## 5. Limitations

This research paper was limited to time from the date of the first diagnosis until the occurrence of the death or end of the study period for 202 stroke patients in case of Karl Hospital, Ilu Ababor Zone.

## Abbreviations

AIC: Akaike's Information Criterion
AIDS: Acquired immune deficiency syndrome
BIC: Bayesian Information Criterion
CT: Computed tomography
HIV: Human immunodeficiency virus
NCD: Noncommunicable diseases
WHO: World Health Organization.

## Ethical Approval

This study was reviewed and approved by Mettu University Research Ethical Committee.

## Consent

As the study was based on retrospective cohort study, informed consent was not needed.

## Conflicts of Interest

The authors declare that there is no competing interest.

## Acknowledgments



## References

[1] D. O. Abegunde, C. D. Mathers, T. Adam, M. Ortegon, and K. Strong, "The burden and costs of chronic diseases in low-income and middle-income countries," *Lancet*, vol. 370, no. 9603, pp. 1929–1938, 2007, PMID: 18063029.

[2] A. A. Alhazzani, A. A. Mahfouz, A. Y. Abolyazid et al., "In hospital stroke mortality: rates and determinants in southwestern Saudi Arabia," *International Journal of Environmental Research and Public Health*, vol. 15, no. 5, p. 927, 2018.

[3] E. S. Donkor, M. O. Owolabi, P. Bampoh, T. Aspelund, and V. Gudnason, "Community awareness of stroke in Accra Ghana," *BMC Public Health*, vol. 14, no. 1, p. 196, 2014.

[4] A. Moran, M. Forouzanfar, U. Sampson, S. Chugh, V. Feigin, and G. Mensah, "The epidemiology of cardiovascular diseases in sub-Saharan Africa: the Global Burden of Diseases, Injuries and Risk Factors 2010 Study," *Progress in Cardiovascular Diseases*, vol. 56, no. 3, pp. 234–239, 2013.

[5] S. Yusuf, S. Reddy, S. Ounpuu, and S. Anand, "Global burden of cardiovascular diseases," *Circulation*, vol. 104, no. 23, pp. 2855–2864, 2001.

[6] A. Misganaw, T. N. Haregu, K. Deribe et al., "National mortality burden due to communicable, non-communicable, and other diseases in Ethiopia, 1990-2015: findings from the Global Burden of Disease Study 2015," *Population Health Metrics*, vol. 15, no. 1, p. 29, 2017.

[7] R. BeLue, T. A. Okoror, J. Iwelunmor et al., "An overview of cardiovascular risk factor burden in sub-Saharan African countries: a socio-cultural perspective," *Globalization and Health*, vol. 5, no. 1, p. 10, 2009.

[8] D. R. Cox and D. Oakes, *Analysis of Survival Data*, Chapman and Hall London Google Scholar, Boca Raton, 1st edition, 1984.

[9] Y. Sun, S. H. Lee, B. H. Heng, and V. S. Chin, "5-year survival and rehospitalization due to stroke recurrence among patients with hemorrhagic or ischemic strokes in Singapore," *BMC Neurology*, vol. 13, no. 1, p. 133, 2013.

[10] D. W. Hosmer, S. Lemeshow, and X. Rodney, *Applied Logistic Regression*, John Wiley & Sons, Inc., New York, 2nd edition, 2000.

# Permissions

All chapters in this book were first published by Hindawi Publishing Corporation; hereby published with permission under the Creative Commons Attribution License or equivalent. Every chapter published in this book has been scrutinized by our experts. Their significance has been extensively debated. The topics covered herein carry significant findings which will fuel the growth of the discipline. They may even be implemented as practical applications or may be referred to as a beginning point for another development.

The contributors of this book come from diverse backgrounds, making this book a truly international effort. This book will bring forth new frontiers with its revolutionizing research information and detailed analysis of the nascent developments around the world.

We would like to thank all the contributing authors for lending their expertise to make the book truly unique. They have played a crucial role in the development of this book. Without their invaluable contributions this book wouldn't have been possible. They have made vital efforts to compile up to date information on the varied aspects of this subject to make this book a valuable addition to the collection of many professionals and students.

This book was conceptualized with the vision of imparting up-to-date information and advanced data in this field. To ensure the same, a matchless editorial board was set up. Every individual on the board went through rigorous rounds of assessment to prove their worth. After which they invested a large part of their time researching and compiling the most relevant data for our readers.

The editorial board has been involved in producing this book since its inception. They have spent rigorous hours researching and exploring the diverse topics which have resulted in the successful publishing of this book. They have passed on their knowledge of decades through this book. To expedite this challenging task, the publisher supported the team at every step. A small team of assistant editors was also appointed to further simplify the editing procedure and attain best results for the readers.

Apart from the editorial board, the designing team has also invested a significant amount of their time in understanding the subject and creating the most relevant covers. They scrutinized every image to scout for the most suitable representation of the subject and create an appropriate cover for the book.

The publishing team has been an ardent support to the editorial, designing and production team. Their endless efforts to recruit the best for this project, has resulted in the accomplishment of this book. They are a veteran in the field of academics and their pool of knowledge is as vast as their experience in printing. Their expertise and guidance has proved useful at every step. Their uncompromising quality standards have made this book an exceptional effort. Their encouragement from time to time has been an inspiration for everyone.

The publisher and the editorial board hope that this book will prove to be a valuable piece of knowledge for researchers, students, practitioners and scholars across the globe.

# List of Contributors

**Clotilde Balucani, Paola Palazzo, Limin Zhao, April Sisson and Andrei V. Alexandrov**
Comprehensive Stroke Center, Department of Neurology, University of Alabama at Birmingham, RWUH M226, 619 19th Street South, Birmingham, AL 35249-3280, USA

**Kristian Barlinn**
Comprehensive Stroke Center, Department of Neurology, University of Alabama at Birmingham, RWUH M226, 619 19th Street South, Birmingham, AL 35249-3280, USA
Dresden University Stroke Center, University of Technology Dresden, 01307 Dresden, Germany

**Myriam Villeneuve and Anouk Lamontagne**
School of Physical and Occupational Therapy, McGill University, Montreal, QC, Canada
Feil and Oberfeld Research Centre, Jewish Rehabilitation Hospital, Research Site of the Montreal Center for Interdisciplinary Research in Rehabilitation (CRIR), 3205 Place Alton-Goldbloom, Laval, QC, Canada

**Ahmad Mirdamadi**
Medical School, Islamic Azad University, Najafabad Branch, Isfahan, Iran

**Mohsen MirmohammadSadeghi**
Hypertension Research Center, Isfahan Cardiovascular Research Institute, Isfahan University of Medical\ Sciences, Isfahan, Iran

**Mahfar Arasteh**
Isfahan University of Medical Sciences, Isfahan, Iran

**Mojgan Gharipour**
Isfahan Cardiovascular Research Center, Isfahan Cardiovascular Research Institute (WHO Collaborating Center), Isfahan University of Medical Sciences, Isfahan, Iran

**Mayra Johana Montalvo**
Neuromodulation Center, Spaulding Rehabilitation Hospital, Harvard Medical School, 96/79 13th Street, Boston, MA 02129, USA

**Muhib Alam Khan**
Department of Neurology, Warren Alpert Medical School at Brown University, 110 Lockwood Street, Suite 324, Providence, RI 02903, USA

**Preema J. Mehta**
Department of Neurology, Howard University Hospital, 2041 Georgia Ave., Washington, DC 20060, USA
Department of Neurology, Howard University College of Medicine, Washington, DC 20059, USA

**Sherita Chapman, Annapurni Jayam-Trouth and Mohankumar Kurukumbi**
Department of Neurology, Howard University Hospital, 2041 Georgia Ave., Washington, DC 20060, USA

**Bhawna Khattar and Alakananda Banerjee**
Department of Physiotherapy and Rehabilitation, Max Super Speciality Hospital, Saket, New Delhi, India

**Rajsekhar Reddi**
Department of Neurology, Max Super Speciality Hospital, Saket, New Delhi, India

**Anirban Dutta**
Department of Clinical Neurophysiology, Georg-August-University, Goettingen, Germany

**Chiaki Takahashi**
Department of Neurosurgery, Takaoka City Hospital, 4-1, Takara-machi, Takaoka, Toyama, Japan

**Salman Assad, Justin Nolte, Dharampreet Singh, Samrina Hanif and Paul Ferguson**
Department of Neurology, Marshall University School of Medicine, Huntington, WV, USA

**Re-I Chin and John J. Monda**
Saint Louis University School of Medicine, 1402 S Grand Blvd, Saint Louis, MO 63104, USA

**Maulik Sheth and Debapriya De**
Department of Internal Medicine, SSM St. Mary's Health Center, 6420 Clayton Rd, Richmond Heights, MO 63117, USA

**William Ogle**
Department of Cardiothoracic Surgery, SSM St. Mary's Health Center, 6420 Clayton Rd, Richmond Heights, MO 63117, USA

**Gloria Merenda**
Department of Pathology, SSM St. Mary's Health Center, 6420 Clayton Rd, Richmond Heights, MO 63117, USA

**Amir M. Torabi**
East Dallas Neurological Services Baylor Medical Center, Garland, TX, USA

**Kathryn Zalewski, Kristina Laundre, Amber Wacek and Melissa Wiedmeyer**
College of Health Sciences, Department of Human Movement Science, Doctor of Physical Therapy Program, University of Wisconsin-Milwaukee, Pavilion 360, Milwaukee, WI 53201, USA

**Julie Kerk**
Neurorehabilitation Unit, Department of Physical Therapy, Froedtert Memorial Lutheran Hospital, 9200 West Wisconsin Avenue, Milwaukee, WI 53226, USA

**Elisa F. Ciceri, Valeria Cuccarini and Luisa Chiapparini**
Neuroradiology Department, Fondazione Istituto "C. Besta", Via Celoria 11, 20133 Milan, Italy

**Veronica Saletti**
Paediatric Department, Fondazione Istituto "C. Besta", Via Celoria 11, 20133 Milan, Italy

**Luca Valvassori**
Neuroradiology Department, Ospedale Niguarda, Piazza Ospedale Maggiore 3, 20162 Milan, Italy

**Brian Malm**
Section of Cardiovascular Medicine, Department of Internal Medicine, Yale University School of Medicine, Yale University, New Haven, CT, USA
Department of Cardiology, VA Connecticut Healthcare System, West Haven, CT, USA

**Paul Hermany**
Section of Cardiovascular Medicine, Department of Internal Medicine, Yale University School of Medicine, Yale University, New Haven, CT, USA

**Alan Morrison**
Warren Alpert School of Medicine, Brown University, Providence, RI, USA

**Ali A. Alsaad and Michael B. Phillips**
Department of Internal Medicine, Mayo Clinic, Jacksonville, FL 32224, USA

**Christopher O. Austin**
Division of Cardiovascular Diseases, Mayo Clinic, Jacksonville, FL 32224, USA

**Maisha T. Robinson**
Department of Neurology, Mayo Clinic, Jacksonville, FL 32224, USA

**G. Thielman**
Department of Physical Therapy, University of the Sciences, Philadelphia, PA 19104-4495, USA

**P. Bonsall**
Department of Occupational Therapy, Magee Rehabilitation Hospital, Philadelphia, PA 19106, USA

**Siva P. Sontineni, Aryan N. Mooss, Venkata G. Andukuri, Susan Marie Schima and Dennis Esterbrooks**
Division of Cardiology, Creighton University, Omaha, NE 68131, USA

**R. Vibo and J. Kõrv**
Department of Neurology and Neurosurgery, University of Tartu, 51014 Tartu, Estonia

**S. Schneider**
Department of Neurology, North Estonia Medical Center, 13419 Tallinn, Estonia

**Scott E. Kasner, Lauren H. Sansing and Steven R. Messé**
Department of Neurology, The Hospital of the University of PA, 3400 Spruce Street, Philadelphia, PA, 19104, USA

**James S. McKinney**
Department of Neurology, The Hospital of the University of PA, 3400 Spruce Street, Philadelphia, PA, 19104, USA
Department of Neurology, Robert Wood Johnson Medical School, University of Medicine & Dentistry of New Jersey, 97 Patterson Street, New Brunswick, NJ 08901, USA

**Bryan A. Pukenas, Sudhakar R. Satti, John B.Weigele and Robert W. Hurst**
Department of Neuroradiology, The Hospital of the University of Pennsylvania, 3400 Spruce Street, Philadelphia, PA, 19104, USA

**Joshua M. Levine**
Department of Neurology, The Hospital of the University of PA, 3400 Spruce Street, Philadelphia, PA, 19104, USA
Department of Neurosurgery, The Hospital of the University of Pennsylvania, 3400 Spruce Street, Philadelphia, Pennsylvania, 19104, USA
Department of Anesthesiology and Critical Care, The Hospital of the University of Pennsylvania, 3400 Spruce Street, Philadelphia, Pennsylvania, 19104, USA

**Tatsushi Mutoh**
Department of Stroke Science, Research Institute for Brain and Blood Vessels-Akita, Akita 010-0874, Japan
Department of Surgical Neurology, Research Institute for Brain and Blood Vessels-Akita, Akita 010-0874, Japan

**Tatsuya Ishikawa and Nobuyuki Yasui**
Department of Surgical Neurology, Research Institute for Brain and Blood Vessels-Akita, Akita 010-0874, Japan

**Akifumi Suzuki**
Department of Stroke Science, Research Institute for Brain and Blood Vessels-Akita, Akita 010-0874, Japan

**Raquel Calvão de Melo and José Carlos Alves**
Department of Psychiatry, Divino Espírito Santo Hospital, 9500-370 Ponta Delgada, Portugal

**Rui Lopes**
Clinic of Psychiatry and Mental Health, São João Hospital, 4200-319 Porto, Portugal

**María Jesús Gómez Ramos, Carmen Sánchez Álvarez and Lisa Ortin Katnich**
Department of ICU, Reina Sofía General University Hospital, University of Murcia, 30.003 Murcia, Spain

**Francisco Miguel González Valverde**
Department of Surgery, Reina Sofía General University Hospital, University of Murcia, 30.003 Murcia, Spain

**Francisco Pastor Quirante**
Department of Pathology, Reina Sofía General University Hospital, University of Murcia, 30.003 Murcia, Spain

**Kachi Illoh**
Division of Neurology Products, Center for Drug Evaluation and Research, U. S. Food and Drug Administration, Building 22, Room 5402, 10903 New Hampshire Avenue, Silver Spring, MD 20993, USA

**Emilio Supsupin and Edwin D. Cacayorin**
Department of Diagnostic and Interventional Imaging, The University of Texas Medical School at Houston, 6431 Fannin Street, MSB 2.130B, Houston, TX 77030, USA

**Hashem M. Shaltoni**
Department of Radiology, Baylor College of Medicine, One Baylor Plaza, Mail Stop BCM360, Houston, TX 77030, USA

**Archana Balachandran, Siddarameshwar Kalyanshettar, Shankargouda Patil and Vijaykumar Shegji**
Department of Pediatrics, Shri. B.M. Patil Medical College Hospital and Research Centre, BLDE University, Vijayapur, Karnataka 586103, India

**Kyaw Kyaw and Sammy San Myint Aung**
Institute for Heart and Vascular Health, Renown Regional Medical Center, 1500 E. 2nd St. No. 302, Reno, NV 89502, USA

**Htun Latt**
Department of Internal Medicine, University of Nevada, Reno School of Medicine, 1155 Mill St. No. W11, Reno, NV 89502, USA

**Jay Babu**
Department of Biology, University of Nevada, Reno, 1664 N. Virginia Street, Reno, NV 89557, USA

**Rajesh Rangaswamy**
Department of Radiology, Renown Regional Medical Center, 1155 Mill St., Reno, NV 89502, USA

**Nneka Schwimmer-Okike, Johannes Niebuhr and Heike Kielstein**
Department of Anatomy and Cell Biology, Faculty of Medicine, Martin Luther University Halle Wittenberg, 06108 Halle (Saale), Germany

**Grit Gesine Ruth Schramek**
Institute for Pathology, University Hospital Halle, 06108 Halle (Saale), Germany

**Stefan Frantz**
Department of Internal Medicine III, University Hospital Halle, 06120 Halle (Saale), Germany

**James R. Agapoff IV**
Department of Psychiatry, University of Hawai'i at Mānoa, John A. Burns School of Medicine, Honolulu, HI, USA

**Marco R Schroeter**
Department of Cardiology and Pneumology, Heart Center, University of Göttingen, Göttingen, Germany

**Wolfgang Schillinger**
Department of Cardiology and Pneumology, Heart Center, University of Göttingen, Göttingen, Germany; Internal Medicine I, Helios Albert-Schweitzer Clinic Northeim, Northeim, Germany

**Daniel N. Kianpour and Thomas M. Nguyen**
Swedish Neuroscience Institute, Seattle, WA, USA

**Arthur M. Lam**
University of California San Diego, USA

**Xiao Ran**
Department of Emergency Medicine, Tongji Hospital, Tongji Medical College, Huazhong University of Science and Technology, Jiefang Avenue No. 1095,Wuhan 430030, China

**Qin Zhang**
Department of Anesthesia, Tongji Hospital, Tongji Medical College, Huazhong University of Science and Technology, Jiefang Avenue No. 1095, Wuhan 430030, China

**Dao Wen Wang**
The Institute of Hypertension and Department of Internal Medicine, Tongji Hospital, Tongji Medical College, Huazhong University of Science and Technology, Jiefang Avenue No. 1095, Wuhan 430030, China

**Christina-Maria Kastorini**
School of Medicine, University of Ioannina, 45110 Ioannina, Greece
Department of Nutrition Science and Dietetics, Harokopio University, 17671 Athens, Greece

**Haralampos J. Milionis and John A. Goudevenos**
School of Medicine, University of Ioannina, 45110 Ioannina, Greece

**Demosthenes B. Panagiotakos**
Department of Nutrition Science and Dietetics, Harokopio University, 17671 Athens, Greece

**Cheung-Ter Ong**
Department of Neurology, Chia-Yi Christian Hospital, 539 Chung-Shao Road, Chia-Yi 60002, Taiwan
Department of Physical Therapy, Shu Zen College of Medicine and Management, Kaohsiung, Taiwan

**Rei-Yeuh Chang**
Department of Cardiology, Chia-Yi Christian Hospital, 539 Chung-Shao Road, Chia-Yi 60002, Taiwan

**Richard Harry Asmah**
Department of Biomedical Sciences, School of Basic and Biomedical Sciences, University of Health and Allied Sciences, Ho, Ghana

**Pomah Sackey, Derek Doku and Marjorie Quarchie**
Department of Medical Laboratory Sciences, School of Biomedical and Allied Health Sciences, University of Ghana, Ghana

**Patrick Adjei and Timothy N. Archampong**
Department of Medicine and Therapeutics, University of Ghana Medical School, Ghana

**Seth Attoh**
Division of Pathology, 37 Military Hospital, Accra, Ghana

**Felix Botchway**
Child Health Department, Korle-Bu Teaching Hospital, Accra, Ghana

**David Adedia**
Department of Basic Sciences, School of Basic and Biomedical Sciences, University of Health and Allied Sciences, Ho, Ghana

**Eric Sampene Donkor**
Department of Medical Microbiology, University of Ghana Medical School, Ghana

**Valeria Silvestri, Vivian Mushi and Billy Ngasala**
Department of Parasitology and Medical Entomology, Muhimbili University of Health and Applied Science, Dar es Salaam, Tanzania

**Jacqueline Kihwele**
Department of Internal Medicine, Muhimbili University of Health and Applied Science, Dar es Salaam, Tanzania

**Deodatus Sabas**
Directorate of Library Service, Muhimbili University of Health and Allied Sciences, Dar es Salaam, Tanzania

**Lorenzo Rocchi**
Department of Medical Sciences and Public Health, University of Cagliari, Cagliari, Italy

**Tissa Wijeratne**
School of Applied Health, Department of Psychology, RMIT University, Melbourne, Australia
Department of Medicine, Faculty of Medicine, University of Rajarata, Saliyapura, Anuradhapura, Sri Lanka
Department of Neurology, Western Health & University of Melbourne, AIMSS, Level Three, WHCRE, Sunshine Hospital, St Albans, 3021, Australia

**Carmela Sales**
School of Applied Health, Department of Psychology, RMIT University, Melbourne, Australia
Department of Neurology, Western Health & University of Melbourne, AIMSS, Level Three, WHCRE, Sunshine Hospital, St Albans, 3021, Australia

**Chanith Wijeratne**
Monash Medical School, Clayton, Victoria, Australia

**Leila Karimi**
School of Applied Health, Department of Psychology, RMIT University, Melbourne, Australia
Department of Neurology, Western Health & University of Melbourne, AIMSS, Level Three, WHCRE, Sunshine Hospital, St Albans, 3021, Australia
Faculty of Social and Political Sciences, Tbilisi State University, Georgia

**Mihajlo Jakovljevic**
Institute of Advanced Manufacturing Technologies, Peter the Great St. Petersburg Polytechnic University, St. Petersburg, Russia
Institute of Comparative Economic Studies, Hosei University Chiyoda, Japan
Department of Global Health Economics and Policy, University of Kragujevac, Serbia

**Wan-Chen Tsai, Hui-Chen Lin, Wen-Neng Chang, Nai-Wen Tsai and Chih-Cheng Huang**
Department of Neurology, Chang Gung Memorial Hospital-Kaohsiung Medical Center, Chang Gung University College of Medicine, Kaohsiung, Taiwan

**Yun-Ru Lai and Che-Wei Hsu**
Department of Neurology, Chang Gung Memorial Hospital-Kaohsiung Medical Center, Chang Gung University College of Medicine, Kaohsiung, Taiwan
Department of Biological Science, National Sun Yat-Sen University, Kaohsiung, Taiwan

**Hung-Chen Wang**
Department of Neurosurgery, Chang Gung Memorial Hospital-Kaohsiung Medical Center, Chang Gung University College of Medicine, Kaohsiung, Taiwan

**Chih-Min Su**
Department of Emergency Medicine, Chang Gung Memorial Hospital-Kaohsiung Medical Center, Chang Gung University College of Medicine, Kaohsiung, Taiwan

**Yu-Jih Su**
Department of Medicine, Chang Gung Memorial Hospital-Kaohsiung Medical Center, Chang Gung University College of Medicine, Kaohsiung, Taiwan

**Wei-Che Lin**
Department of Radiology, Chang Gung Memorial Hospital-Kaohsiung Medical Center, Chang Gung University College of Medicine, Kaohsiung, Taiwan

**Ben-Chung Cheng**
Department of Biological Science, National Sun Yat-Sen University, Kaohsiung, Taiwan
Department of Medicine, Chang Gung Memorial Hospital-Kaohsiung Medical Center, Chang Gung University College of Medicine, Kaohsiung, Taiwan

**Cheng-Hsien Lu**
Department of Neurology, Chang Gung Memorial Hospital-Kaohsiung Medical Center, Chang Gung University College of Medicine, Kaohsiung, Taiwan
Department of Biological Science, National Sun Yat-Sen University, Kaohsiung, Taiwan

**Fikru Tsehayneh and Abenet Tafesse**
Department of Neurology, Addis Ababa University School of Medicine, Addis Ababa, Ethiopia

**Yangyang Miao, Xinru Zhang, Jing Jin and Xingyu Wang**
Key Laboratory of Advanced Control and Optimization for Chemical Processes, Ministry of Education, East China University of Science and Technology, Shanghai, China

**Shugeng Chen and Jie Jia**
Department of Rehabilitation, Huashan Hospital, Fudan University, Shanghai, China

**Ren Xu**
Guger Technologies OG, Austria

**Ian Daly**
Brain-Computer Interfaces and Neural Engineering Laboratory, School of Computer Science and Electronic Engineering, University of Essex, Colchester, Essex CO4 3SQ, UK

**Andrzej Cichocki**
Skolkowo Institute of Science and Technology (SKOLTECH), 143026 Moscow, Russia
Systems Research Institute PAS, Warsaw, Poland
Nicolaus Copernicus University (UMK), Torun, Poland

**Tzyy-Ping Jung**
Institute for Neural Computation and Institute of Engineering in Medicine, University of California San Diego, La Jolla, CA, USA

**Ahsan Rao and Paul Aylin**
School of PublicHealth, Faculty ofMedicine, Dr. FosterUnit, 3 Dorset Rise, London EC4Y 8EN, UK

**Emily Barrow, Sabine Vuik and Ara Darzi**
Centre for Health Policy, Institute for Global Health Innovation, Imperial College London, QEQM, St Mary's Hospital, Floor 10, Praed Street, London W2 1NY, UK

**Dereje Gebeyehu Ababu and Azmeraw Misganaw Getahun**
Department of Statistics, Faculty of Natural & Computational Science, Mettu University, Ethiopia

# Index

www.ingramcontent.com/pod-product-compliance
Lightning Source LLC
LaVergne TN
LVHW060059220926
848484LV00008BA/2248